# *Strategic Management of Nurses*

## A Policy-Oriented Approach

# Strategic Management of Nurses

## A Policy-Oriented Approach

### Lois Friss, RN, Dr PH

THE
AUPHA
PRESS

*Published by*
National Health Publishing
99 Painters Mill Road
Owings Mills, Maryland 21117
(301) 363–6400

*A division of Williams & Wilkins*

The AUPHA Press is a joint venture between
the Association of University Programs in Health Administration
and National Health Publishing.

*Printed in the United States of America*
*First Printing*

*Acquisitions Editor:* Brigitte Pocta
*Developmental Editor:* Cindy Konits
*Production Coordinator:* Karen Babcock
*Copyeditor:* Michael Treadway
*Designer:* Sandy Renovetz
*Compositor:* National Health Publishing
*Printer:* Edwards Brothers

ISBN: 1-55857-006-3
LC: 88–063328

I dedicate this book to the major heroes,
the hospital staff nurses,
who shape intelligent careers
in a system without a career structure.

# Contents

## Section II    Management Issues

# Foreword

*Hospitals exist to provide nursing care.* Indeed, if patients did not require the round-the-clock care of professional nurses, all health care services would be provided in the home, physician offices, and same-day diagnostic/treatment centers. Even though the nursing function is the raison d'etre of hospitals, many administrators know far too little of nurses, nursing, or the professional and career issues which influence the provision of effective and efficient nursing care in hospitals.

Little work on nursing (whether theory or empirical research) finds its way into the most read general management and health administration journals, and administrators rarely read the nursing management literature. Accordingly, this book could fill an important void. In it health care administrators have access to credible thinking and a summary of research regarding: the nature of nursing work; the organizational/managerial parameters that influence nursing service performance; and selected policy issues that mediate the relationship between the nursing profession and health care organizations.

I am confident that the book will stimulate dialogue and health debate among policy analysts/makers, executives, nurse managers and nursing care professionals. Like good work in any area, the book raises far more questions than it answers.

This treatment is particularly credible given Professor Friss' breadth of education and experience. She is trained in both clinical nursing and health administration, has held a variety of staff nursing and nursing management positions, and has taught health care management and policy for the past twenty years.

Dennis D. Pointer, Ph.D.
Arthur Graham Glasgow Professor
Department of Health Administration
Medical College of Virginia
Virginia Commonwealth University
Richmond, Virginia

# Foreword

Lois Friss has provided a valuable resource in this book for leaders, managers, and health policy lobbyists and analysts. She combines a scholarly approach to the literature with her original and provocative perspective so that the reader has an excellent resource for thought, discussion and action. Faculty in professional programs in the health field will find the book as useful as practitioners.

The nursing shortage has plagued this nation and others for decades. While earlier versions of the shortage were episodic in nature, the current situation already appears to be more lasting and pervasive in scope. Many chapters in the book offer insights into the shortage of nurses and practical solutions aimed at both recruitment and retention of nurses. Chapter 2 on the practice of nursing offers an abridged, encyclopedic approach to understanding the nursing field. Usually such an approach militates against the author's fresh insight or provocative exploration of the issue or its future resolution. One would not expect to find in such content any mention, no less discussion, of some of the current controversies of the field which have immediate implications for educators, practitioners and managers. Her discussion of documentation is a case in point and was of considerable interest to me.

Midway through my own clinical career in psychiatric nursing I helped introduce into practice extensive interpersonal recording (now termed documentation). While documentation has become increasingly important, the dilemma faced by nurses regarding the time demands of extensive documentation has caused many administrators and nurses in both hospitals and home care to question the relevance and value of the type of documentation in current use. Such questions have ramifications for educators who must teach both theory and practice regarding documentation and managers who must implement such practices.

Certainly the view of "steady state" nurses presented is original and points to problems regarding the image of such nurses within the profession and within the larger society. Cues for management aimed at increasing the career views of this large group have value in the hospital microcosm as improvement in the steady state nurses' self image will alter positively their presentation of themselves, which in turn may have positive effects on recruitment to the profession, rewards, and other variables. The importance of the steady state worker cannot be overstated. One of the assets of this book is that Friss approaches this group with understanding, wit, and depth. She offers practical help to managers in "reframing" the questions that arise in contemplating this group.

The question of priorities in hospital management concerns many of us whose contact with hospitals is extensive but out of the line of authority. While many hospital board members stress bottom line issues, more are troubled by what they see as the "hospital is run like any business" philosophy. Board members have a more difficult time articulating their philosophy of the hospital as caring and nurturing, which is not surprising considering the low value placed on these characteristics. Articulation of these values usually occurs in either praise or protest following a personal experience. At that time the hospital's nature is carefully assessed. However, rarely in my personal experience has the major function of the hospital been articulated as goal with the bottom line aspects included as strategic planning for meeting that goal. Rather the business means of ensuring a viable organization so that the nature of the enterprise can be realized have, more often than not, become the ends or upper level goals with care relegated to an assumption. It is the kind of assumption which is covered by the expression "it goes without saying . . ." and is usually used to excuse an omission that definitely does require saying.

The question of whether nurses are victims and oppressed by the conditions of their employment is of considerable interest as one examines the reasons given for dissatisfaction with employment over most of this decade. The behavior of nurses has attested to the picture of an oppressed group. While conditions of employment have kept nurses down, their participation in these conditions has played a major role in sustaining them. Most groups in our society have risen in protest to unfair practices and many have influenced positive movement in their lives through such protest. Nurses have for too long depended on others to influence positive movement in their lives and their participation in change, at least for the steady state workers, has been minimal. Where we are seeing the negative effects of such behaviors is in the drop in applicants to nursing programs. These young people are not willing to participate in what they believe is an unrewarding, masochistic field. The satisfactions of being a nurse have for too long been cloaked by negative self images, passivity, complaining without positive action, and tacit acceptance of broadscale media derogation. It is the downsizing of nursing school classes that seems to have the most potential for changing this situation as even the most insensitive nursing and health field managers have come to realize that the revolving door, disposable nurse will not be there to fill their entry level jobs without massive change in all the factors cited.

The hospital's mission of caring for those too sick to be cared for at home, or in need of medical technology impossible to provide in the home cannot be accomplished without the active and positive participation of educated, competent nurses. *The Strategic Management of Nurses: A Policy-Oriented Approach* provides the help the administrator needs to make the necessary organizational changes to foster the growth and development of the major resource a hospital (or home health care agency) has to achieve its mission.

Claire Fagin

# Preface

This book does not attempt to provide a comprehensive review of the literature written by economists, sociologists, psychologists, organization theorists, nurses, and other social scientists on the problems of nursing management and policy. Instead, I have used my own knowledge and familiarity with management and nursing education to select those topics that seem most pervasive, persistent, problematic, and prejudicial. My purpose is to encourage dialogue among nurses, managers, and policy analysts about the organization of nursing work, nursing careers, managerial initiatives, and the future of nursing.

The work force issue for the next decade, in hospitals especially, will be the shortage of full-time competent professional workers. Because nurses comprise the largest group of these professionals, hospital managers will need to understand nursing duties, the career structure of nursing, and research on nursing management if they are to manage successfully for both the short and the long term. It is appropriate to focus on hospital nursing because two-thirds of nurses work in hospitals, and because hospitals both establish the wages paid other nurses and set boundaries on the potentials for reform of nursing education and licensure.

As a final note, this book refers to nurses in the feminine gender because 97% of nurses are women, and the history of nursing is inextricably linked with the status and role of women in society. It is not my intent to neglect the concerns of male nurses, who also play a key role in hospital settings. Indeed, my approach uses analytical techniques applied to understanding the work of men. The solutions proposed, if put into practice, will make nursing a more attractive career for talented men and women.

# *Acknowledgments*

---

Careers are shaped and books are written with the advice and support of many individuals. My most consistent supporter and confidant has been my husband, Gerald. My daughter Leslie has provided excellent research assistance and graphics support. Norma Peal, a doctoral student at the University of Southern California, and Constance Sullivan, a classmate at Syracuse University, have been thoughtful readers and critics. Artimese Porter, word processing manager at the USC School of Public Administration, has shown more patience during the preparation of this manuscript than any author deserves.

# A Personal Statement

This selective review of the literature with its policy and managerial recommendations is the culmination of two decades of education and experience. So that the reader may understand my perspective, I offer the following information about my career.

The foundation for my career was laid by my high school guidance teacher, who recommended that I attend the BSN program at Syracuse University rather than the diploma program in my hometown. This was a revolutionary and extravagant recommendation at the time, which was made possible through the New York State Regents scholarship program.

The dean of the Syracuse University School of Nursing, Edith Smith, now deceased, educated nurses like other undergraduates and deftly taught us how to be feminine, assertive, and, in retrospect, oblivious to historical baggage. For example, when we asked why physicians and other nurses were upset when we did not open the door for physicians, she acted somewhat puzzled and said that etiquette required that whoever got to the door first should hold it for the next one to enter.

Other career determinants are items not included in the usual satisfaction questionnaires. Among the incidents that shaped my career were when my salary was reduced with my promotion to head nurse because I was no longer working evenings; when my supervisor told me that as a head nurse I was not paid to think but to put out the work; when the education instructor explained that I was being paid substantially more for being a clinical instructor because I was being paid for what I knew, not what I did; when I was asked to approve the tenth renewal of a critical care nurse training program in a metropolitan area because of the "shortage," on the rationale that military wives were transient workers.

It was in the master's degree program in public health that I learned, much to my surprise, that nursing was a low-status occupation among those influential in health care. Again a mentor, Milton Roemer, M.D., provided a useful insight: Consider nursing as an applied social science.

In terms of the career theory presented in this book, my anchors are service, autonomy, creativity, and variety. My career style is spiral, which I am now practicing in a compatible steady-state environment. After a few years of clinical practice, I stayed home to raise my family. On my return, I worked part-time, obtained my graduate education, and explored community-based health activities. None of these were job changes from my perspective—they were all based on the same anchors and my desire to negotiate a career. At the end of an exploratory period, I became a university faculty member, where the norms of academia have shaped my steady-state career.

Although academic life and its norms do indeed foster autonomy, variety, service, and creativity, as I mature the security aspects are also appreciated and will undoubtedly influence my future career choices.

As an Associate Professor at the University of Southern California School of Public Administration, where I teach in the programs in Health Services Administration, my primary research interest is in work force policy, with emphasis on the impact of macro policies, such as educational funding, on the micro issues of managing registered nurses in hospitals. Before writing the present volume, I published both conceptual and empirical studies of turnover in hospitals, job satisfaction, organization, and job involvement of both staff nurses and directors of nursing services.

In all my academic work, my experience as a head nurse, a nursing instructor, a board member for a comprehensive health planning agency, an assistant director of a regional medical program responsible for work force education, and a continuing education specialist in health policy has been of immense value.

# Section I

# Generic Issues

# Chapter 1

# Career Perspectives

A good manager . . . isn't worried about his own career but rather the career of those who work for him. My advice: Don't worry about yourself. Take care of those who work for you and you'll float to greatness on their achievements.

(H. M. Burns in Kent 1985, 210)

The organization career in a work-centered society motivates members to enact organizational performances. It also offers control potentials . . .

(Blankenship 1977, 398)

A career approach provides a framework for understanding the work commitments of all workers, whether technical, professional, or managerial. The career model overcomes the limitations of previous models in which household-related factors (e.g., marital status, family income, husband's attitudes toward work, number of children) were used to explain the work behavior of women, and organizational characteristics (e.g., pay, promotional opportunities, and organizational climate) were used to understand the work behaviors of men. Four major career styles were identified by Driver (1979), who studied a sample of male executives and later applied his findings to other workers. Career anchors, used to understand individual values and motives, were first identified by Schein (1971, 1975, 1978) in a

1

longitudinal study of MBA graduates. Later studies suggest that the concept is applicable to women and professionals (DeLong 1982a,b, 1983), and career anchors predict career transitions from employee to manager among engineers, who, like nurses, practice in organizations (Rynes 1987).

## Career Negotiation

A career is not necessarily a tidy progression of jobs with increasing responsibility that leads to a predetermined end. Indeed, most careers are best understood through hindsight review rather than through advance planning. Formal career planning is not common among either men or women, nor is it necessarily related to the level of formal education.

Women, and an increasing number of men, fashion careers based on contingencies. That is, many workers like to remain open to many possibilities. Since they expect to mesh different interests, women especially try to remain flexible and adaptable, as the timing of marriage, children, and other family responsibilities is not entirely predictable. However, employment decisions reflect both career and family values, which vary in intensity over time. For example, for women aged 22 to 44 years, a combination of career and family values predicts employment; for women between 45 and 64 years, career values alone are the best predictors of paid employment (Faver 1982). A study of age differences in the work involvement of men and women concluded that these differences are more complex than previously thought (Lorence 1987). Work autonomy has the most consistent and strongest impact on job involvement for both men and women. Job reward rather than age seems most important for explaining the job involvement of men, probably because older males have better jobs and higher pay. Among women, however, job involvement is higher among older women even when one controls for family characteristics, personal traits, and work rewards. Job mobility for women, as contrasted with men, increases with age (Hall 1986).[1]

Contrary to common perception, women's plans for labor force participation have a much greater effect on plans for childbearing than vice versa (Department of Labor 1975, 28). Thus, career decisions are not one-time events. It is important to realize that careers are not static. As opportunities arise, successes are achieved, constraints change, and the career is modified. In occupations such as hospital nursing, where pay is often not high enough to make a full-time continuous commitment worthwhile, careers are especially fluid, and the importance of organizational experiences on career development is masked.

Unfortunately, researchers are unable to identify the predictors of career commitment (Blau 1985). Male careers have been investigated more thoroughly because their careers have been more predictable, with age and career stages occurring together. Understanding female careers is more difficult because life stages do not match organizational career stages as closely. It is difficult to determine if job expectations and satisfaction are related to female workers' age and the life problems they face or to the job itself.

We do know that some women are more work oriented than others. A few never work for pay. Other women work for a short time, drop out for a brief period of child raising, and then return to work full-time. Other women have a continued series of interruptions. Many women work full-time throughout their lives. Women with more continuous career histories are more likely to invest in education and training based on long-term goals than are those with interrupted careers. In nursing, workers with the latter orientation are the essential core for hospital practice as it becomes more intensive and extensive.

Demographic variables (e.g., marital status, number of children, educational level) have an effect on career orientation but do not specifically identify the career-oriented individual. Although one can argue about the major influences on career development, researchers believe that education, occupational prestige, age, commitment to continue working, and work experiences are more important than sex as predictors of job preferences, intellectual development, and participation (Lacy, Bokemeier, and Shepard 1983; Miller et al. 1979; Haber, Lamas, and Green 1983).

Entrants use the experience of senior personnel as their model of future expectations. If the wage profile remains too flat, the organization eventually becomes less attractive not only to beginners but also to those nurses who are planning a lifetime career.

Nurses are expert career negotiators. Over a lifetime, they usually work the hours of their choice and in the settings they prefer, despite complaints. One of the reasons nurses choose their occupation so much earlier than other women may be the occupation's reputation for "meshing potential"—the ability to get a job almost any time, any place, with a selection of shifts that can accommodate special demands. The significant policy problems are not so much those of individual nurses but the related organizational and societal impacts—too many day workers and too few expert nurses to care for patients in hospitals.

Instead of viewing nurses as a homogeneous group whose job attachment is determined by sex role, analysts and executives need a method of thinking about motivation and job satisfaction for different groups of nurses. Although nurses may not be able to describe their career strategies, executives can study career histories and rethink their assumptions and strategies for attracting and retaining enough nurses. It is important for executives to take a career approach because they are in competition with other industries for talented workers. Continuing to ignore the work expectations of career men and women will mean that nursing will attract workers mostly from the noncareer residual pool, who may be cheaper by the hour but much more expensive by the case, as they require more training and supervision and cause the hospital to incur higher replacement costs.

## Career Styles

The following observed patterns can assist executives in designing work systems and incentives to attract and retain workers with the right mix of career styles: steady-state, linear, entrepreneurial, transient, and spiral. Achieving organizational objectives requires that policies and procedures be designed for individuals with diverse career orientations.

### Steady-State Orientation

> The majority of nurses with a long work history in clinical practice can best be described as steady-state workers who value the norms of the profession.[2] They have little desire for movement except to a higher income or level of professional skill. These nurses expect to meet accepted standards for providing nursing care to patients. Steady-state nurses with a full-time lifetime commitment are the backbone of the nursing service.

Research suggests that workers motivated by professional expectations are characterized by:

- Expertise—specialized education in a body of abstract knowledge

- Autonomy—a perceived right to make choices that concern both means and ends

- Identification with the profession and with fellow professionals
- Ethics—a felt obligation to render service without concern for self-interest and without becoming emotionally involved with the client
- Collegial maintenance of standards with a perceived commitment to help police the conduct of fellow professionals (Kerr, Von Glinow, and Schriesheim 1977).

Steady-state nurses are likely to value access to clinical data, adequate equipment, and opportunities for patient contact and continuing education. Those who look beyond the organization value professional certification and respect for nursing as a profession. To the extent that they conform to the "clinical mentality" syndrome as described in a landmark study by Freidson (1970), steady-state nurses have a preference for action, feel personal (rather than communal) responsibility for their work, believe in what they are doing, trust firsthand experience, and emphasize uncertainties caused by differences among patients.

Frequently overlooked sources of dissatisfaction to steady-state nurses are related to their having too much responsibility (because of inadequate staffing), incompetent allied personnel, and poor interpersonal relationships with subordinates (Cronin-Stubbs 1977). Because hospitals have been accustomed to employing efficient nurses who were well indoctrinated during their apprentice training, hospitals tend to give new graduates too much responsibility too soon. The career impact of this legacy is hard to identify but is undoubtedly significant. Another management practice working against the development of steady-state nurses is the use of nurse registries and incentives to work fewer hours for higher per diem pay.

There are those who denigrate the clinical aspirations of steady-state nurses. Others say they cannot understand why anyone would want to stay in one department doing the same thing indefinitely. These observers confuse their own motivations with the motivations of others. The ecclesiastical phrase *nolo episcopari* ("I am content to be a parish priest and do not want to be made a bishop") could apply to these nurses who are not alone among professionals in valuing their primary work. To the steady-state nurse, although there may be unpleasant tasks, the challenges come from the work itself. The identification with nursing holds primary importance. The nurse with a steady-state orientation, without middle-management interest, should not be written off as devoid of ambition, aspiration, or intellectual curiosity. Achievement for steady-state nurses is derived from patient care; it is an important source of job satisfaction and dissatisfaction for staff nurses; it is not defined by supervisory promotions.

Despite the widely held belief that practicing professionals in organizations experience conflict with the bureaucratic structure of the organization, this is a simplistic notion that needs to be set aside. Professionals who are most involved in their work tend to gravitate to the most effective organizations. Contemporary professionals are not committed to outdated solo practice or bureaucracy models (Blankenship 1977). Nurses with a high professional and organizational orientation are most valued in hospitals (Kramer 1970). The symbiosis between nurses and hospitals should not be surprising, since in some respects, professions are like bureaucracies: Both are oriented toward an impersonal functional purpose, written records, a high level of accountability, and organizational integrity. Bureaucratic structures that enhance professional growth, promote coordination, and provide access to resources and information without interfering with professional autonomy decrease rather than increase conflict. Professional and organizational memberships are continuous, overlapping, and usually complementary, but occasionally conflicting.

**Managerial Implications.** Career satisfaction for steady-state individuals will be enhanced by a work environment where professional work is held in high esteem by the employer and where the employee can relate to the employer's goals and objectives. It also implies that abilities should be both well utilized and recognized. Further, the environment should allow for self-determination of practice issues—timing, work organization, and staffing. Opportunities for personal growth and job challenges that will be valued are those that do not threaten job security. A superb technique for achieving work satisfaction and quality practice is to provide feedback about client outcomes. Two models designed to minimize conflicts between management and clinicians are primary care nursing and decentralization. General management can assist in making these models successful by developing policies to promote both physician-nurse involvement in patient care decisions and organizational loyalty, the latter by rewarding competence and tenure.

Since steady-state nurses are more oriented to tasks than to organizational goals, they may not view their jobs as a career in the conventional sense, especially when they are young. Executives can help by identifying role models for them, publicizing reentry policies, and voicing their awareness that nurses have high work force involvement over a lifetime.

The executive's role is to shape and guide the professional system, being careful to neither ignore it nor extend too far into clinical practice issues. Rather than stressing organizational incompatibility, clinical managers should give advice based on technical knowledge and principles of application.

By respecting the individual nurse's professional orientation and using the control and authority systems advisedly, executives can encourage professionalism and self-control. Professional influences minimize the amount of education and surveillance that the organization has to provide. Even though career advancement opportunities, in the traditional sense, may seem limited within the hospital, career satisfaction is still possible. Nurses are likely to respond to a sense of belonging, a feeling of challenge, a sense of personal significance, and the perception that their talents are being properly used. Nurses' need for achievement can be channeled to patient care concerns, which are certainly not incompatible with physician or organizational goals.

Because nurses frequently work alone with the client, and there are few opportunities for direct observation, natural learning and group interaction opportunities are few. Yet interaction with colleagues has been found to be the positive critical variable in performance among physicians, the occupational group that nurses use for their clinical model (Freidson 1970). Executives can use this insight when working with nurses. Initiating clinical career ladders requires dialogue about practices and standards that have intrinsic value. To be successful, career incentives should match the level of competence and responsibility of the nurses to whom they are offered. A good test for this is to observe whether the incentives are strong enough to stimulate the nurses to invest in their own advanced education.

The current emphasis on "running hospitals like a business" has dangers that outside consultants may not fully appreciate. Instituting formal systems to increase accountability and efficiency may centralize authority, limit flexibility, and lead to role stress as well as unanticipated, but expensive, outcomes, especially for the steady-state nurse. Professional workers in the for-profit sector of the economy enjoy higher wages, more benefits, and greater promotion opportunities than workers in not-for-profit organizations (Mirvis and Hackett 1983). If we take away the advantages in challenge, variety, and autonomy hospital workers now have over private-sector workers, how long can we expect hospital nurses to accept the lesser material rewards and tolerate the pressures to emphasize quantity rather than quality? This is not to argue that hospitals should not be well managed. It does, however, argue against industrial-type control systems, developed separately from practice priorities, if the aim is to develop a stable core of cost-effective nurses. Another business rule should not be forgotten. Productivity gains should be shared with the workers.

## Linear Orientation

Nurses pursuing a linear career model adopt a hierarchical orientation in which there is a steady climb to jobs of increasing administrative, professional, or political responsibility. These nurses traditionally have aspired to be nursing supervisors and directors of nursing services. Now there are opportunities for upwardly oriented nurses in professional associations, politics, and health corporations as well. Linear nurses are consultants to legislators and lawyers as well as administrators of non-hospital-based agencies. Some work for consulting firms, whereas others serve as executive-branch policy advisors. These nurses seldom complain of the blocked mobility or limited authority attributed to hospital nursing administrators. Nor do employers complain that nurses in these leadership jobs are ineffectual. Just as all women now have a wider range of occupational choices, so those with upward aspirations have new career alternatives.

There has been both popular and research interest in the career motives, aspirations, and dilemmas of female managers, especially those in nontraditional occupations (Terborg 1977). Despite the large and increasing number of nurse executives, little documentation exists about the career dilemmas in traditional occupations. It is reasonable to assume that nurse managers are not an idiosyncratic group who differ from all other managers. Until proven otherwise, it seems sensible to apply findings from nonnurse managers to nurse managers. It seems that:

1. The skills women managers need are the same as those needed by men; the same kinds of life experiences, interests, and skills are needed for success (Ritchie and Moses 1983; Donnell and Hall 1980).

2. The career anchor is the best measure for differentiating students who aspire to be managers from those who seek to become practicing professionals (Rynes 1987).

3. Managerial motivation is related to managerial success (Miner 1974).

4. Among management recruits, managerial motivation does not differ between men and women (Howard and Wilson 1982).

5. Managerial success is influenced considerably by having a challenging first job (Buchanan 1974; Hall 1976; Hall and Fukami 1979).

6. Women, as compared to men, experience a relative decline in satisfaction as they acquire more training, get older, and advance to upper management levels—suggesting insufficient integration into top management (Forsionne-Guisseppi and Peeters 1982).

7. Today's young managers, both male and female, are less motivated by success, less optimistic, and less committed to large organizations than previous generations were (Howard and Wilson 1982).

8. The factors important for job involvement are different for managers and nonmanagers (McKelvey and Sekaran 1977).

9. The desire for promotion is a function of workers' expectation of promotion (Walker, Tausky, and Oliver 1982).

Staff nurses may or may not have management potential. The folk wisdom is that nurses, like other professionals, dislike administration and are not good at it. This is true for some. However, the nature of the work in most hospitals requires many staff nurses to bear first-line managerial responsibility without the ability to hire, fire, or even provide performance evaluations for their assistants for whom they are held legally accountable. It may be that nurses assume they do not like management and make strong statements about disliking administration because they are not given the requisite authority and power to meet the managerial responsibilities they have.

In organizations where a high degree of conformity is required, a core of unoriginal, inflexible middle managers may evolve. This phenomenon is so pronounced in some hospitals that it can be described as a cadre of senior nurses with long tenure who supervise a larger revolving segment of young nurses. When upper management accepts this mode of operation, it implies that the costs of low morale, resistance to change, and high turnover among new nurses are affordable—that the price is worth the gain. The gain might be lower payroll costs or the avoidance of conflict among the senior nurses, medical staff, and other support staff. In this situation, there is little need to study the motivations of the staff nurses, but considerable need to study the motivations of the executives.

**Managerial Implications.** Hospital executives need to invest in management development programs for nurses, or they will fall behind the competition and lose a generation of managers. Certainly, with almost a million nurses employed in short-term general hospitals, there are enough who like administration (as distinguished from routine paperwork) to fill the available positions. It seems reasonable to assume that, when employers want upgraded nursing executives, they will act like executives in other industries. That is, employers will identify individuals who want to manage, give them responsibility for a problem that they can manage, help them define the problem, and, as necessary, help them find a solution. Employers will value and reward both education and competence with increased salary and responsibility.

A close examination of work histories will often show that, contrary to common business practice, nurses who have been given increased responsibility have not received increased salary, status, or benefits. Not surprisingly, many nurses with management potential and savvy leave hospital nursing. When this happens, the residual managerial pool may well have a disproportionate number of nurse managers who lack innate management attitudes and who exhibit symptoms of blocked development, including passive resistance to change, insecurity, hostility, alienation from management, and lack of educational credentials.

Primary responsibility rests with senior management to (1) modify the management selection and development system, and (2) reward competent nurse executives, managers, and supervisors. When management development systems are beyond the capacity of individual hospitals (where promotion opportunities are few), the professional associations could play an essential role by developing assessment centers, obtaining funds for tuition reimbursement for management education, and providing for paid internships.

The first two career orientations, steady-state and linear, can be described as traditional. They are in essence emotionally based. That is, the career is guided by internalized norms of the organization or the profession. Both professional and managerial career patterns are understood throughout our culture, but the remaining ones are not. Other individuals shape their careers with less reliance on shared beliefs or professional or organizational expectations. These styles, which are less clearly articulated, are the entrepreneurial career, the transient career, and the spiral career.

## Entrepreneurial and Transient Styles

Workers with an entrepreneurial career style choose to go into business for themselves. For example, a few nurses, especially those with an interest in mental health, primary care, or consulting, have established private practices. Some of these entrepreneurial nurses desire staff appointments, but others do not. In a modified form of private practice, a group of nurses may contract to provide staffing for a clinical service such as critical care. The growth patterns for these experimental forms cannot be predicted with certainty.

Those workers with a transient career pattern have a work history that makes little sense to the outsider. The worker seems to hold a series of unrelated jobs of relatively short duration. This appears to suggest a lack of commitment to both the organization and the profession. This pattern characterizes the early career period for many male and female professionals, and it may continue for others throughout most of their working lives.

Two subgroups of transient career workers were found to exist among a study sample of executives: those who were highly paid and those who were low paid (M. Driver, University of Southern California School of Business Administration, personal communication, 1982). The highly paid executives were troubleshooters who were adept at solving complex problems. However, once the challenge was over, they moved to other areas. Within nursing, there are consultants and a few directors of nursing services who serve as troubleshooters, but there are many more of the second type, those who work when it is convenient in order to achieve a target income or enhance their personal situation when opportunities arise.

Transient nurses are often viewed as opportunists, working when necessary at the jobs that best fit their personal requirements. Transitory workers are essentially day workers, willing to do a day's work for a day's pay. As such, they are scorned by some nursing leaders who promote professionalism. Yet there is no reason to believe that they are less competent than any other worker. Both independent and part-time workers can be motivated by intrinsic features, even though their initial reason for working may be economic or social. Although executives may find it hard to accept, independent workers may even have a greater work commitment than regular employees (Kohn and Schooler 1973).

Transient workers are useful. Some provide care to patients while studying for other jobs. University hospitals, in particular, may depend on short-term nurses to staff the night shifts. Transient nurses are part of the on-call pool that allows the hospital to accommodate fluctuating occupancy. They also comprise a reserve pool that can be attracted back to work by higher salaries when employers want more nurses.

The prevailing emphasis on home-career conflict as the root determinant of nurse work force participation fosters, whether consciously or not, an increase in the number of nurses with a transient orientation to work. Hospitals are often caught in a circular process of attracting nurses who expect to have short tenure, tailoring rewards to them, perpetuating short tenure, and as a result having few nurses of long tenure who can provide the needed continuity, stability, and clinical expertise.

Flextime is a popular remedy for overcoming the nursing shortage without increasing pay, but it probably increases the proportion of transient nurses. Evaluation of flextime schemes suggests that the long-term consequence may be to increase rather than decrease alienation and cynicism among employees who value intrinsically rewarding work (Rainey and Wolf 1981). This may be mitigated when employees with emotional needs for self-actualization participate in the decision to implement flextime in such a way that jobs are simultaneously enriched (Latack and Foster 1985). Insofar as productivity is concerned, it would appear that flextime has a positive effect when limited physical resources are being shared by a work group (Ralston, Anthony, and Gustafson 1985). An evaluation in Canadian hospitals found that the extended workday, another attempt to give employees more time off, resulted in a decrease in the amount of patient care. Turnover and absenteeism rates were not reduced, even though the nurses had increased leisure time (Staples and Curtis 1975).

**Managerial Implications.** If hospitals decrease the number of permanent full-time staff in favor of a larger float pool or part-time staff to achieve variable staffing levels, without simultaneously investing in core nurses, the pool of remaining hospital nurses will consist primarily of transient day workers. In the long run, most applicants will come from the group of women desiring modest work commitments. As cost containment artificially constrains wages, career-oriented nurses will prepare for out-of-hospital careers. By suboptimizing, as many hospitals did when prospective payment was introduced in 1983, hospitals sow the seeds of future shortages of professionally and organizationally committed workers.

Without denigrating the contribution of entrepreneurial and transient workers, managers need to differentiate clearly between the rewards offered them and those available to core steady-state and linear workers. Organizationally committed workers should have a greater voice in organizational and practice decisions, and pay and benefits should reflect their greater value to the organization in the long run. Meanwhile, in the new health care environment, many opportunities exist for entrepreneurial nurses to develop, market, and profit from new product development.

## Spiral Orientation

The fifth career style is the spiral career. It is described as rational, because the individual has assumed more independent responsibility for shaping the career independently of either the organization or the profession. These individuals usually have a five- to seven-year period of employment that engages their talents, interests, and personal involvement. This is followed by other relatively long periods of work that provide new career challenges. To the outsider, this career may be difficult to fathom, but to the individual nurse it makes sense.

The spiral career style works well for nurses who are preparing for out-of-hospital careers as well as for those who cherish traditional female values and work. Nurses expect to care for others and to provide sustenance. Having received an education and worked for pay for a few years, has a nurse changed or abandoned her career when she opts to stay home to have children? Is it surprising when, having mastered the homemaker challenge, she returns to the hospital to reexamine her options and reestablish a paid career? Should we believe that there is something wrong with nursing or the educational system when she chooses other socially useful work over underpaid or unsatisfactory hospital employment? The nurse whose primary career orientation is spiral seeks opportunities for self-development. Although salary may not be a primary motivator, nurses with this orientation are likely to find well-paid service-oriented jobs and will not settle for being poorly paid.

Spiral career workers, when asked what their career plans are, feel embarrassed. They may deny that they are fashioning a career or, at best, say they want an interesting or fulfilling job. Managers and counselors who only understand professional and hierarchical careers are confused by such a response. Questions such as, "Where are you going?" and "What is your long-range plan?" are inappropriate for these individuals; advice appropriate for steady-state and linear individuals is also inappropriate.

**Managerial Implications.** To deal with individuals who are committed to shaping a spiral career, one should abandon hopes to "psych out" or manipulate the individual. The best approach for this as perhaps for all the other career styles is to configure a specific job that needs doing, agree on both the terms and the length of the commitment, and keep your promise. These employees need clear time frames and challenging initial job assignments. They will probably respond well to a management-by-objectives program. Other strategies are to provide horizontal transfers to new jobs, or even sabbaticals for highly valued individuals.

## Career Anchors

Individual motives and values can be visualized by using career anchor concepts. A career anchor is the combination of perceived needs, values, and talents that guide and constrain individual career decisions. The premise of career anchors is that the constellation of what people are good at and what they are seeking from work, together with the kind of organization they want to be associated with, stabilizes with work experience. The primary anchor then becomes the constellation of features that the individual is least likely to forego.

Eight career anchors have been identified: service, managerial competence, autonomy, technical or functional competence, security, identity, variety, and creativity (DeLong 1982a).

1. *Service.* Service-oriented people are concerned with helping others and seeing the change their efforts make. They want to use interpersonal skills in the service of others. Their rewards come from seeing others change because of their efforts.

2. *Managerial Competence.* Individuals with a managerial orientation perceive that their competencies lie in interpersonal skills and the ability to analyze problems and to remain emotionally stable in the face of challenges. They hope to advance in the organizational hierarchy and have the potential for high income.

3. *Autonomy.* Individuals with an autonomy orientation are concerned primarily with their own sense of freedom. They may find organizational life too restrictive. When employed by organizations, they will seek situations where they have autonomy to pursue professional or technical-functional competence.

4. *Technical-Functional Competence.* Those persons who are motivated by the work itself (for example, critical care nursing, financial analysis, or medical technology) are concerned with technical or functional competence. They seek job challenge and personal recognition for their talents.

5. *Security.* People with a security orientation tie their careers either to a specific company or to a specific geographic location. They are concerned with long-term stability and benefits and are more likely to let the organization define their careers. Many of these individuals want to spend time with their families or pursue personal interests and will sacrifice upward advancement to work established hours.

6. *Identity.* Persons whose anchor is identity are guided throughout their careers by the status and prestige of belonging to prestigious or powerful employers. They are unlikely to be attracted to low-profile organizations and likely to identify with visible organizational accomplishments.

7. *Variety.* Variety-oriented individuals seek many challenges rather than routine and predictable tasks and settings. They can be motivated by changing assignments, such as the float pool and ad hoc task forces.

8. *Creativity.* Individuals who are creativity oriented need to develop something of their own. They like new endeavors and projects. As their career progresses, they may leave the organization to go out on their own. They comprise the smallest group in organizations that have been studied, probably because organizations have difficulty providing enough freedom for this group.

All of these categories are essentially self-descriptions, not identifications that are assigned arbitrarily. To that extent, they are biased and may not reflect objective reality. This is not a serious disadvantage in the context used here, since supervisors are interested in understanding professional job attitudes and employee perceptions of their work and life space, rather than the "facts" as determined by an unbiased observer.

Within occupations, individuals describe differing constellations of anchors. It is unlikely that all nurses will be primarily guided by one career anchor alone. A review of the studies that have been done on other occupational groups suggests that subclustering occurs. Among dentists, for example, there were four distinct groups with similar career values and orientations (DeLong 1983).

In the future, we can expect researchers to link career anchors with career styles (Friss 1982). The spiral career style, for example, may well be linked with the creativity anchor (Prince 1979). The steady-state career seems likely to be rooted in the security and technical-functional anchors, whereas the linear careerist might hold the managerial competence and variety anchors.[3]

## Career Stage

Research on career stages, which began in the 1940s and 1950s, had a developmental focus that has resulted in several models of occupational choice and development. Although the models differ as to time periods, labels, and emphasis, the premise is that careers develop in predictable stages. Unfortunately, theorists assumed that only males with steady-state or linear styles had staged careers. Therefore, career stage and life stage were parallel concerns. This is not necessarily true for women. Despite the difficulty in understanding the complex stages of women's careers, attention to stage is essential. This is especially true in understanding nurses because full-time hospital nurses tend to be young. The employment structure, especially in community hospitals, encourages mature nurses to work part-time or seek employment in nonhospital settings. Thus, studies of hospital nurses are in fact studies of nurses in early career stages.

For example, in a well-designed, theory-based study, five tenure categories were identified (Seyboldt 1983): entry (under six months), early (six months to one year), middle (one to three years), advanced (three to six years), and later (over six years). Seyboldt described these categories as (1) raw recruits, (2) "Young Turks" who were interested in performance outcomes, (3) skeptics about supervisory expectations, (4) burn out candidates who needed feedback from their work, and (5) career-satisfied or "old guard" workers.

These categories are much more compressed than the divisions career researchers have generally used. Workers in other organizations are described as passing through an exploratory phase, which is followed by establishment, maintenance, and decline stages that parallel maturation.

The corresponding ages are 15 to 24 years, 25 to 44 years, 45 to 65 years, and over age 65. The establishment phase is subdivided into (1) preentry and entry; (2) basic training and initiation; (3) first regular assignment and promotion or leveling off; (4) second assignment; (5) tenure, termination, and exit; and (6) postexit.

The interest in reality shock, or the transition from school to work, stems from in-depth study of the exploratory phase, where it is believed that group values and norms most influence a new member's behavior. It is during this time that the skills and values acquired in school or in other organizations must be adjusted to the demands of the job. Although reality shock occurs in most occupations where education occurs away from work, the theory has been best tested in nursing (Kramer 1974).

During the entry stage, the goals should be to provide a realistic preview of the job, linkage with inside peers (mentors), and an early collaborative appraisal process, and to initiate a proactive socialization process (Wanous 1978; Louis 1980). The failures that can occur are (1) A high-potential recruit rejects a job offer, (2) a high-potential recruit joins but soon leaves, (3) a high-potential recruit joins but loses motivation and becomes a marginal performer, or (4) a recruit seems to have high talent but actually has low talent or motivation, or values that are incompatible with those of the organization (Schein 1978).

To avoid these negative outcomes, it is important that recruitment and selection activities be well integrated with job placement and early supervision, as well as human resource planning and development strategies. Likewise, supervisors of new employees must be chosen carefully. The supervisor's responsibilities are to minimize assignments that are either too hard or too easy, provide assignments that are meaningful, provide early and frequent feedback, and transmit values and norms. Supervisors can expect that new workers' expectations will be inflated, except regarding pay (which is concretely defined), and that with increased experience, individuals will be less satisfied (Wanous 1977). The aims of a coordinated entry program are to moderate expectations and reduce turnover without reducing recruitment success.

Whether the tournament career model, in which early career successes are associated more strongly with career outcomes than are later competitions, applies to steady-state nursing careers has not been verified. Critical-incident studies are needed to ascertain the effect of early jobs on later organizational and career commitment.

The factors that facilitate career development during the establishment phase are:

1. Career development courses
2. Behavior modeling training for supervisors
3. Supervisors who provide high support with autonomy and who set high expectations
4. Challenging initial job assignments (Hall and Fukami 1979).

The following facilitate continued growth in middle and late career: (1) continued career exploration, (2) effective personnel policies, (3) periodic job changes, (4) a good communications climate, (5) rewards for performance, (6) participative leadership, (7) matrix structures, and (8) lateral and downward job moves (Hall and Fukami 1979).

As the person's organizational career progresses, tenure becomes an important moderating variable for job satisfaction for both men and women (Katz 1978a, b). The timetables for organizational socialization are not fixed and probably vary within and between organizations. Diagnostic studies of nurses demonstrate that organizations can assess their reward structure by tenure category to obtain useful information (Feldman 1976).

An alternative model of career stages for (steady-state) professionals suggests four organizational career stages: learning, contributing, training, and shaping the organization (Thompson, Dalton, and Price 1977). During the learning stage, the primary relationship is that of an apprentice, and the major psychological issue is dependence. During the next phase the worker is an individual contributor whose primary relationships are with colleagues; the major psychological issue is independence. During the third phase, the central activity is training. The primary relationship is one of being a mentor, but not a manager, who assumes responsibility for others and becomes an informal idea person. The final stage is that of influencing organizational direction. The primary relationship is as a sponsor; the major psychological issue is exercising power. At this time, the individual has the expertise and influence necessary to institute innovations.

Other models exist, but the central theme is that employees are continuously negotiating and remodeling their perspective toward the organization and their own roles in it (Katz 1980). There is reason to believe that differences in worker satisfaction are at least as great within occupational categories as between them (Van Maanen and Katz 1976). More attention will be given to clarifying multiple measures of work commitment, job involvement, organizational commitment, and intent to remain, and matching them to different career stage dimensions such as age, organizational tenure, and position tenure (Morrow and McElroy 1987).

Careers for the talented will be shaped differently from those of the average and below-average employee. A perpetual dilemma for supervisors is to establish the balance between treating workers equally yet rewarding those with special talent. Hospitals affiliated with universities and teaching programs will have more challenging advanced clinical positions for the many talented who, as a result, will gravitate to that setting. Multihospital systems can provide opportunities for talented workers at other sites more easily than can free-standing hospitals.

Regardless of the setting, the careers of the talented should receive high priority for two major reasons: First, talented aspiring nurses must be able to foresee challenging careers in nursing, or they will select other college majors. Second, talented nurses are needed to invest in nursing as a career and assume leadership positions in research, clinical practice, administration, and teaching. Otherwise, future executives will be faced with a shortage of qualified staff nurses and middle managers. Having said this, it is important to remember that, in their daily work, subunit supervisors spend time influencing the productivity and commitment of nurses, not all of whom are extraordinarily gifted or skilled.

Regional associations of hospitals have much to gain by advertising lifetime opportunities in clinical nursing, and encouraging employer actions that will minimize the churning that results from an abundance of transient and spiral workers. The multihospital systems have an advantage here, because they may have not only more expertise in human resource management but also more career opportunities to offer.

## Life Cycle

Life cycle theory suggests that there is a complex interaction among basic talents, motives, values (career anchors), opportunity structures, and the totality of life roles (Bailyn and Schein 1976). Circumstances related to life cycles affect the work behaviors of both men and women. Traditional career expectations have been built on the traditional male life cycle: focus on a career with neglect of family life in the early years followed by a period of reevaluation of priorities and a resolution, with more attention to personal needs later in life. Much of the tension in career development comes from (1) the lack of acceptance of different family life and career cycle models and (2) the disjuncture between career and life cycles, which occurs more often among women than among men.

The overall life role of women has been described as an orderly and developmental one, which can be divided into sequences according to the preeminent task in each stage (Zytowski 1969). This is the basis for the stereotype of nursing work: a few years of full-time work followed by either retirement or years of part-time work and early withdrawal from hospital work. Although this may sound archaic, one must recall that nursing attracts primarily women who assume responsibility for shaping paid and nonpaid careers simultaneously. Although female nurses, along with other women, are modifying their career patterns, as evidenced by their early return to the work force after childbearing, no evidence exists that women are abandoning their basic strategy of seeking work and family satisfaction (Regan and Rowland 1985). Indeed, nursing may be the prototype profession for models of female work force participation.

A common mistake is to assume that these marriage and family variables are exogenous variables, ones that occur independently of work force decisions. Basic work force decisions, such as whether to take chemistry in high school to meet nursing admission requirements, are made before rather than after marriage and childbearing decisions. Marital status is influenced by the same factors that influence the labor supply: age, education, income, and the state of the economy. It seems that life and career satisfaction are intimately linked (Kavanagh and Halpern 1977). Those who emphasize that a woman's paid career is dependent on the husband's approval forget that these decisions are interdependent. A career-committed woman is unlikely to choose or remain with a mate who does not share her preferences.

Two other studies of women have expanded on the life cycle approach. Andrisani's (1978) study, using national labor force data, failed to support the common belief that women who are reentering the work force pay above-average psychic costs. He found that reentering women were more satisfied than those who have been continuously employed. Andrisani speculated that women who are deeply committed to work have high self-esteem and attach importance to the intrinsic aspects of work. Whether this is true of nurses is not known.

What is known is that nurse refresher programs, which are instituted during times of work force shortages (based on the presumption that the returning worker is emotionally fragile), are universally unsuccessful. The nurses who participate in them do not continue in hospital employment, although they may use the education as a springboard for employment in other areas of nursing. Such behavior supports the belief that mature women with employment alternatives do not find the employment practices in the hospitals compatible with their career expectations. Although hospitals need to offer orientation programs to new workers, the premise of many reentry programs—that nurses are insecure and technologically obsolete—may be based on paternalism instead of reality.

The other study addressed value transition in adult women (Ryff 1979). Noting that women as compared to men have shown changes in lifestyle or personality between middle age and old age, Ryff found that, during middle age, women have a heightened personal emphasis on mastery, competence, control of the environment, and being instrumental. That is, there is a movement away from service to others toward concern with one's own position (Sheehy 1976; Gould 1978). Furthermore, when the middle-aged person has to face a major discrepancy between personal and societal or organizational value systems, the contradictions are difficult to reconcile. The fact that older nurses with experience are less likely to work implies that the stimulus for a changed reward system is not coming solely from young workers who want autonomy and expanded use of their talents, but also from mature workers who want higher pay and more influence. In a university teaching hospital study, Weisman (1982) found that mature nurses were more likely than young nurses to leave when they were dissatisfied.

Reinterpretation of data from a seminal study of commitment of teachers and nurses, by Hrebiniak and Alutto (1972), shows that younger employees who were uncertain about what was expected of them were least committed to staying with their current employer, whereas younger employees who knew their obligations and older employees regardless of their uncertainties were all highly committed (Salancik 1977). Deutsch (1985), found that younger nurses preferred the extended workday. As the work force ages, researchers and managers will have more need to consider the work-related impacts of age and the life cycle.

## Organizational Implications

A reasonable question that managers ask, given the complexity of career development, is whether work-related experiences are important.

There are those who argue that professional education determines the career structure. Others argue that the influences of peers and the professional organizations are paramount (Light 1980). In practical terms, few managers would argue that their own careers were shaped independently of job-related rewards. It is unlikely that nursing careers are either. At a time when nursing is losing its attractiveness, as evidenced by the decline in nursing school enrollments and the test scores of applicants, it is imperative that executives take a detailed career process perspective when viewing staffing and quality problems.

Organizations benefit from having employees with differing career orientations: steady-state, linear, spiral, and transient. Executives can modify work force practices that cause an imbalance, whether it be too many or too few steady-state, transient, spiral, or linear nurses. Rather than thinking about what motivates nurses as a group, executives can ask what the organization needs and then establish the policies necessary to obtain the right nursing mix. It would be misleading to suggest that this process is either exact or easy. Once senior management commits itself to a career-based employment system, many practical guides are available (Burack and Mathys 1980; Schein 1978; Hall 1976; Gibson and Dewhirst 1986). Tables 1-1 and 1-2 list the motives underlying each career style and suggest organizational strategies.

Managers need adopt neither an overly optimistic nor an overly pessimistic view of their own abilities to reward individuals and influence

**Table 1-1** Strongest Motives for Each Career Style

| Spiral | Linear | Steady-State | Transient |
|---|---|---|---|
| Novelty | Money | Competence | Novelty |
| Prestige | Recognition | Stability | Other people |
| Money | Prestige | Autonomy | Creativity |
| Self-development | Self-development | Achievement | Power |
| Recognition | Management | Recognition/ | Achievement |
|  | Power | organization |  |
|  | Achievement | contribution |  |
|  | Competence |  |  |

Source: Driver, M. 1981. Demographic and societal factors affecting the linear career crisis. Unpublished manuscript, Department of Management Organization, University of Southern California.

**Table 1-2** Suggested Management Strategies for Each Career Style

| Career Style | Management Strategies |
|---|---|
| Steady-state | Permanent specialty assignments<br>Authority to make work-related decisions<br>Precise job descriptions<br>Job security, good benefits<br>Emphasis on quality care, patient service, feedback on outcomes<br>Respect and professional recognition<br>Continuing education opportunities<br>Shared governance<br>Differentiated practice |
| Linear | Opportunities for upward mobility<br>Job descriptions more flexible as pyramid is climbed<br>Recognition, status, and power for achievement<br>Less supervision with high responsibility<br>Pay for performance<br>Opportunities for skill training |
| Spiral | Job rotation, enlargement<br>Negotiated, evolving job descriptions based on mutual need<br>Matrix organization or autonomous teams<br>Encouragement of creativity, interpersonal closeness, training others |
| Transient | Clearly defined duties and responsibilities<br>Appropriate assignments, immediate feedback<br>Bonuses, job rotation, flextime<br>Clear reentry policies<br>Clear career lines to encourage transition to other career styles |

behavior. Granted that the individuals have greater knowledge of their own career goals than the organization has, organizations can seek opportunities to reward the best performing workers or those most likely to fit the organizational goals.

Career terminology itself allows employees to recognize different alternatives, respect their own patterns, seek out appropriate models, and weigh conflicting advice given by well-meaning individuals. Experience has shown that individuals can identify their own career style and the job changes accompanying a shift in career anchors. The use of career terminology can help staff members understand each other's similarities and differences, and clarify why some things are important and others are not. This is particularly important in a field where there has been little career awareness, in spite of a high level of work involvement. Since no one career type is presented as inherently better than any other, the tendency to disparage individuals who follow a different pattern is reduced. This, in turn, facilitates worker acceptance of targeted rather than global work force improvement plans.

Career concepts provide a check on a common work force error, namely, a tendency for employers to hire persons with similar backgrounds based on a common belief that homogeneity will increase organizational stability and survival. For example, a department that uses high developmental potential as the criterion for hiring, training, and promoting soon finds that turnover is high and morale is low. As the organizationally independent nurses develop self-confidence, they search for new challenges elsewhere. Other facilities, such as government hospitals that offer considerable job security and high fringe benefits, may find that both staffing and supervisory style are unnecessarily rigid. They may need to structure policies that permit use of supplemental agencies, or, if they need rejuvenation, they might experiment with a few fixed-term contracts to encourage spiral workers.

Pressures for short-term operating efficiencies often lead to narrowly conceived solutions. An organizational philosophy that develops a revolving-door culture by hiring too many transient nurses (because they provide more flexibility and are cheaper than raising wages for all workers) may be enhancing a downward spiral that will affect quality of care and the ability to attract and retain either clinically expert or administratively experienced nurses. When conditions improve, these hospitals will have lost the best nurses, be understaffed, and find that their competitors have an edge. This, in turn, will fuel the next round of catch-up pay raises, reliance on more inexperienced or part-time workers, and less than optimal productivity. Enlightened employers jointly foster employment security and productivity during both lean and expansive times. Retrenchment is always difficult, but executives with good competency assessment programs can use lean times as an opportunity for replacing marginal employees with a tenuous career commitment to achieve a better mix.

The recurring cycles of nurse shortages suggest that, collectively, employers have neglected the development of steady-state workers through a combination of low pay, short pay ranges, a lack of seniority-related benefits, and limited professional development opportunities. These deficiencies, coupled with strategies that encourage the development of transient workers—such as part-time work, flexible schedules, and low fringe benefits—leave the hospitals vulnerable in the future. Cure depends not so much on new techniques as on a changed perspective. If an industry is not getting a fair share of professional workers who will work continuously over a lifetime, what do managers need to do differently? Are they understating the importance of salary, compacted salary schedules, salary reduction programs, pensions, continuing education, and participation in organizational decision-making for a key group of workers?

As employers develop a disaggregated career awareness, they become more concerned about how their individual actions shape the career patterns of nurses. In a competitive environment such as currently exists, as employers have cut back indiscriminately on steady-state or linear career incentives, they have sown the seeds of work force shortages in the future for all employers of nurses. Executives with long-term vision and concern are well advised to increase industry efforts to identify and reward careers in hospitals lest they lose a generation of those most difficult to replace. Even though it may not be possible for one employer to monitor or change the employment practices of poor employers, self-interest requires that enough employers be concerned about the long-range quality and quantity of the shared pool of workers to maintain the reputation of hospitals as a desirable place to work.

## Advantages

Among the advantages of using the career framework are that (1) it can integrate the useful insights of various disciplines, (2) it can be applied to both men and women, (3) it encourages an understanding of the relationships between paid and nonpaid work, (4) it is compatible with the idea that both employees and employers seek the best fit of work expectations and rewards, and (5) comprehensive texts are available to assist with implementation.

Much of the organization design literature assumes the traditional stance, that is, that executives and supervisors assess the environment, establish goals, set priorities, and control workers to achieve objectives. The static nature of most approaches fails to provide supervisors with a framework that is compatible with current cultural trends toward a fluid life cycle and an age-irrelevant society. Gradually, the rational approach has been tempered by an awareness that individual values permeate the organization and that the combined values of employees and employers give organizations a unique personality or culture. A career-oriented approach to interpreting individual behaviors is a dynamic approach that encourages interactive rather than manipulative or coercive control methods. As more people seek to lead integrated lives in which their family lives and their work lives are mutually reinforcing, executives and supervisors will need to be more attuned to the changing aspirations and desires of workers.

Most other concepts used to distinguish workers from one another are difficult, if not impossible, to link with organizational strategies, policies, or long-term planning. It is difficult to link intrinsic motivation to alternative career profiles, for example. Furthermore, it is difficult to translate the changes that are occurring in personal preferences among nurses into work-related concerns. Thus, although it is interesting to know that among nursing students the profiles on deference needs and autonomy are changing, such that nurses do not differ from other students, this information does not help a supervisor modify the reward structure (Kahn 1980).

The career concepts approach gives managers a structure for exploring career commitments and encourages them to avoid treating workers as a homogeneous group whose behavior is bounded by family interests. Employers can use the framework to reflect on how they fared during previous cycles and examine their current work force policies on hiring, training, counseling, transferring, and terminating employees. The question to ask is whether the incentive structure needs to be modified to attract or retain a particular career type based on the organization's future plans and projections.

Career concepts can also diminish the usual gap between what supervisors think employees want and what employees really want. The intent is not for supervisors to mold individuals toward their own preference or the needs of the organization. Instead supervisors can be encouraged to provide differential rewards appropriate for the present, with a concern for future career development. This can give steady-state nurses an opportunity to evaluate clinical equipment prior to purchase, work with physicians on quality control, or have budgets for equipment repair or replacement, for example. They can give spiral career-oriented nurses an opportunity to face new challenges by working on new or short-term projects. Career concepts can help determine whether proposed solutions are the best for the work force problem at hand. Career differentiation gives employers a practical way to tailor incentives that is not discriminatory. This step precedes modifying employment practices to obtain workers with different orientations.

In addition to clarifying different types of careers, career concepts are compatible with the four major thrusts of career theory, which suggests that careers are related to (1) social class, (2) individual psychological traits, (3) life cycle, and (4) career stage (Sonnenfeld and Kotter 1982). Further research should clarify hypothesized relationships between career types and measures of job satisfaction. Future research should enable us to link career concepts with organizational practices. Until then, the concepts can serve useful functions by specifying career diversity and encouraging the development of career strategies that target resources for the future without jeopardizing the present.

## Objections to Career Concepts

Staw (1980) argued against making career management rational on the grounds that informed workers will become aware of alternatives and become dissatisfied or leave the organization. The implied assumptions are that workers can be isolated from information and that the employer is better served by a docile, captive work force. The first assumption is an impossibility, and the second is both questionable and unlikely. Staw also assumes that career management awareness involves a career education component for all employees. These are in fact separate options. Employers are free to use career theories and frameworks without instituting career development programs for workers. Even more important, hospital nurses need guidance not on how to negotiate a career to achieve personal goals, but on the possibilities for developing a career within the industry, if not within the specific institution.

Although it may not be to employers' advantage to embrace career education as a primary objective, employers are responsible for determining work requirements and designing incentive systems to attract and retain the right mix of workers without paying so much that the employer becomes financially nonviable. Organizational career planning is related to individual planning, but the two should not be confused. Organizational career management has the following components: assessment of potential, appraisal of performance, career planning connection, career ladders, succession planning, a personnel information system, career information, counseling, and a functioning personnel system (Burack and Mathys 1980). The issue is not losing employees, but losing the right kind while encouraging others to make a career commitment. It may even be advantageous, as well as affordable, to lose two temporary workers to encourage the tenure of one skilled clinician.

Another concern is that the categories can be used to label people or pigeonhole them. The career framework does provide a labeling terminology. It is human nature to cluster people and things in an effort to simplify complexity, and to predict more of people's behavior more of the time. However, the career concepts terminology does not carry the negative connotation that goes with the usual professional versus nonprofessional dichotomy. Moreover, in an era when many more women than before are opting for careers, managers need contemporary language and images. These concepts are based on a review of past actions rather than on a subjective assessment of motivations, social pressures, aspirations, or attributes (such as age, race, and sex). In the past, problems associated with sex were not separated from problems related to age. Faced with nurse shortages, employers and analysts tend to seek solutions to the problems of women with young children (i.e., young women). The career perspective encourages new questions. Where are the women without children? women with career commitments? mature women who work full-time?

Another objection to a career focus argues that it is not feasible because climates and benefits must apply to all equally, especially if one wants to encourage a shared, patient-focused culture. That is, diversity is not feasible without unfair discrimination. On the contrary, career concepts are most compatible in an environment where management does have a shared vision of promoting service to clients and encouraging the professional growth of employees. What it requires are some universal policies, not only in the obvious areas of rule compliance, base pay, and benefits, but also in individualized approaches for individuals and groups related to tasks and goal identification—areas specifically related to careers. One universal strategy in a field dominated by women who do not have a highly developed career orientation and who plan to mesh paid and nonpaid work is a specific and widely known procedure for reentry. The commitment to career clarification, with incentives tied to organizational needs, can be applied universally. Nurses shape different careers. The problem is that they do it independently of the hospital in many cases. The challenge is for the organization to use differentiated career systems in ways that keep hospital nursing an attractive career.

# Summary

This chapter takes a career approach to understanding the work motivations of nurses, rather than adopting previously used models of motivation, which assumed that gender-related differences were paramount. Career progression is unpredictable, and careers for all workers are not static but fluid. Not all nurses can be expected to be full-time bedside nurses, nor would hospitals, individually or collectively, find that desirable. Management policies, however, should be to design career structures so that enough nurses (and potential nurses) with a full-time career orientation will find nursing a worthwhile career. It is difficult to predict career commitment, but many agree that a flat wage profile leads many current and potential nurses to perceive bedside nursing as unattractive. The emphasis on flexibility of hours and shifts attracts and encourages nurses with a part-time and temporary orientation. As successful as this may be in the short term, this very feature may lead to the demise of a core of experienced, clinically competent bedside nurses.

Five basic career styles have been identified. The steady-state workers are the backbone of the profession. Their main focus is excellence in patient care. Nurses who pursue linear careers have upward career aspirations. These first two types represent traditional nurses' careers. The third is that of the entrepreneurs who choose to go into business for themselves. The fourth is the transient career pattern, which is characterized by working in a series of brief, unrelated jobs. The final career style is the spiral career. It is characterized by workers staying five to seven years in a job and then moving to a new career challenge. Each type of career style presents both problems and opportunities for managers.

Career anchors, which are a combination of needs, values, and talent, influence career decisions. Possible anchors include service, security, variety, and autonomy, among others. Although research does not yet link specific anchors to career styles, managers can use the two concepts to clarify their assumptions about motivation and reward strategies. Another important concept is that of career stages based on length of time in the job. Workers have different needs during the different stages of job tenure, as distinguished from needs attributed to chronological age. Life cycle theory revolves around the interaction of career anchors, opportunities, and life roles. Managers of nurses, like managers of workers generally, need to consider not only young nurses' home commitments, but also the needs of reentering nurses and of mature nurses.

Since work-related behavior is heavily influenced by the perceptions individuals have of career structures, employers must send clear signals to attract and retain the mix of nurses necessary to achieve their strategic objectives. Short-term fixes may enable marginal hospitals to survive in the short run but are expensive to the industry in the long run and should be avoided. In the current climate, there is a special need in most hospitals to make steady-state careers attractive.

Some researchers see flaws in the career concepts, but these can be overcome. Overall, career theory is less sex-biased than other models of motivation, such as hierarchy of needs, intrinsic versus extrinsic motivation, and home-career conflict. It is also more appropriate than the professional-bureaucratic conflict model. Overall, it is vital that managers cluster their human resource management approaches to encourage the career mix suitable for their organization without damaging the career image of steady-state nurses.

## Endnotes

1. For a full discussion of age-related differences in work attitudes and behavior, see Rhodes (1983); for a discussion of both age and gender dimensions of work, see Hall (1986).

2. Throughout this text nursing is called a profession. This conforms to contemporary usage (Evans and Laumann 1983). The professions do not necessarily constitute a set of high-status occupations meeting a narrowly specified set of defining characteristics. Rather, the professions are those occupations specializing in the development, transmission, and application of the technical, systematic components of knowledge. Therefore, these occupations stand particularly close to core parts of the cultural system.

   It is not necessary here to debate degrees of professionalism in relation to other occupations. Generally, the more an individual invests in education to become a member of an occupation, the more likely the individual is to identify with occupational norms and work. Except for law, medicine, pharmacy, and dentistry, none of 23 occupations (including nursing) studied by Evans and Laumann (1983) offer even a majority of its incumbents a lifetime of work. Thus, limited upward mobility and fluid career structures are not idiosyncratic to nurses or to women in general.

In traditional terms, many nurses are local in orientation rather than cosmopolitan. This means that the value system that was shaped during their education is supported and influenced by work and life experiences more than by professional associations or external peers. The challenge for managers is to build organizational loyalty among members with an established occupational loyalty (Van Maanen and Barley 1984).

3.  When I have used the DeLong (1982b) career anchor instrument in management classes, I have never had a student score high on the technical-functional competence anchor. I tell these students that, in all probability, they are surrounded by individuals who are not representative of the majority of hospital workers. Nor are they being taught theories of motivation that are appropriate for women or professional service workers (Friss 1986).

# References

Andrisani, P. 1978. Job satisfaction among working women. *Signs* 3: 588–607.

Bailyn, L., and E. Schein. 1976. Life/career considerations as indicators of quality of employment, in A. Bederman and T. Drury, eds., *Measuring work quality for social reporting.* New York: Wiley, pp. 151–68.

Blankenship, R., ed. 1977. *Colleagues in organization.* New York: Wiley.

Blau, G. 1985. The measurement and prediction of career commitment. *Journal of Occupational Psychology* 58: 277–288.

Buchanan, B. 1974. Building organizational commitment: the socialization of managers in work organizations. *Administrative Science Quarterly* 19: 533–546.

Burack, E., and N. Mathys. 1980. *Career management in organizations: a practical human resource planning approach.* Lake Forest, IL: Brace Park.

Cronin-Stubbs, D. 1977. Job satisfaction and dissatisfaction among new graduate staff nurses. *Journal of Nursing Administration* 7(10): 44–49.

DeLong, T. 1982a. Reexamining the career anchor model. *Personnel* 59 (3): 50–61

DeLong, T. 1982b. The multi-dimensional career orientations of women. *Clinical Preventive Dentistry* 4: 23–26.

DeLong, T. 1983. Dentists and career satisfaction: an empirical view. *Journal of Dentistry for Children* 50: 179–185.

Department of Labor. 1975. *Birth expectations and working plans of young women: changes in role choices.* Washington, DC: Government Printing Office.

Deutsch, B. 1985. *A comparison of leisure activities and levels of derived satisfaction between nurses working on a traditional and restructured work-week schedule.* Unpublished doctoral dissertation, New York University.

Donnell, S., and J. Hall. 1980. Men and women as managers: a significant case of no significant difference. *Organizational Dynamics* 8 (4): 60–77.

Driver, M. 1979. Career concepts and career management in organizations, in C. Cooper, ed., *Behavioral problems in organizations.* Englewood Cliffs, NJ: Prentice Hall, pp. 79–139.

Evans, M., and E. Laumann. 1983. Professional commitment: myth or reality? *Research in Social Stratification and Mobility.* 2: 3–40.

Faver, C. 1982. Women, careers, and family: generational and life-cycle effects on achievement orientation. *Journal of Family Issues* 2: 91–112.

Feldman, C. 1976. A contingency theory of socialization. *Administrative Science Quarterly* 21: 433–452.

Forsionne-Guisseppi, A., and V. Peeters. 1982. Differences in job motivation and satisfaction among female and male managers. *Human Relations* 35: 101–118.

Freidson, E. 1970. *Profession of medicine.* New York: Harper and Row.

Friss, L. 1982. Hospital nurse staffing: an urgent need for management reappraisal. *Health Care Management Review* 7 (1): 21–28.

Friss, L. 1986. *Let's rethink motivating women.* Working paper, University of Southern California School of Public Administration.

Gibson, L., and H. Dewhirst. 1986. Using career paths to maximize nursing resources. *Healthcare Management Review* 11 (2): 73–82.

Gould, R. 1978. *Transformations: growth and change in adult life.* New York: Simon and Schuster.

Haber, S., E. Lamas, and G. Green. 1983. A new method for estimating job separations by sex and race. *Monthly Labor Review* 106 (6): 20–27.

Hall, D. 1976. *Careers in organizations.* Pacific Palisades, CA: Goodyear.

Hall, R. 1986. *Dimensions of work.* Beverly Hills, CA: Sage.

Hall, D., and C. Fukami. 1979. Organizational design and adult learning. *Research in Organizational Behavior.* 1: 125–168.

Howard, A., and J. Wilson. 1982. Leadership in a declining work ethic. *California Management Review* 24 (4): 33–46.

Hrebiniak, L., and J. Alutto. 1972. Personal and role-related factors in the development of organization commitment. *Administrative Science Quarterly* 17: 555–573.

Kahn, A. 1980. Modifications in nursing attitudes as measured by the EPPS: a significant reversal from the past. *Nursing Research* 29 (1): 61–63.

Katz, R. 1978a. The influence of job longevity on employee reactions to task characteristics. *Human Relations* 31: 703–725.

Katz, R. 1978b. Job longevity as a situational factor in job satisfaction. *Administrative Science Quarterly* 23: 204–223.

Katz, R. 1980. Time and work: toward an integrative perspective. *Research in Organizational Behavior* 2: 81–127.

Kavanagh, M., and M. Halpern. 1977. The impact of job level and sex differences on the relationship between life and job satisfaction. *Academy of Management Journal* 20: 66–73.

Kent, R., ed. 1985. *Money talks.* New York: Facts on File.

Kerr, W., M. Von Glinow, and J. Schriesheim. 1977. Issues in the study of professionals in organizations: the case of scientists and engineers. *Organizational Behavior and Human Performance* 18: 329–345.

Kohn, M., and C. Schooler. 1973. Occupational experience and psychological functioning: an assessment of reciprocal effects. *American Sociological Review* 38: 97–118.

Kramer, M. 1970. Role conceptions of baccalaureate nurses and success in hospital nursing. *Nursing Research* 19: 428–439.

Kramer, M. 1974. *Reality shock*. St. Louis: C.V. Mosby.

Lacy, W., J. Bokemeier, and J. Shepard. 1983. Job attitude preference and work commitment of men and women in the United States. *Personnel Psychology* 36: 315–329.

Latack, J., and L. Foster. 1985. Implementation of compressed work schedules: participation and job redesign as critical factors for employee acceptance. *Personnel Psychology* 38: 75–92.

Light, D. 1980. *Becoming psychiatrists: the professional transformation of self.* New York: Norton.

Lorence, J. 1987. Age differences in work involvement. *Work and Occupations* 14: 533–557.

Louis, M. 1980. Surprise and sense making: what newcomers experience entering unfamiliar organizational settings. *Administrative Science Quarterly* 25: 226–251.

McKelvey, B., and U. Sekaran. 1977. Toward a career based theory of job involvement: a study of scientists and engineers. *Administrative Science Quarterly* 22: 282–305.

Miller, J., C. Schooler, M. Kohn, et al. 1979. Women and work: the psychological effects of occupational conditions. *American Journal of Sociology* 85: 66–94.

Miner, J. 1974. Motivation to manage among women: studies of business managers and educational administrators. *Journal of Vocational Behavior* 5: 197–208.

Mirvis, P., and E. Hackett. 1983. Work and work force characteristics in the nonprofit sector. *Monthly Labor Review* 106: 3–11.

Morrow, P., and J. McElroy. 1987. Work commitment and job satisfaction over three career stages. *Journal of Vocational Behavior* 30: 330–346.

Prince, J. 1979. *An investigation of career concepts and career anchors*. Paper presented at the Western Academy of Management meeting, Portland, OR, April 1979.

Rainey, G., and W. Wolf. 1981. Flex-time: short term benefits, long term . . . . ? *Public Administration Review* 41: 52–62.

Ralston, D., W. Anthony, and D. Gustafson. 1985. Employees may love flextime, but what does it do to the organization's productivity? *Journal of Applied Psychology* 70: 272–279.

Regan, M., and H. Roland. 1985. Rearranging family and career priorities. *Journal of Marriage and the Family* 47: 985–992.

Rhodes, S. 1983. Age-related differences in work attitudes and behavior: a review and conceptual analysis. *Psychological Bulletin* 93: 328–361.

Ritchie, R., and J. Moses. 1983. Assessment center correlates of women's advancement into middle management: a seven-year longitudinal analysis. *Journal of Applied Psychology* 68: 227–231.

Ryff, C. 1979. Value transition and adult development in women: the instrumentality-terminality sequence hypothesis, in Rokeach, ed., *Understanding Human Values.* New York: Free Press, pp. 148–153.

Rynes, S. 1987. Career transitions from engineering to management: are they predictable among students? *Journal of Vocational Behavior* 30: 138–154.

Salancik, G. 1977. Commitment and the control of organizational behavior and belief, in B.Staw and G. Salancik, eds., *New directions in organizational behavior.* Chicago: St. Clair Press, pp.1–54.

Schein, E. 1971. The individual, the organization and the career: a conceptual scheme. *Journal of Applied Behavioral Science* 7: 401–426.

Schein, E. 1975. How career anchors hold executives to their career paths. *Personnel* 52 (3): 11–24.

Schein, E. 1978. *Career dynamics: matching individuals and organizational needs.* Reading, MA: Addison-Wesley.

Seyboldt, J. 1983. Dealing with premature employee turnover. *California Management Review* 25(3): 107–117.

Sheehy, G. 1976. *Passages.* New York: McGraw-Hill.

Sonnenfeld, J., and J. Kotter. 1982. The maturation of career theory. *Human Relations* 35: 19–46.

Staples, S., and B. Curtis. 1975. Extended work day—two years later. *Hospital Administration in Canada* 17(1): 32–34.

Staw, B. 1980. Rationality and justification in organizational life. *Research in Organizational Behavior* 2: 45–80.

Terborg, J. 1977. Women in management: a research review. *Journal of Applied Psychology* 62: 647–664.

Thompson, P., G. Dalton, and R. Price. 1977. The four stages of professional careers: a new look at performance by professionals. *Organizational Dynamics* 6:(11): 19–42

Van Maanen, J., and S. Barley. 1984. Occupational communities: culture and control in organizations. *Research in Organizational Behavior* 6: 287-365.

Van Maanen, J., and R. Katz. 1975. Individuals and their careers: some temporal considerations for work satisfaction. *Personnel Psychology* 29: 601–616.

Walker, J., C. Tausky, and D. Oliver. 1982. Men and women at work: similarities and differences in work values within occupational groupings. *Journal of Vocational Behavior* 21: 17–36.

Wanous, J. 1977. Organizational entry. Newcomers moving from outside to inside. *Psychological Bulletin* 84: 601–618.

Wanous, J. 1978. Realistic job preview: can a procedure to reduce turnover also influence the relationship between abilities and performance? *Psychology* 3: 244–258.

Weisman, C. 1982. Recruit from within: hospital nurse retention in the 80s. *Journal of Nursing Administration* 12(5): 24–31.

Zytowski, D. 1969. Toward a theory of career development for women. *Personnel and Guidance Journal* 47: 660–664.

# Chapter 2

# The Practice of Nursing

---

You must know your materials. Study them. Know everything about them—what they can do, their history, what they can do in the future.

(Leopold C. Silberstein in Kent 1985, 147)

## Definitions of Nursing Practice

### Federal Definitions

The U.S. Department of Labor lists titles and characteristics for 282 occupations. Since the Department of Labor has key responsibilities for conducting wage and salary surveys and cooperating with the Office of Personnel Management in designing position classification standards, its job descriptions and classifications are significant. Nursing is described as an occupation in which educational level is a matter of personal preference (Dillon 1975). Jobs are scattered widely and involve helping and working with people; the nurse is part of a team. The work involves much detail and is scrutinized closely. Nurses direct the work of others with a high level of responsibility. Overtime and shift work are usually required.

For all nurses in federal employment, salary is determined by the factor evaluation system of the Civil Service Commission. The 17 benchmark job descriptions are based on an occupational analysis. The points that are assigned to the nine factors described in the analysis are summed and converted into a pay grade. Salaries of nurses working for the Veterans Administration are higher, but are linked to the GS-9 Civil Service pay grade (Friss 1981).

The nine factors, which are common to all classifications, are the knowledge required by the position, supervisory controls, guidelines, complexity, scope and effect, personal contacts, purpose of contacts, physical demands, and work environment. Trainee nurses are classified at GS-4 or GS-5; general medical surgical staff nurses and intensive care nurses are classified at GS-9. Community health nurses, operating room nurses, psychiatric nurses, and occupational health nurses are also classified at GS-9. Nurse practitioners, specialists, midwives, and anesthetists are classified at GS-11. The highest classification assigned is to an advanced nurse practitioner at the GS-12 level (Civil Service Commission 1977). (The 1988 salary schedule for GS-6 employees ranges from $16,851 to $21,909, GS-9 salaries range from $22,907 to $29,783, and GS-12 from $33,218 to $43,181 with 10 steps in each grade. The corresponding Veterans Administration nurse schedule ranges are from $16,851 to $21,909, from $22,907 to $29,783, and from $33,218 to $43,181. In areas where it is difficult to recruit nurses the Veterans Administration has special entrance salary rates.)

The Department of Labor also develops projections about the availability of jobs. By the year 2000 there will be an estimated 612,000 new jobs for nurses, which is a 44% increase over the 1.4 million positions that existed in 1986.

## Legal Definition

State guidelines for nurses are developed as a result of a social contract. The scope of nursing practice is defined legally in each state by the state's nurse practice act. These acts define nursing within the state, establish legal boundaries, and state specific roles and activities that nurses may perform. These definitions are the basis for licensing and educational standards; they prohibit unqualified and incompetent persons from practicing. The independent practice of nursing includes observation, care, and counseling of the ill, injured, or infirm; the maintenance of health and the prevention of illness in others; and the supervision and teaching of other personnel. Outsiders are most familiar with the dependent practice component of nursing, or that aspect of practice that stems from other professionals, such as the administration of medicine and treatments prescribed by physicians. The boundaries of the two practice components, dependent and independent, are often unclear. Ultimately, the courts define nursing's status as a profession. The judicial system regards nursing as an occupation that possesses a body of knowledge that is not known to laypersons. However, since physicians also possess this knowledge, nurses do not have a monopoly, and physicians are allowed to testify in cases about nurses' actions. Courts are confused about the relative independence of nurses and are reluctant to find nurses liable when they are following physicians' orders. The trend, however, is to expect nurses to take affirmative steps to protect patients from the negligent acts of physicians and to hold nurses to a standard of care separate from that of physicians (Murphy 1987).

Since 1971, more than 35 states have revised or redefined nursing practice. This redefinition was prompted by the pressures of federal legislation (Medicare requirements), the upgraded educational preparation of nurses, the reality of nursing work in complex care settings, and the general trend in society toward equality and autonomy of workers. The American Nurses' Association (1984) has stated that the primary purpose of licensing is to protect the public by setting standards to provide for safe and effective nursing practice. The New York State definition has served as a model for nursing as a profession independent from medicine. The statute (New York State 1972) defines nursing as follows:

> The practice of the profession of nursing as a registered professional nurse is defined as diagnosing and treating human responses to actual and potential health problems through such service as case finding, health teaching, health counseling, provision of care supportive to or restorative of life and well-being, and executing medical regimens prescribed by a licensed or otherwise legally authorized physician or dentist. A nursing regimen shall be consistent with and shall not vary any existing medical regimen.

Where states did not simply expand the basic definition, the effect of changes has been similar, allowing for either joint action of medical and nursing boards or delegation by individual physicians (Bullough 1976). Most states require specialized education, judgment, and skill based on knowledge of scientific principles (Durbin 1981). The usual activities identified include:

1. Case finding, teaching health care, and counseling patients and their families about health needs

2. Making nursing diagnoses and treating human responses to actual and potential physical and emotional problems

3. Administering medications and treatments prescribed by a doctor or dentist

4. Working with the health team to deliver planned health care

5. Providing care to support or restore life and well-being

6. Teaching and supervising other persons in any of these activities.

Legal restraints are sometimes cited as justification for continuance of outdated policies and practices. History has shown that when there is a need for change, nursing, physician, and hospital associations work with the legislature and regulatory boards to change laws and regulations. Presently, legislators in some jurisdictions are under pressure to expand the authority of qualified nurse practitioners to encompass prescribing medications (other than narcotics) under a standardized procedure.

States administer the licensing examination (NCLEX-RN) developed by the National Council of State Boards of Nursing. Under the 1978 Federal Uniform Guidelines in Employee Selection, such tests must be based on a current and appropriate job analysis to prevent an adverse impact on blacks, Hispanics, Asians, and the physically handicapped. The current licensing test meets these criteria. The council also has responsibility for reviewing periodically the statutory definitions of professional and practical nursing as well as reviewing and proposing model practice laws. The council also recommends a passing score, which all states have adopted. On this basis, nurses have geographical mobility. States either agree to honor each others' licenses by reciprocity or examine individual qualifications and endorse the nurse from another state to practice.

Since 1982, a criterion-referenced approach has been used; each candidate's test performance is compared to a consistent standard or criterion judged by experts to represent acceptable nursing competence. The questions, developed with the assistance of experts in testing, education, and practice, cover five nursing behaviors, eight categories of nursing functions, and four client needs categories.

The five nursing behaviors are assessing, analyzing, planning, implementing, and evaluating. Each area has equal weight in the examination.

The eight categories of human functioning include protective functions; sensory-perceptual functions; nutrition; growth and development; fluid-gas transport; elimination; psychosocial and cultural functions; and comfort, rest, activity, and mobility. These topics correspond closely to nursing tasks and the informing functions.

The four client needs categories are a safe and therapeutically effective care environment, physiological integrity, psychosocial integrity, and maintenance and promotion of health. These domains stem from a 1984 job analysis of new graduates; the new test plan became effective in July 1988. The new test plan will result in changes in nursing curricula as colleges prepare their students for modified examinations and clarify the expected competencies of entry-level nurses.

## Professional Definitions

Professional definitions originate with individual nurses and professional organizations. No single definition has been universally accepted by the nursing profession, but professional definitions can be more flexible and often precede statutory changes. In other situations professional definitions may impede changes.

For example, the 1955 model definition of nursing practice by the American Nurses' Association (ANA) concluded by stating, "The foregoing shall not be deemed to include any acts of diagnosis or prescription of therapeutic or corrective measures" (American Journal of Nursing 1955). This limited definition was unworkable from the beginning. Accommodating mechanisms, called "joint statements," were developed by nursing and medical associations to overcome the self-imposed limitations. Educators were hesitant to teach beyond safe limits. Working nurses were intimidated by the results handed down by state attorneys general stating that it was illegal for nurses to diagnose or treat patients.

The 1970 ANA revision of the definition of nursing practice modified the diagnosis and prescription limitation, legitimized the expanded role of the nurse, and set the stage for the increase in expanded practice laws. Currently, the ANA defines nursing as the diagnosis and treatment of human responses to actual or potential health problems. (Refer to Appendix 2A at the end of this chapter for a definition and examples of human responses.)

The ANA does not restrict itself to defining nursing practice. The professional nursing code (see Appendix 2B) calls for a nondiscriminatory approach to patients (referred to in the code as clients) and a respect for their privacy. Not only are nurses responsible for their own actions, but they should use informed judgment in accepting responsibilities and delegating work to others. Within the scope of practice, nurses should act to safeguard the client from the incompetent, unethical, or illegal practice of others.

Other issues referred to in the code are the responsibilities for maintaining competence, participation in professional activities to improve standards and employment, and collaboration with others to meet the health needs of the public. Individual nurses choose to ignore, selectively follow, or embrace this charter, just as do members of other professions. The culture of nursing fosters egalitarian values, social responsibility, and professional oversight of others. Although none would argue that all nurses are egalitarians acting on social values, many nurses do not embrace managerial values or believe that the central role of nursing is to carry out hospital and physician orders.

Professional definitions do not have the force of law, but are the ultimate tools of self-governance. Further, nursing standards that flow from professional definitions will be used by the courts in the determination of liability and the resolution of malpractice suits (Eccard 1977). The National Labor Relations Board and the courts reinstated a head nurse who was fired for reporting to the Joint Commission on Accreditation of Hospitals (JCAH) that there were serious deficiencies in the quality of patient care and in working conditions at the hospital where the nurse was employed. This decision was made without the help of unions or channels outside the immediate employee-employer relationship.  The supporting rationales were that the nurse was required, as a condition of employment, to join with others to meet public health needs and to comply with the ANA code. Since the code mandates nurses to act to improve standards, the employee was deemed to have acted properly (Moskowitz and Moskowitz 1984).

The National League for Nursing (NLN), another major national nursing association, stresses improvement of nursing through accreditation of educational programs, consultation, testing, research, and publication. Its major impacts have been through accrediting nursing schools and encouraging the development of a State Board Test Pool Examination. Together, these two activities have established a threshold for educational standards, minimum national competency levels, and licensure by endorsement among the states. In the process, examination, rather than years of education or degree, allows entry into nursing practice. The NLN, along with the ANA, has adopted a policy position that professional nursing practice should require the minimum of a baccalaureate degree with a major in nursing. However, the baccalaureate representatives do not have a plurality of votes in the NLN and have been unable to take an advocacy position.

Progress is being made in developing competency statements for ADN- and BSN-educated nurses; this is an important first step in differentiating licenses and job descriptions (Midwest Alliance 1987; Primm 1986). Refer to Appendix 2C for copies of the most widely distributed competency statement.

Certification as a method of recognizing nurses with special aptitudes was first used by public health nurses early in this century. Now there are 13 certifying organizations for specialist nurses of all types (ANA 1988; Swansburg and Swansburg 1984). Certification validates, through predetermined standards, a nurse's qualifications, knowledge, and practice in a defined nursing area. As in all professions, the professional associations have taken the lead, since they possess the expertise to devise the examinations and have the motivation to set standards for advanced practice.

The certifying organizations certified 69,140 nurses in 1982, of whom 13,593 are nurse practitioners and midwives (Institute of Medicine 1983, 253–259). Specialty roles are being extended in primary care, acute care, and long-term care. The ANA offers certification in 17 areas of nursing practice and two lines of nursing administration and by 1988 had certified 48,000 nurses. Of these areas of certification, the primary ones for nurses in short-term general hospitals are medical-surgical nurse, clinical specialist in medical-surgical nursing, high-risk perinatal nurse, child and adolescent nurse, and general nursing practice plus the medical-surgical clinical specialist. Educational requirements vary considerably. Community health and nursing administration require a baccalaureate degree for certification. The Nursing Administration Advanced classification, the nurse practitioner programs, and the clinical specialist programs require a master's degree or a specialized training program. Other certification areas interest those who wish to give primary care, work in an ambulatory or mental health setting, or limit their practice to either the young or the old patient.

The trend toward state certification began about 1975 when states reviewed laws pertaining to nurse anesthetists and midwives. Now clinical specialists are being added. The usual practice is for states to use professional certifying associations as the testing bodies for state certification. The current trend to certify specialists suggests that the advanced level of nursing practice is the specialty level, rather than the bachelor's degree. Increasingly, the trend is toward master's degree education for nurse practitioners and other specialists. Thus, educational preparation for nursing starts at one year for the practical nurse, a minimum of two years for the registered nurse, and six years for a specialty level. Bullough stated "from the point of view of the law, the baccalaureate level is a way station on the path toward a nursing specialty rather than a major endpoint in and of itself" (Bullough 1983, 285). If this is true, hospitals that expect to employ specialists will need to establish policies that foster educational upgrading of diploma and associate degree nurses (ADN) so that there are a sufficient number of baccalaureate applicants who qualify for graduate education.

This trend toward certification mirrors the societal tendency to rely less on formal education and more on professional standing to advance professionally. Certification will encourage nurses to invest in their careers, help them achieve professional recognition, define the scope of practice, exert an upward pressure on salaries, and promote mobility. Since credentials will be verifiable, certification will decrease mobility for those who do not invest in advancement. To the extent that the credential becomes the norm of practice, employers will have less ability to substitute less qualified nurses.

## Nursing Education

The major educational pathways for entry into practice are diploma programs in hospital schools of nursing, associate of arts degree programs located in community colleges, and baccalaureate (bachelor's of science in nursing, or BSN) programs in four-year colleges and universities.

The transition from apprentice education to college-based education occurred after the nursing equivalent of the Flexner Report was written by Lucille Brown in 1948 for the Russell Sage Foundation. This report recommended upgrading the requirement for registered nurse (RN) status to the bachelor's degree and that for practical nurses to a technical nursing education at a community college. Instead, both community and four-year colleges educated RNs while practical nurse education remained a one-year dead-end. Although many physicians and administrators regret the gradual loss of diploma graduates, the transition was inevitable. After World War II, men and women looked to community colleges for preparation for local jobs, and bright women wanted a college education along with their male classmates.

Traditionally, the diploma programs require three calendar years. The ADN programs require two (up to three) academic years, and the BSN programs require four (up to five) academic years. Graduates from each level receive a generalist education in nursing and take the same standard national examination. It has been estimated by the U.S. Department of Health and Human Services (DHHS) that the highest degree held by 22.8% of nurses was an ADN, 45.3% had diplomas, and 25.5% baccalaureates (DHHS 1988, 10–16). Because of rapid and continuing shifts by entering students, new nurse graduates are now prepared in academic settings—87% in 1985–1986 (NLN 1988, 38). Since this trend away from apprentice education is recent, only 32.7% of practicing nurses have a baccalaureate degree or higher (DHHS 1986, 46).

Each program establishes its own goals and curriculum just as do other college programs. The philosophy of the host institution and the desire to be accredited by the NLN influence these goals and curricula. All programs educate nurses to meet the minimum safe level of practice established by the state. Beyond that, diploma programs have usually emphasized hospital practice. In college-based programs, the curriculum tends to be based on a generic model of practice, with the expectation that graduates will work in a number and variety of nursing situations. Increasingly, faculty in baccalaureate programs are encouraging students to prepare for employment outside acute care hospitals.

In 1985–1986, there was an overall 14.7% decline in fall admissions and a 11.1% drop in enrollments over 1983 (NLN 1988, 1). The five-year trend shows that baccalaureate graduations dropped by 4.5% (NLN 1988, 38), which is contrary to the general trend for women (Figure 2-1) Although prospective nurses are shunning generic BSN programs, existing nurses endorse the bachelor's degree; during the past 10 years there has been a 111% increase in the number of graduates from special RN programs, so that the overall increase in the baccalaureate supply was 23.1% even though generic student graduates accounted for only a 7.3% increase (NLN 1988, 45). Regional differences in the number of graduations from diploma, ADN, and BSN programs determine local supply and RN mix.

The quality of the nursing work force is also important. College Board data indicate that the SAT scores of high-school students interested in

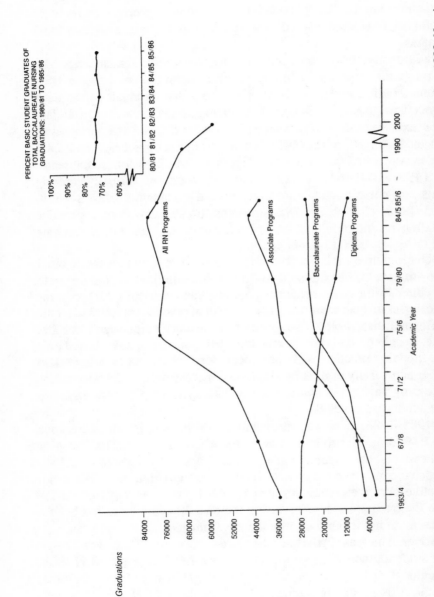

**Figure 2-1**  Registered nurse program graduates by program type. Source: National League for Nursing. 1988. *Nursing Student Census.* New York: National League for Nursing, p. 39, 46. Data for the years 1990 and 2000 from Department of Health and Human Services. 1985. *Health United States.* Washington, D.C.: Government Printing Office, p. 111.

nursing careers were well below the average for college-bound students. Further, the gap between prospective nurses and nonnurses has been widening (Aiken and Mullinix 1987). In 1983–1984, only 84% of graduates came from accredited programs (NLN 1988, 38). Although nearly all graduates of diploma and BSN programs came from NLN-accredited schools, only 71.6% of ADN graduates came from professionally accredited schools.

Projections for the total nurse work force in 1990, by type of education, are shown in Table 2-1. Employers who are dependent on diploma nurses will need to consider incentives to attract an older work force and can anticipate lower work force participation, since labor force participation drops sharply after age 55. In general, as the level of education increases, a higher percentage of nurses work full-time (Levine and Moses 1982, 486). Thus, the drop-off in basic BSN nurses will have a greater effect on working hours than the decline in numbers alone would indicate. Among hospital nurses, 43% had a diploma education; ADN-educated nurses comprised 29%, and 26% had a baccalaureate degree in 1984 (DHHS 1986, 10).

The lack of an educational prerequisite for licensure is the primary cause of ambiguity about the professional status of nursing. The diverse educational backgrounds make it difficult for nurses who favor educational upgrading to overcome the objections of others who are afraid that being "grandfathered in" (allowed to continue practice without the degree) will lead to lower status. It is easy to understand that the many practicing nurses from technical programs, who experienced a demanding apprentice education with emphasis on skill development, have difficulty accommodating to the large number of young nurses who value problem-solving approaches and expect to become technically proficient on the job. Conversely, nurses

**Table 2-1**   Projected Supply of Employed Registered Nurses, 1990, by Type of Education (Intermediate Projection)

| Type | Number | Percent of Total | Median Age |
|------|--------|------------------|------------|
| Diploma nurse | 614,000 | 35.9 | 45 |
| Associate nurse | 475,000 | 27.8 | 35 |
| Baccalaureate or higher | 621,000 | 36.3 | 32 |

Source: Institute of Medicine. 1983. *Nursing and nursing education: Public policies and private actions*. Washington, DC: National Academy Press, pp.77–78.

who received their education in an academic setting have difficulty accepting the task orientation and lack of intellectual stimulation that pervades many nursing units.

Some critics blame educators for changing nursing performance and expectations. However, these changes were inevitable given the social changes that affected the expectations of nursing school applicants. Like other students, nurses expect to receive college credit for their courses. Even so, although the educational standards of nursing have been rising, standards in the larger community have been rising faster.

Professionals from other disciplines where educational standards for entry are uniform find nursing's multiple educational pathways confusing. Nursing is often berated for not establishing the bachelor's degree as a requirement for entry into practice or for gaining more power in relation to managers or physicians. The critics ignore some realities: Physicians control the flow of specialized knowledge and the downward delegation of new tasks; administrators want to retain flexibility to contain labor costs; and auxiliary workers resist codification that limits their career aspirations.

Educational preparation is not related to pay differentials within the hospital. Those in a position to pay more to nurses with higher education argue that the duties performed by nurses from each of the programs are the same. Therefore, educational preparation seems irrelevant as a pay determinant. The problem is circular and mutually reinforcing. As employers fail to differentiate by giving those with educational credentials more complex assignments, preparatory educational differences are muted or lost. Educators then lack practice differences to use as a basis for upgrading the curriculum. When potential students and counselors cannot perceive curricular and entry-level job differences in such a system, students choose programs based on convenience or price rather than intellectual rigor or career aspirations. In the long run, hospitals lose their ability to attract recruits with college and career aspirations, and thus reinforce the original difficulty of differentiating among applicants. The industry faces a major challenge in effecting the alignment of education, responsibility, and pay needed to bring nursing into conformity with current cultural expectations of women.

## Nursing as a Career

Social scientists have described nursing as an ambiguous profession with a symbolic heritage of female roles: mother, sex object, angel of mercy, heroine, and careerist (Williams 1983). This ambiguity is attributed not only to the diversity of educational preparation but also to the fact that nurses come from all social classes and work in a wide range of organizations with diverse responsibilities. Although the trend does favor clinical advancement, hospital nurses still tend to become administrative specialists with low occupational prestige as compared with other professionals, even though their subordinates and families see them as having high status.

Nursing is not a closed occupation. That is, nursing can neither control the labor supply nor define or monopolize a distinct set of roles (Levi 1980). Nurses know that they are jacks-of-all-trades and masters of none (Kron and Durbin 1981). The high level of substitutability among nursing aides, licensed practical nurses, and levels of RNs makes it virtually impossible for nurses to initiate a successful job action, a reserved power that industrial relations experts believe is essential to improve working conditions.

## Labor Force Supply and Participation

The following data indicate that the nurse supply is expanding much faster than the population, that nurses are working, and that a higher proportion of nurses are working at the bedside. Temporary agencies are encouraging nurses to work more hours.

1. Between 1977 and 1984, the number of nurses increased by 55%, while the population grew by only 8% (Aiken and Mullinix 1987).

2. Among all nurses, the proportion employed in nursing in 1984 was 78.7%, up from 76.4% in 1980 (DHHS 1986, 29; Levine and Moses 1982, 484). In contrast, the labor force participation of all women between the ages of 20 and 54, the years with the highest participation, has never been above 70% (Population Reference Bureau 1981).

3. Only 2.2% of employed nurses were working through temporary agencies in 1984, and many of these nurses were probably using them for a second job (DHHS 1986, 35).

4. In 1984, only 14.6% of all nurses were not employed in nursing and not seeking a job, down from 27.2% in 1977. Almost three-quarters of these nurses were over 50 years old or had children less than six years of age (DHHS 1986, 61). The unemployment rate was only 2%.

5. The proportion of hospital nurses working as staff nurses has increased to 73.3% in 1984 from 71.9% in 1980 (DHHS 1986, 42; Levine and Moses 1982, 491).

6. Of the 5% of all nurses employed in nonnursing occupations, over one-third were in other health-related occupations (DHHS 1986, 69).

In addition, the proportion of males in nursing doubled between 1977 and 1982 and is now 3% (DHHS 1986, 9).

Hospital-specific data are less encouraging, however. In 1984, 68% of employed nurses worked in hospitals, down from 68.6% in 1980 and 70.6% in 1977 (DHHS 1986, 38; Levine and Moses 1982, 488). Further, the proportion of nurses working part-time in hospitals has increased to 31.8% from 30.8% in 1980 and 29.4% in 1977 (DHHS 1986, 40; Levine and Moses 1982, 487; DHHS 1982, 14). These date combined with the educational trends suggest that career-oriented women are opting out of hospital work, leaving a larger reservoir of less-educated part-time workers.

The easiest way to fill budgeted vacancies would be to encourage steady-state nurses to take full-time work. However, this conflicts with current practices, which assume that productivity comes from flexible staffing strategies and a compacted salary structure. Actually, productivity is related to total payroll, which may be less with fewer, relatively well paid, productive workers than with more workers who require much supervision and are less productive.

Concerning future supply, the *Sixth Report to the President and Congress on the Status of Health Personnel in the United States* (DHHS 1988) concluded that the supply of and requirements for RNs taken as a whole throughout the country would not be seriously out of balance in the year 2000. However, distributional imbalances of RNs in local areas and regions in some selected or specialty areas of practice currently exist and may continue into the future. The data indicate that in the year 2000 the supply of associate-degree nurses will be significantly greater than requirements, whereas the requirements for baccalaureate graduates will be 43% greater than the supply. For nurses with graduate degrees, the requirements are estimated to be almost three times greater than the supply throughout the projection period—the years 2000 to 2020.

## Where Do Nurses Work?

Nursing became a salaried occupation rather than a fee-for-service occupation during the depression of the 1930s, when private-duty nursing almost disappeared. The technological changes during and after World War II made independent practice obsolete. Of the 1.9 million nurses at work in 1984, 68% were employed in hospitals. The remainder were employed in nursing homes, public health, ambulatory services, student health services, nursing education, occupational health, federal and state governments, and private duty (Table 2-2).

Since 1980, the number of nurses working in nursing education, occupational health, student health, and nursing homes has declined; the increases have occurred primarily in hospitals, but also in public health and ambulatory services. All but 7.5% of nurses employed in hospitals work in nonfederal short-term hospitals. Within hospitals, the core clinical areas are obstetrics, pediatrics, medicine, surgery, operating room, emergency care, and intensive care (medical and surgical). Specialty medical and surgical units and psychiatric, geriatric, and ambulatory services are found in larger hospitals.

Little is known about the characteristics of nurses who choose and remain in a particular area, even though unit characteristics vary considera-

**Table 2-2** Nurse Employment Settings

| Practice Setting | Number | Percent of Total |
|---|---|---|
| Hospitals | 1,011,955 | 68.1 |
| Nursing homes | 115,077 | 7.7 |
| Public health | 101,430 | 6.8 |
| Ambulatory services | 97,374 | 6.6 |
| Student health services | 43,144 | 2.9 |
| Nursing education | 40,311 | 2.7 |
| Occupational health | 22,890 | 1.5 |
| Private-duty | 22,675 | 1.5 |
| Other self-employed | 9,214 | 0.6 |
| Other | 21,450 | 1.6 |
| Total | 1,485,725 | 100.0 |

Source: Department of Health and Human Services. 1986. *National sample survey of registered nurses, 1984: summary of results*. Rockville, MD: Division of Nursing, Department of Health and Human Services, pp. 32, 39.

bly. Operating room nurses have specific duties, give advice when asked, and are expected to provide quick, reliable assistance. Surgical units are less structured and rule oriented than medical units. They also provide more potential for job discretion and opportunities to use technical skills. Patients on medical wards have longer stays than those on surgical units, are more likely to die, and place greater affective demands on nurses.

Employers benefit when nurses remain generalists and are thus amenable to staffing changes, but as technology has become more complex, specialization enables nurses to feel confident that the patient is receiving quality care. Therefore, nurses increasingly resist (often without success) assignment to clinical areas where they do not believe they are competent to practice. The lack of uniform educational prerequisites and the increase in credentialing enable managers and nurses within organizations to adopt their own policies and standards for assigning nurses to clinical areas. Evidence exists that job satisfaction is higher when vocational interests are related to the clinical assignment (Hener and Meir 1981).

## Career Ladders

During the past several years, employers have developed career ladders consisting of titles with successively higher salaries, status, and sometimes greater autonomy or more responsible assignments. Nurses within facilities have established criteria for differentiating competency levels. The purpose is to retain career nurses at the bedside rather than lose them to teaching or administrative positions. Clinical ladders can allow for lateral mobility to other clinical specialties or to the management ladder, although ladders are usually designed for varying levels of clinical competence within a specialty. The process varies by practice setting and medical staff acceptance. A common complaint is that it is difficult to observe differences among nurses, since tasks are similar and superior judgment is hard to document.

Hospital career ladder programs began as a vehicle for recruitment and maintenance of staff nurses. Currently they are being advocated as a motivational tool to enhance productivity. In one such case, three levels of staff nurses were established, with the two pay differentials totaling 7% above the first level (Vestal 1984). Nurses in these three levels comprised 30% of the RN staff. The other 70% had administrative, educational, or clinical specialist titles. The sixth and highest level paid 20% more than the third level, which is not enough to constitute a real career ladder. A bona fide career ladder requires that the incentives match the level of competence and responsibility. A good test for this is whether or not the differences are enough to stimulate nurses to invest in their own advanced education. As it is, the federal government must subsidize graduate education to achieve even a small increase in supply.

It is easy to overlook the obvious: Ours is a society in which the core element of a career ladder is transferable college credit. Nurses with baccalaureate degrees are more likely to work in public health, teaching, research, and administration than are graduates from other programs. Even so, 50% of practicing nurses with the bachelor's degree remain as staff nurses. Nurses who graduated from diploma programs often have few, if any, transferable college credits. Therefore, their careers are blocked. Diploma nurses usually work in hospitals, physicians' offices, and long-term care facilities. In contrast, ADN graduates have transferable college credits, and they can study for two to three more years and receive a BSN. However, if upper-division nursing programs in the area do not have "second-step" programs, it may be difficult to get a BSN. Without the BSN degree it is difficult to qualify for better hospital jobs or obtain higher education in nursing.

## Hospital Staff Nursing

The number of RNs employed in community hospitals rose by more than 100,000 from 1981 to 1985, for a total of 851,827, a 13% increase. In addition, the number of full-time equivalent RNs per 100 adjusted average daily census in 1985 was 87, up from 73 per 100 in 1981. During this time there was relatively little change in the number of total employees in community hospitals. Nursing personnel represented 38% of total personnel in community hospitals in 1985; of these, 60% were RNs. The nursing personnel mix has been changing toward a higher percentage of RNs and a lower percentage of LPNs and nurse aides. The separation rate of RNs rose from 4% to 6% per quarter in 1985 over 1983 (DHHS 1988, Chapter 10, 23–24).

Thus, nurses are the largest and most unstable group within the hospital. The instability stems from the reward system and the historical isolation of the nursing department from general administration and physicians. This isolation was at one time so severe that it was referred to as a caste system (Katz 1969). In effective hospitals nurses are integrated into the hospital at all levels.

Many nursing functions are resources to the physician and hospital rather than to patients. In fact, when any professional works for an organization, the employer can be considered the primary client. The professional assumes that the services rendered to the employer ultimately benefit the consumer and the public at large.

Contrary to prevailing beliefs, professional and bureaucratic roles may not be in opposition. Early on, nurses rated successful by their supervisors were those who integrated both roles (Kramer 1970). Among hospital nurses, bureaucratic role orientation was associated with both career and job satisfaction (Hurka 1972). Theorists challenge the prevailing but outmoded concept that there is inherent conflict between the professional and the employing organization. Instead hospitals should be viewed as collegial organizations, as places where there are parallel processes of professional membership and organizational experience with continuous overlapping—sometimes complementary, sometimes conflicting—roles.

Nurse specialization patterns follow those of clinical medicine and its hierarchy. Nurses work independently of their colleagues, as do other professionals, but closely with the client. In caring for a patient, nurses have considerable discretion, bounded by a standard body of knowledge, skills, indoctrination, and peer review. Hospital nurses also serve the organization by controlling and harnessing knowledge for solving problems and coordinating work. Patients do view nurses as intelligent and necessary, but as being controlled by physicians (Swansburg 1983).

In technological terms, nursing is an intensive technology. Intensive technologies are characterized by a variety of techniques, which are drawn upon to achieve a change in some specific object. The selection, combination, and order of application are designed by the worker based on feedback from the object itself (Thompson 1967). A continuing challenge exists in hospitals to manage departments with production line technologies and inert inputs, such as dietary, housekeeping, and maintenance, simultaneously with departments with intensive technologies and active input, such as nursing. This complexity, along with the values orientation of the workers, distinguishes hospitals from manufacturing businesses.

Some believe that staff nursing in hospitals is inherently stressful or unsatisfying. Although both stress and satisfaction are important subjects, we do not know whether the practice of nursing in hospitals is more stressful or less satisfying than other occupations.

A study based on a stratified random sample of workers in Finland looked at job dissatisfaction and work-related exhaustion in male and female workers and ascertained that nursing was not a high-stress job (Kauppinen-Toropainen, Kandolin, and Mutanen 1983). In another study, a sample of Midwestern nurses reported a moderate level of satisfaction, but the level was lower than in other occupations, such as university faculty, administrative personnel, elementary school teachers, and clerical workers. Nurses, however, were more satisfied than police officers, factory workers, and factory foremen. The determinants of job satisfaction were the same for all groups, but only factory workers reported lower levels of task autonomy and salary than nurses, whereas only police officers reported a lower level of supervisory assistance (Mottaz 1988).

This section discusses four main aspects of nursing practice:

- Client interaction
- Tasks
- Processes
- Roles

## Dynamics of Client Interaction

Despite the popular misconception, the nurse of the Florence Nightingale era was not the warm and empathetic mother depicted as the symbolic heritage of nursing. Early nursing content was organized around three focal points: a body of skills, rules for sanitation and hygiene, and a philosophy of nursing that included a code of ethics. Skills were identified by a job analysis based on the practices and requirements of employers caring for patients with acute illness (Wadle and Munns 1983). In those more authoritarian times, the nurse's role was to repress subjectivity, "have the answer," and do the job. Nursing routines have even been described as a defense against anxiety—a protective mechanism and a barrier to patient interaction (Menzies 1970). It is even postulated that nursing history is being rewritten to conform to current perceptions that nursing was originally a caring and mothering activity (Armstrong 1983).

It is only in recent decades that both patients and nursing itself have changed (Preston 1979). The traditional dependent patient role is obsolete, but the desired changes are not clearly defined. Some patients want to submit to omniscient providers, whereas others want to cooperate with skilled and knowledgeable nurses and physicians. These preferences, which vary with the patient's social class, personality, and medical condition, may lie on a continuum, but if so, the criteria have not been identified. Instead, patients tend to give global praise or express specific complaints when asked what makes a good nurse.

Nursing has both caring and curing functions. Meeting the psychosocial needs of patients remains more of an art than a science. All therapists must demonstrate trust and competence; the relationship must be instantly functional but not sentimental, personal, or one of kinship. This is especially difficult to achieve in nursing because many of the procedures utilized are intensely personal and require detachment on the part of the nurse to preserve objectivity. Nursing problems also vary according to the health focus and unit of service (Orem 1985).[1] For instance, clients in rehabilitation units exert a different influence on the nursing work system than do patients in critical care units.

Patients relate to nurses differently than they relate to all other providers. Nurses are the built-in social structural linkage between the consumer and other providers (Birenbaum 1981). Nurses respond to patient requests but also initiate action when they know the patient needs attention. The nurse is expected to initiate contact even if the patient has not asked for it. According to the concept of "shared power," whoever is physically and/or psychologically closest to the patient at the time of need and has the skill to supply the need can act without going through a hierarchy of professionals.

In contrast, the patient approaches the physician when seeking a cure and maintains a social distance in the relationship. All other providers approach the patient after the doctor requests the visit. Most of the other providers require the assistance of the nurse to approach the hospitalized patient.

When nurses vehemently state that patient needs must come first, they are reflecting an ingrained understanding of the basic source of their legitimacy. Within the patient-nurse relationship, patient expectations and reactions can be ignored only briefly or with considerable risk. It is not enough that the public provides nurses with a license to perform and a mechanism for accountability. Nurses must continually meet service expectations and earn the right to intrude on the individual's space and body.

The work system on hospital units is more than the sum of individual patient needs and expectations. Patients (and most work force analysts) view nursing practice from the perspective of what was done to or for them. Almost without exception, nurse-client relationships are conceptualized according to the private-duty model. The quality of care is judged on the basis of what was done (or not done) or by the outcome for an individual patient. This model does not recognize that a group of nurses are making simultaneous decisions about many patients. Although it is unrealistic to expect the sick to ponder how the nurse makes choices about service priorities, it is obligatory for others to understand that viewing work from the perspective of the single patient differs from what nurses are paid to do, that is, care for multiple patients, so that appropriate care for one may be sacrificed to provide more essential care for another. Concurrently with any task under way, the nurse is withholding desirable services from others based on an internal calculation of client need. Nurses may not have a formal understanding of opportunity costs, but their professional lives are a continuous series of investment choices, trade-offs, and estimates of probable benefits.

Finally, patients can be visualized as the raw material of the firm, the input to the process (Perrow 1965). Although the words have a demeaning connotation, the concept is important. Within the context of the nursing units, the goal is to change the health state of the patient. In technological terms, this is the equivalent of transforming the raw material. The raw material, rather than being inert, is characterized by uncertainty (the degree to which patients' conditions are not fully understood), instability (the number of emergencies and nursing observations required), and variability (the extent to which nursing care must be individualized) (Overton, Schneck, and Hazlett 1977).

Competition among hospitals is causing executives to reassess organization-patient relations. There is an increased interest in assessing markets and patient satisfaction with services (Jenna 1986). There is also an awareness that patients have a greater influence on their choice of hospitals than was previously acknowledged (Okorafor 1983; Peters and Wacker 1982). An emphasis on patient relations is compatible with the traditional literature, which has established that the needs and expectations of clients become the goals of the organization and the determinants of work patterns (Rosengren 1970).

## Tasks

An essential element of nursing practice is meeting the physical needs of patients. The widely accepted "Rush-Medicus" Nursing Process structure lists nine physical needs that should be met: protection of the patient from (1) infections and (2) accident or injury, and attention to the needs for (3) rest, (4) hygiene, (5) nutrition, (6) oxygen supply, (7) elimination, (8) activity, and (9) skin care (Hegyvary 1979). Until the 1950s, mastery of procedures to meet these needs efficiently was the test of a good nursing education. Even though these basic tasks have become fragmented through specialization and departmentalization, patients, physicians, administrators, and nurses are likely to agree that this prime responsibility rests with the nursing staff. A key criterion for continuing hospitalization is whether the patient, in order to respond to medical treatment, needs nursing care services not available elsewhere (e.g., at home or in an outpatient clinic).

A seminal study of nursing tasks identified 306 tasks in six functional areas (Wood 1972). The functional areas were (1) assisting, (2) comfort and safety, (3) nutrition and elimination, (4) medications and treatments, (5) observation and communication, and (6) administration and coordination. Detailed understanding of these tasks and their relative criticality enabled educators to design a core curriculum for nursing occupations, especially for the nursing assistant and technical nursing categories. Unfortunately, the finding that many nursing tasks could be performed by those with less than a professional nursing education has been misapplied in the practice setting. Since neither judgment nor decision-making can be delegated, nurses must determine the boundaries of independent practice and determine the priorities between nursing tasks and dependent practice (responsibilities delegated from physicians). Within hospitals, nurses have established procedures for delegating tasks and responsibilities to aides and licensed vocational nurses.

Just as physicians remain accountable for delegated work, so nurses remain accountable for their independent practice and for work delegated to subordinates. Since events that require judgment cannot be scheduled in efficient blocks of time, nurses must be available at all times. This means that there is a practical limit to task delegation. It is not inefficient to pay RNs to perform some simpler tasks when they are needed to make judgments and there is insufficient work requiring their professional attention.

In contrast with medicine, which has a 400-year history of describing the basic elements of its practice, nursing has only a 25-year history (Norris 1982). Such basic phenomena as vomiting, constipation, diarrhea, and their remedies are only now being researched for practice implications. Although this research emphasis may seem trivial in an era of fascination with change and technological advances, the expectation of patients, doctors, and hospital nurses is that these unchanging physical and emotional needs will be met (Yura and Walsh 1988). This lack of a scientific base also explains why nursing educators want to prepare students for graduate study and research careers. Until nursing becomes less of an art and more firmly grounded in the physical and behavioral sciences, it will remain difficult to explain and monitor practice. During the 1970s, leaders in nursing education and service emphasized the necessity of developing a nursing care plan and documenting related activity for each patient. To an outsider, this may seem as simple as deciding which patient record form (e.g., Kardex) to order. To those involved, it is a major exercise in group process that challenges the value systems of the participants, increases professional identification, and protects the integrity of patient care decisions. Since Florence Nightingale organized nursing content around a philosophy of nursing, along with a body of skills, rules for sanitation and hygiene, and a code of ethics, nurses have concerned themselves with the principles of practice. Nurses see their philosophy and beliefs about health, illness, and disease as critical issues that determine the assumptions that underlie the basic principles of care, the relevance of nursing methods, and nursing as a profession.

Those who believe that this emphasis is much ado about nothing should recognize that nursing interventions, under other circumstances, could result in lawsuits under assault-and-battery statutes. Because nursing activities are often performed privately, and thus not easily observed or documented, everyone depends on the nurses' ethical system to exert the necessary self-control when providing therapeutic services. Furthermore, the shared sense of mission that results from dialogue among nurses with differing values may not be nonproductive activity but the bedrock for a successful business as well (Peters and Waterman 1982). Although task performance is and has been essential, patients increasingly desire a therapeutic model that offers more collaboration between themselves and care providers. As a consequence, nurses are compelled to see clients as more than a collection of body systems.

## Processes

The process of nursing assumes that the nurse is a knowledge worker—one who thinks as well as performs. This distinction becomes important when establishing pay policies. The income of knowledgeable workers will not necessarily be determined by supply, demand, or productivity (Drucker 1982). Stated more concisely, the nursing process consists of assessing patient needs, implementing the planned nursing action, reassessing patient needs, and reapplying the nursing action, in a cyclic pattern (Brodt 1978). Reassessment implies evaluation; the framework most commonly used is that of assessing, planning, implementing, and evaluating (Stevens 1980).

Terminology is important. "Assessment" seems less threatening than the more direct term "nursing diagnosis." Yet as educational theorists, clinicians, and administrators construct and refine models of practice to better organize education and research, progress is being made on codifying nursing diagnoses. At an international conference of nurses on this topic, 30 physical and psychological nursing diagnoses were approved (Kim and Mority 1982). Although the list of diagnoses has not been validated in its present form, research continues (Gordon 1985; Turkoski 1988).

Nursing diagnoses are separate from nursing goals and problems as well as from medical diagnoses and treatments; they are not restricted to the patient's symptoms. Assessment, or diagnosis, is continuous; it changes as the patient's condition changes; and it leads directly to nursing action and alters previous interventions (Kron and Durbin 1981).

The cyclic nature of patient assessment merits further discussion. Physicians concern themselves with physiology and the diagnosis of underlying pathologies. Their time frame for responding to patient reactions is usually on a two-times-a-day basis for a hospitalized patient, unless called on by another doctor or nurse to intervene more frequently. When providing care, the physician sees patients sequentially and allocates as much time as necessary to each. Nurses do not approach patients sequentially but "dovetail" their work. An initial detailed assessment may be scheduled, but continuing assessments occur with each patient encounter. This explains why delegating nursing tasks can be counterproductive. Even though an assistant may perform a procedure competently, if the cyclic reassessment has not yet occurred, the patient may not be cared for appropriately. That is, the nurses make nursing diagnoses and modify nursing care plans as they go.

For example, a nurse confronted with a hemorrhaging patient and a crying patient must make a choice; without calling a physician, the nurse will treat the hemorrhaging patient before the crying one. This is a simplified example of the nurse's independent practice. In reality, the nurse is responsible for medical and nursing interventions for many patients with simultaneous nursing and medical needs.

Yet nurses often have almost no scheduling authority; they must adjust their workloads to meet the schedules of other departments—x-ray, dietary, and housekeeping—as well as physicians. The nursing process emphasizes judgment, timing, and priority setting—otherwise known as problem solving. In addition, the nurse, in contrast with most other providers, must ensure continuity; at a set time the nurse will depart, and her duties must be picked up without a misstep by another nurse. The nurse's role and managerial control are profoundly affected by the obligation to ensure continuity of care over time.

## Practice Models

Among nursing schools there are five to seven predominant models of nursing practice that influence how the nursing care plan is made and modified (Silva 1987; Fawcett 1984). Each allows for the expression of the patient's feelings, the maintenance of patient independence, and the inclusion of common interventions. Four of the models also include health education (Riehl and Roy 1980). Reaching consensus on philosophy, objectives, and course content is not easy for nursing school faculties, but their task is probably not as formidable as that of hospital nurses. Unable to avoid the service demands of patients and doctors, nurses, with their different models of practice, cannot quickly develop a consensus about nursing education. This is especially so when the staff must also integrate the views of those mature nurses whose education emphasized following orders with the views of younger nurses educated toward more independent practice.

One often-overlooked problem that complicates discussions about nursing work is that the profession has not learned how to deal effectively with fallibility. The history of swift and severe punishment for nursing errors makes it difficult for nurses to seek help, share confidences, or consult with each other (Manthey 1980). This is substantially different from the management culture, where the expectation is not that every decision and action will be perfect, but that together workers will achieve a credible result. The many prescriptions for improving the management of nursing services do not alert managers to the problems of designing control systems to offset the "terror of error" problem. Encouraging errors to surface by creating a climate of support and training is difficult, since the organization fears malpractice suits and nourishes personal responsibility, which is a necessary component of clinical practice.

In most models, the informing process has been inadequately articulated. Several models of practice include a patient education component and a psychosocial emphasis that encourages communication. Other models emphasize the importance of authority and leadership, since successful nursing requires cooperation with many other groups. But providing information is an integral part of the decision-making process, and it goes beyond teaching, providing emotional support, and linking with both the health care team and community agencies.

Additional attention must be given to how the nurse generates new information, processes it, assigns priorities, and decides how to proceed. Let us take the example of laboratory reports. Physicians review lab reports for each patient they have admitted, and write orders for tests, medicines, and procedures as necessary. Nurses also look at the reports for the patients for whom they are responsible. Since all patients do not have the same physician (in community hospitals), the nurse must factor in how each physician prefers to handle exceptional findings. The nurse then decides whether to carry out a nursing procedure, follow a conditional medical order, repeat a test, notify the physician, or discuss the results with the patient. Simultaneously, the nurse determines the degree of urgency for each activity. Independent actions depend on policies that set boundaries on independent practice. These boundaries, in turn, are derived from the philosophy of nursing practice.

Time-and-motion studies have difficulty capturing the decisions that accompany procedures. Posting lab reports is a clerical activity that can be delegated. However, in order to process the reports and take action, the nurse must read them. Certainly it is inefficient to have nurses performing nonnursing tasks. Yet generating information, processing it, transmitting it with the appropriate degree of urgency, and documenting it are an integral part of nursing. The tools of information are paper, phone, and computer terminal. The obsession with the elimination of clerical duties for nurses and bureaucratic requirements for unnecessary reports may impede the efficient practice of nursing. However, the two should not be confused.

Documentation, in the form of charting, has always been an integral part of nursing practice. Now, with reimbursement changes exerting pressures for early discharge of patients, documentation has become more precise and more important than in the past. Documentation verifies personal accountability and influences the practices of other providers. The decline in the use of ancillary services in New Jersey after providers adapted to prospective payment mechanisms is attributed to physician acceptance of recorded nurse observations. Documentation is more than a bureaucratic requirement, since it influences professional practice. However, the proliferation of documentation requirements is believed by many to be burdensome, costly, and of questionable value.

Among nursing educators, the emphasis on the process of nursing has probably passed its zenith. Comprehensive guidelines for general nursing care and specialty units, with an emphasis on outcomes, are now well developed (Duke University Hospital 1983). The advancement of nursing science will continue to emphasize improved practice and theories of nursing care. Since this can only be done by nurses, these activities will continue to be the focus of nursing education and practice.

## Overlapping Roles

Much research has been done on nursing roles and their socialization (Conway 1983). Topics frequently addressed are role conception, autonomy, role clarity, role conflict, and role strain. To date no clear connection has been found between expected or actual competencies and type of educational program. The primary sources of role stress are ambiguity, lack of autonomy, and the limitations imposed on the development of the nurses' professional role by the competing demands of the work setting and by other professionals (physicians). Future studies need to explore the organizational context (e.g., task and skill variety, feedback, participation, formalization, level, and leadership) to better understand both role conflict and role ambiguity (Jackson and Schuler 1985).

### Levels of Nursing

**Primary Care.** Primary care, where one nurse is responsible for all nursing care for an individual patient, is the most recent attempt to reduce both the ambiguity of overlapping nursing roles and the costs of coordination among workers. While on duty, one nurse completely assesses, plans, and implements the care of the patients assigned to her. The nurse accepts authority, autonomy, and accountability for a small caseload of patients throughout their hospitalization. When the primary care nurse is absent, an associate nurse gives total care to the nurse's patients. The goals are to provide continuous, comprehensive, coordinated, individualized, patient-centered care. Primary care has the potential for fostering an "It's not my patient" attitude. Primary care does not solve the problem of overlapping physician roles or of nurses performing inappropriate medical tasks, although having one nurse accountable may help existing problems to surface and be resolved.

In addition, primary care provides opportunities for using new specialists. During the past few years the new roles of nurse practitioner, nurse clinician, expanded-role nurse, and physician's assistant have presented both opportunities and problems.

**Nurse Practitioner.** A nurse practitioner is one whose education extends beyond the basic requirements for licensing to a formally planned program for expanded functions in the diagnosis and treatment of patients. In 1981, 2,000 nurse practitioners graduated, for a total of 20,000 now in practice.

The nurse practitioner evolved in response to a shortage of primary physicians. The six nurse practitioner specialty areas, besides anesthesia, are pediatrics, midwifery, maternity, family practice, adult care, and psychiatric care. In 1980, 17,000 nurses identified themselves as nurse practitioners or nurse midwives, and 15,000 as nurse anesthetists. The largest proportion of these practitioners did not have a bachelor's or master's education. A bachelor's degree is not a requirement for entry to those programs (half of the total) that do not require a master's degree. Programs vary in length from 3 to 20 months, with the master's degree programs having a consistently higher average time requirement than the certificate programs. The reasons given as influencing the decision to enter the program are, in rank order, greater influence on patient care, additional learning opportunities, challenge of the work, frustration of former work, more independence, more responsibility, collaboration with physicians, increased salary, and increased status (Department of Health, Education, and Welfare 1976).

Nurse practitioners may practice either as members of an interdisciplinary health team or in solo practice. They can handle about 67% to 71% of the caseload of a primary care physician (Bullough and Bullough 1977). When they practice in hospitals, there is much controversy about how they should relate to other nurses. A 1984 study revealed that, within six months of graduation, two-thirds of nurse practitioner graduates were employed as providers of primary care in ambulatory clinical practices. More than half of their patients were in the low-income category (DHHS 1984). A review of 100 nurse-physician teams, also described as joint practice, found that enhanced economic status was neither contemplated nor achieved (Roueché 1977). There is no obvious explanation for this contradiction other than deeply entrenched custom.

An early study of the job satisfaction of nurse practitioners found that, although nurse practitioners had intrinsic and overall satisfaction scores that were higher than those of nonspecialists, more of the nonspecialists were satisfied with nursing as a career and would choose it again (Bullough 1974). The explanation offered was that the lag between increased responsibilities and basic rewards such as pay, job security, and better working conditions did not satisfy nurse practitioners' needs for salary, security, and good working conditions so that they could fully appreciate the intrinsic rewards. Alternatively, as they confronted the reality of limited career potential, regardless of personal investment and ability, they may have concluded that nursing was not a desirable choice for those committed to a career.

In July 1988, New York State passed a law that allows qualified RNs to use the title "nurse practitioner." Nurses so certified may diagnose illnesses and physical conditions and perform therapeutic and corrective measures within a specialty area of practice. The new privileges will apply to nurse practitioners working in hospitals as well as those in private practice. To qualify, RNs must be certified by a national certifying body or complete a program approved by the state education department. No physician may collaborate with more than four nurse practitioners who are not on the same physical premises as the physician.

**Clinical Specialist.** A clinical specialist is usually a nurse with a master's degree and expertise in a designated field. The clinical specialist program was designed originally by educators, who became concerned that nursing was becoming too task oriented to deal with the social and psychological needs of hospitalized patients. However, as employers were reluctant to pay for this level of care when direct patient care was included, the task requirements were retained (Bullough and Bullough 1977). When caring for individual patients, clinical specialists tend to be used as staff nurses rather than as consultants to primary care nurses or planners for patients with complex problems.

Integration of clinical specialists with other nurses poses problems. If nurses with additional competence are to achieve their potential for enhancing the practice of nursing, organization design must allow for consultation and flexible staffing. This is difficult to accomplish in traditional organizations, which stress tight staffing parameters. Ultimately, specialists come to believe they are poorly utilized.

Some analysts predict the demise of clinical specialists under the dual impact of the physician surplus and stringent reimbursement policies. This may happen, but the number of clinical specialists is increasing, and federal funds are supporting clinical nurse specialists. Many educational programs prefer to educate clinical specialists for out-of-hospital settings. Pilot projects demonstrate that clinical specialists can manage patients with chronic conditions more cost effectively than physicians can, without jeopardizing quality of care. If clinical specialists are to thrive in hospitals, it will be necessary to gain physician cooperation, expand salary ranges, and provide administrative support for collaboration among nurses.

**Expanded-Role Nurse.** An expanded-role nurse is one who has a higher level of autonomous practice than a staff nurse. The work usually includes history taking and diagnostic responsibilities. For example, a coronary care nurse would be described as having an expanded role in that subspecialty area. Hospitals may also have nurses employed by the physicians, who have staff privileges (Rustia, Wilson, and Quinn 1985). Each of these special nursing groups needs to be integrated into the administrative and clinical management system of the hospital, since the hospital has ultimate responsibility for the quality of care.

Given these various ways of viewing nursing work, a logical question arises as to how nurses themselves view their work. Responses from a study group, consisting of graduates from Connecticut nursing schools within three years after graduation, revealed that upon graduation an RN should be competent in six areas (Bradley 1983). In rank order of importance, these were (1) nursing process, (2) leadership, (3) skills, (4) research, (5) change, and (6) nursing as a community problem. The primary area (process, or caring for individual patients) stressed the design of nursing care plans, problem solving, and communication with patients and their families. Leadership meant supervision and direction of the nursing care team. Research and skills were approximately equal in importance. Research was valued as important to the profession as a whole; nurses believed that it was important for nurses to read journals and apply research findings in their practice. Technical skills were seen as being acquired on the job. The head nurse rather than the new graduate was the focal point for change. Understanding the health care system was accomplished through health referrals and the use of home care coordinators.

## Physician's Assistants

The majority of physician's assistants (PAs) are male nonnurses, whose duties are delegated by the physician, although the proportion of females is increasing. (Note the apostrophe in the title. A physician is approved to have an assistant, but the assistant must locate a sponsor physician. This arrangement limits career mobility). Some believe that physicians have more anxiety about physician's assistants than about nurse practitioners. This anxiety is attributed to a belief that nurses know what the proper relationship between a physician and an assistant ought to be, have a sense of their own limitations, and are less likely to go off on their own in all directions (Record and Greenlick 1975). PAs have less job mobility than nurses because they are not licensed (except in Colorado) and, in general, are paid more than nurses (Beall vs. Curtis et al. 1982). Organizations that hire both nurse practitioners and PAs are vulnerable to lawsuits on the grounds that jobs that score the same number of points on job evaluation studies should be paid the same (comparable worth). Cases have been filed in several states on these grounds.

A review of the literature indicates that both nurse practitioners and PAs in primary practice are more likely than physicians to practice in rural or inner-city areas (Lawrence 1978). Both nurse practitioners and PAs have a high level of consumer acceptance, generate enough revenue to offset costs in fee-for-service settings, and do not cause a decrease in process or quality outcomes. Because PAs are usually employed directly by physicians, they seldom are hired to work with community hospital staff nurses. Health maintenance organizations are more likely than other employers to hire both types.

## Physicians

Physician and nurse practice cannot be separated. In California, for example, the legislative intent section of the state law governing business and professionals explicitly states that it recognizes the existence of overlapping functions between physicians and RNs (California Business and Professional Code 1977). Nurse-physician relationships are more important than ever. For example, courts are finding that nurses have a legal responsibility to report doctors' orders that are not in accordance with accepted medical practice. The courts expect nurses to exercise independent judgment in implementing physician orders and even to take affirmative steps to protect patients from the negligent acts of physicians (Murphy 1987). Recent findings that patient deaths are related to a lack of communication among critical care nurses certainly underscore the need for administrative leadership in fostering physician-nurse communication (Georgopoulos 1985). Evidence that poor communication with physicians gets translated into negative attitudes toward patients is another indicator of how central nurse-physician relations are to hospital success (Nievaard 1987).[2]

In general, nursing care will not conflict with or contradict physicians' orders. It would help if nursing models were more explicit about integrating the medical plan with the nursing plan to encourage more collaborative practice. However, when medical care and nursing care are not easily complementary (and in a percentage of cases they will not be), nurses are being urged by society and their instructors to exhibit more autonomy. The administrators have the responsibility for designing and supporting a collegial peer review system that will protect the patient's interest, advance nursing practice, and resolve conflicts between the nursing and medical staffs. Interestingly, in this era of marketing, the physician has been described as a nursing service customer (Luciano 1985). Since the goals of the physician and nurse are the same—to deliver quality care and discharge the patient as soon as possible—good nurse-physician relations can lead to better outcomes, higher occupancy, greater financial stability, and satisfaction for both nurses and physicians.

Nurses routinely perform tasks that were formerly reserved for physicians. Among the most common are monitoring cardiac arrhythmias and electrolytes and administering intravenous medications. In intensive care units and specialty services, where the interface between physicians and nurses is well defined and timely decisions are critical, both groups have worked together effectively. In noncritical care units, the authority of nurses to make decisions is more contentious. This is not because nurses want to usurp the doctor's role. Actions such as changing inappropriate special diets, modifying medications when indicated (including dosage and mode of administration), rescheduling diagnostic procedures when indicated by the patient's condition, changing surgical dressings, deciding on the frequency of vital signs monitoring, inserting catheters for patients unable to void, and contributing to decisions on hospital discharge are examples of judgments that, if not made in a timely fashion, can result in discomfort for patients and diminished productivity (Mechanic and Aiken 1982).

Although there is a widely shared belief that nurses are dissatisfied with their participation in the clinical decision-making process, this may have been overestimated. A study of 90 patient care units in six cities found that nurses, especially in the small, specialized, and critical care units, were generally satisfied with their involvement in clinical decisions (Prescott, Dennis, and Jacox 1987). Physicians, however, resisted nurses having greater freedom.

Resolving practice conflicts is crucial to quality service; it is where the legal responsibility of the hospital board of trustees and the administration intersects with the professional accountability of physicians, nurses, and other caregivers. Credential committees may examine qualifications and limit the scope of physician practice, tissue committees may examine organs, and nurses may have the required license and continuing education, but care of a patient is the joint function of the medical and nursing regimes implemented through the hospital employee, namely, the nurse. Mutuality between nurses and physicians is undeniable, and their surveillance of one another is unavoidable. Their independence creates a necessary tension, especially since nurses, patients, and physicians do not necessarily agree on which functions are most important.

Collaborative practice has been proposed as a formal method of dealing with the shifting boundaries of overlapping duties. Many states and hospitals use joint practice committees. These were stimulated by the National Joint Practice Commission that resulted from the Lysaught Report on Nursing (National Commission for the Study of Nursing and Nursing Education 1970). Collaboration is not an ad hoc effort. The National Joint Practice Commission, before disbanding in 1981, established guidelines for joint practice. There are five essential elements: (1) integrated nursing and medical notes on the patient record, (2) primary nursing care, (3) support of nurse decision-making, (4) a joint practice committee, and (5) joint care review. The goals are essentially to provide personalized care to patients, require less supervision by physicians but achieve better coordination, increase the organizational commitment of bedside nurses, and use the staff to increase patient satisfaction with the hospital.

There is little doubt that some physicians, along with nurses, are taking the lead in encouraging the new behaviors—taking risks, being assertive, intervening autonomously, and being accountable—that are necessary for collaborative practice.

Efforts by the American Medical Association to create a new group of bedside workers, called registered care technologists, undermines the concept of collaborative practice. Nurses view this innovation as an intrusion into their domain of educating and licensing workers for whom they will be responsible. They argue that the costs of coordination will more than offset the labor savings, if any, of less-educated workers. Further, they contest the rationale that delegating physical tasks reduces much of the workload, because the nurse must still be present to adjust patients' care to changing conditions.

## Other Hospital Workers

The relationships among hospital workers are paradoxical. The wide range of education and the variety of credentials workers have lead to a highly stratified work force. Job titles, which are strongly associated with social status, education, sex, and pay, make it easier to clarify work domains, assign work, hold individuals accountable, and develop a shared understanding of jobs. However, job stratification often inhibits rather than enhances patient care. Frequently, employed workers closest to the patient do not have much input into clinical decisions and the ultimate outcome. Licensed practical nurses and nursing assistants are often frustrated, especially when they have more experience and organizational knowledge than their superiors. Driven by an egalitarian service ethos which holds that each patient should get care and service based on medical needs, workers reporting to RNs are often limited by their own status boundaries. Their low position in the hierarchy means that direct care providers are unable to get the attention of higher status professionals or to obtain the resources from other departments necessary to meet observed patient needs.

Workers from many other hospital departments visit, serve, and treat patients on the nursing unit. Nurses usually have limited ability to schedule or supervise these activities. Nursing work is performed around countless scheduled and unscheduled interruptions. The amount of energy and satisfaction among individuals from all the involved departments is a measure of the relative success the organization has achieved in developing a common culture, shared goals, and departmental integration. Table 2.3 summarizes the dimensions and characteristics of nursing practice in hospitals.

**Table 2-3** Dimensions and Characteristics of Nursing Practice in Hospitals

| Dimensions | Characteristics |
|---|---|
| Client | Dependent but not passive |
| | Expects nurse to initiate contact |
| | Clinical conditions are uncertain, unstable, and variable |
| | Continuing needs of patients are not synchronized |
| Tasks | Custodial and therapeutic |
| | Partially delegated |
| | Partially self-initiated |
| Processes | Diagnose (assess) |
| | Plan |
| | Implement |
| | Evaluate |
| | Inform |
| | Document |
| | Defined by statute, regulation, profession, and employer |
| | Intrarole conflict |
| | Interrole conflict, role conflict, role overload |
| | Overlap with physicians, allied workers, other nurses |
| | Supervisory responsibility without authority |
| Overall | Employees |
| |    Freedom to structure own work |
| |    Demands from multiple sources |
| |    Accountable for work performed by others |
| |    Career paths hard to discern |
| | Employers |
| |    Able to substitute among levels of RNs and assistants |
| |    Depend on others for evaluation |

## Quality of Care

Patient satisfaction is often used as an indicator of quality of nursing care. Although important, it should not be the sole evaluation measure. Some good nursing interventions, such as teaching patients to deal with their illness and health status, may produce dissatisfaction in some patients (Eriksen 1987).

The release of hospital-specific mortality data by the Health Care Financing Administration, together with changes in accreditation guidelines by JCAHO, will ultimately focus more attention on quality of nursing care. Nursing has a long history of interest in and concern with quality of patient care, but, as in other professions and the entire system, the definition of quality is a matter of debate. In a review of empirical studies of nursing quality, Lang and Clinton (1984) used the Donabedian structure-process-outcome model to place nursing studies in perspective. Instruments to measure the individual competency of nurses exist, but they are used primarily for research purposes. In the future, nurse researchers will undoubtedly focus their efforts on clinical issues. Managers within health care organizations, both general managers and nursing administrators, will have the primary responsibility, along with physicians, for establishing peer review and feedback mechanisms as well as concurrent studies necessary to monitor quality of nursing care.

## Organizational Responsibilities

There is a pressing concern among executives to design the systems necessary to attract and retain professional workers throughout the economy (Von Glinow 1988). Hospitals, although not unique in this respect, have a special challenge because of the lingering stereotypes about female workers, the legacy of an ambiguous educational system, and competition from other industries for talented individuals with an interest in science and service. What is involved, other than attention to professional practice norms and career structures, is managing the organization's culture, designing appropriate structures and decision-making opportunities, and ensuring that professional and financial outcomes are appropriate. These issues are the focus of the next chapters.

## Summary

Nursing is one of 282 jobs described by the U.S. Department of Labor. Federally employed nurses range in classification from GS-4 to GS-12. In general, however, the scope of nursing practice is defined legally in each state by the state's nurse practice act. These definitions have changed greatly since 1971 as a result of many factors, such as Medicare requirements and a general trend toward equality of workers. New York's definition of nursing has served as a model for other states. Two current areas of controversy center around prescribing medications and linking education to licensure.

Actual licensing is performed by the states on the basis of a standardized examination. The test looks at five basic areas of nursing, eight categories of nursing functions, and four client need categories. National coordination of licensure ensures easy geographical mobility. Certification of nurses, which is done by the American Nurses' Association, validates a nurse's proficiency in a specialized field. Certification is especially important as it leads to investment by nurses in their own careers.

Nursing work, in addition to being bounded by law and professional associations, is determined by custom and by employers. Nurses practice independently, dependently, and collaboratively with other professionals and aides. Practice is also influenced by changing conditions and demands of clients, the competence of subordinates, and by physicians.

Practice includes both tasks and processes, including direct patient service, record keeping, and making nursing diagnoses. Making a nursing diagnosis is different from making a medical diagnosis, and requires much planning and reevaluation, tasks made difficult by lack of control in many areas. Also, nurses work with a "terror of error" in patient care decisions. As nurses are responsible for total patient care, it is sometimes appropriate for them to do clerical and other unglamorous duties.

Nurses have a high level of work force participation, especially when they are young, and a large majority work in hospitals as bedside nurses. Expectations about the relationships among the many workers involved with nursing are divergent. Evolving professions, including nurse practitioners, clinical specialists, expanded-role nurses, and physician's assistants, lead to further lack of clarity about the roles of the various care providers. In addition to this role confusion, the relationship between nurses and doctors is often a source of tension.

Three basic educational pathways exist for entry into nursing, although there has been movement away from the diploma programs for decades as well as a serious loss in graduations from baccalaureate nursing programs during the 1980s. This educational diversity leads to philosophical differences. Fortunately, models exist to appeal to individuals with diverse educational aspirations and qualifications. Failure to systematize the links between education and licensure perpetuates the recurring cycle of problems in recruiting and maintaining nurses in hospital employment.

Although other professionals may label nursing as a low-status occupation, nursing has traditionally been an avenue of upward mobility and enjoys high status in many families and among female-dominated occupations. The best generalization is that nursing will mirror the education, career expectations, and problems of women in the surrounding society.

## Endnotes

1.  According to Orem, the seven health foci, which can assist nurses in classifying nursing situations, are related to life cycle, recovery from a specific disease, illness of undetermined origin, defects of a genetic or developmental nature, regulation through active treatment of a disease or injury, restoration of disrupted vital functions, or terminal illness.

2.  See Sowell and Alexander (1988) for a case study in which upgrading the image of nurses among physicians increased occupancy in a cardiac telemetry unit.

## References

Aiken, L., and C. Mullinix. 1987. The nurse shortage: myth or reality? *New England Journal of Medicine* 317(10): 641–646.

American Journal of Nursing. 1955. ANA board approves a definition of nursing practice. *American Journal of Nursing* 55: 1474.

American Nurses' Association. 1984. *Nursing legal authority for practice.* Kansas City, MO: American Nurses' Association.

American Nurses' Association. 1988. *The career credential professional certification.* Kansas City, MO: American Nurses' Association.

Armstrong, D. 1983. The fabrication of nurse-patient relationships. *Social Science and Medicine* 17: 457–460.

Beall, F. vs. Curtis et al. 1982. Civil Action No. 81-12-ATH in the United States District Court for the Middle District of Georgia, Athens Division.

Birenbaum, A. 1981. *Health care and society.* Montclair, NJ: Allanheld, Osmun.

Bradley, J. 1983. Nurses attitudes towards dimensions of nursing practice. *Nursing Research* 32(2): 110–114.

Brodt, D. 1978. The nursing process, in N. Chaska, ed., *The nursing profession: views through the mist.* New York: McGraw-Hill, 256–268.

Brown, E. 1948. *Nursing for the future.* New York: Russell Sage Foundation.

Bullough, B. 1974. Is the nurse practitioner role a source of increased work satisfaction? *Nursing Research* 23: 14–19.

Bullough, B. 1976. The law and the expanding nursing role. *American Journal of Public Health* 66: 249.

Bullough, B. 1983. Introduction—nursing practice law, in B. Bullough, V. Bullough, and M. Soukop, eds., *Issues and strategies for the eighties.* New York: Springer, 279–291.

Bullough, B., and V. Bullough. (eds). 1977. *Expanding horizons for nurses.* New York: Springer.

*California Business and Professional Code.* 1977. Section 2725(d) (West, 1977 Suppl.).

Civil Service Commission. 1977. *Position classification standards: series GS-610.* Washington, DC: Government Printing Office.

Conway, S. 1983. Socialization and roles in nursing. *Annual Review of Nursing Research* 1: 183–207.

Department of Health, Education, and Welfare. 1976. *Longitudinal study of nurse practitioners.* Washington, DC: Government Printing Office.

Department of Health and Human Services. 1984. *Study of nurse practitioners.* Washington, DC: Government Printing Office.

Department of Health and Human Services. 1986. *National sample survey of registered nurses.* Rockville, MD: Bureau of Health Professions.

Department of Health and Human Services. 1988. *Sixth report to the President and Congress on the status of health personnel in the United States.* Washington, DC: Government Printing Office.

Dillon, D. 1975. Towards matching personal and job characteristics. *Occupational Outlook Quarterly.* 19: 2-18

Drucker, P. 1982. *The changing role of the executive.* New York: Times Books.

Duke University Hospital. 1983. *Guidelines for nursing care: process and outcome.* Philadelphia: Lippincott.

Durbin, E. 1981. Legal aspects of nursing practice, in T. Kron and E. Durbin, eds., *The management of patient care,* 5th Ed. Philadelphia: Saunders, pp. 10–13.

Eccard, W. 1977. A revolution in white: new approaches in treating nurses as professionals. *Vanderbilt Law Review* 30: 839–879.

Eriksen, L. 1987. Patient satisfaction: an indicator of nursing care quality? *Nursing Management* 18(7): 31–35.

Fawcett, J. 1984. *Analysis and evaluation of conceptual models of nursing.* Philadelphia: F. A. Davis.

Friss, L. 1981. Work force policy perspectives: registered nurses. *Journal of Health Politics, Policy and Law* 5: 696–719.

Georgopoulos, B. 1985. Organization structure and the performance of hospital emergency services. *Annals of Emergency Medicine* 14(7): 677–684.

Gordon, M. 1985. Nursing diagnosis. *Annual Review of Nursing Research* 3: 127–146.

Hegyvary, S. 1979. Nursing process: the basis for evaluating the quality of nursing care. *International Nursing Review* 26: 113–116.

Hener, T., and E. Meir. 1981. Congruency, consistency, and differentiation as predictors of job satisfaction within the nursing occupation. *Journal of Vocational Behavior* 18: 304–309.

Hurka, S. 1972. Career orientations of registered nurses working in hospitals. *Hospital Administration* 17(Fall): 26–33.

Institute of Medicine. 1983. *Nursing and nursing education: public policies and private actions.* Washington, DC: National Academy Press.

Jackson, S., and R. Schuler. 1985. A meta-analysis and conceptual critique of research on role ambiguity and role conflict in work settings. *Organizational Behavior and Human Decision Processes* 36: 16–78.

Jenna, J. 1986. Toward the patient-driven hospital. *Healthcare Forum* 2: 18–19.

Katz, F. 1969. Nurses, in A. Etzioni, ed., *The Semi Professions.* New York: Free Press, pp. 54–81.

Kauppinen-Toropainen, K., I. Kandolin, and P. Mutanen. 1983. Job dissatisfaction and work-related exhaustion in male and female work. *Journal of Occupational Behavior* 4: 192–207.

Kent, R., ed. 1985. *Money talks.* New York: Facts on File.

Kim, M., and D. Mority. 1982. *Classification of nursing diagnosis.* New York: McGraw-Hill.

Kramer, M. 1970. Role conceptions of baccalaureate nurses and success in hospital nursing. *Nursing Research* 19: 428–439.

Kron, T., and E. Durbin. 1981. *The management of patient care*, 5th Ed. Philadelphia: Saunders.

Lang, N., and J. Clinton. 1984. Assessment of quality of nursing care. *Annual Review of Nursing Research* 2: 135–163.

Lawrence, D. 1978. Physician assistants and nurse practitioners: their impacts on health care access, costs, and quality. *Health and Medical Care Services Review* 1(2): 2–12.

Levi, M. 1980. Functional redundancy and the process of professionalization: the case of registered nurses in the United States. *Journal of Health Politics, Policy and Law* 5: 333–353.

Levine, E., and E. Moses. 1982. Registered nurses today: a statistical profile, in L. Aiken, ed., *Nursing in the 1980s*. Philadelphia: Lippincott, pp. 475–499.

Luciano, K. 1985. The physician as a nursing service customer. *Journal of Nursing Administration* 15(5): 17–19.

Manthey, M. 1980. A theoretical framework for primary nursing. *Journal of Nursing Administration* 10(6): 11–15.

Mechanic, D., and L. Aiken. 1982. A cooperative agenda for medicine and nursing. *New England Journal of Medicine* 307: 747–750.

Menzies, I. 1970. *The functioning of social systems as a defence against anxiety* (Tavistock Pamphlet no. #3). London: Tavistock.

Midwest Alliance in Nursing. 1987. *Associate degree nursing: facilitating competency development*. Indianapolis: Midwest Alliance in Nursing.

Moskowitz, S., and L. Moskowitz. 1984. Protecting your job. *American Journal of Nursing* 84(1): 55–58.

Mottaz, C. 1988. Work satisfaction among hospital nurses. *Hospital and Health Services Administration* 33: 57–74.

Murphy, E. 1987. The professional status of nursing: a view from the courts. *Nursing Outlook* 35(1): 12–15.

National Commission for the Study of Nursing and Nursing Education. 1970. *An abstract for action*. New York: McGraw-Hill.

National League for Nursing. 1988. *Nursing student census with policy implications, 1987*. New York: National League for Nursing.

New York State Educational Law, Title VIII, Article 139, Section 6902. 1972.

Nievaard, A. 1987. Communication climate and patient care: causes and effects of nurses' attitudes to patients. *Social Science and Medicine* 24: 777–784.

Norris, C. 1982. *Concept clarification in nursing*. Rockville, MD: Aspen.

Okorafor, H. 1983. Hospital characteristics attractive to physicians and the consumers: implications for public general hospitals. *Hospital and Health Services Administration* 28(2): 50–65.

Orem, D. 1985. *Nursing concepts of practice*, 3rd Ed. New York: McGraw-Hill.

Overton, P., R. Schneck, and C. Hazlett. 1977. An empirical study of the technology of nursing subunits. *Administrative Science Quarterly* 22: 203–219.

Perrow, C. 1965. Hospitals: technology, structure, and goals, in J. March, ed., *Handbook of Organizations*. Chicago: Rand McNally, pp. 910–971.

Peters, J., and R. Wacker. 1982. Hospital strategic planning must be rooted in values and ethics. *Hospitals* 56(12): 90–98.

Peters, T., and R. Waterman. 1982. *In search of excellence*. New York: Harper and Row.

Population Reference Bureau. 1981. U.S. women at work. *Population Bulletin* 36: 2.

Prescott, P., K. Dennis, and A. Jacox. 1987. Clinical decision making of staff nurses. *Image* 19(2): 56–62.

Preston, R. 1979. *The dilemmas of care.* New York: Elsevier.

Primm, P. 1986. Entry into practice: competency statements for BSNs and ADNs. *Nursing Outlook* 34: 135–137.

Record, J., and M. Greenlick. 1975. New health professions and the physician role: a hypothesis from the Kaiser experience. *Public Health Reports* 90: 241–246.

Riehl, J., and Sister C. Roy. 1980. *Conceptual models for nursing practice,* 2nd Ed. New York: Appleton-Century-Crofts.

Rosengren, W. 1970. The career of clients and organizations, in W. Rosengren and M. Lefton, eds., *Organization and clients.* Columbus, OH: Merrill, pp. 117–135.

Roueché, B. 1977. *Together: casebook of joint practices in primary care.* Chicago: National Joint Practice Commission.

Rustia, J., C. Wilson, and J. Quinn. 1985. Use of physician-hired nurses. *Journal of Nursing Administration* 15 (9): 35–40.

Silva, M. 1987. Conceptual models of nursing. *Annual Review of Nursing Research* 5: 229-246.

Sowell, R., and J. Alexander. 1988. A model for success in nursing administration. *Nursing and Health Care* 9(1): 25–30.

Stevens, B. 1980. *The nurse executive.* Wakefield, MA: Nursing Resources.

Swansburg, F. 1983. The consumer's perception of nursing care, in B. Bullough, V. Bullough, and M. Soukop, eds., *Nursing issues and strategies for the eighties.* New York: Springer, pp. 105–114.

Swansburg, R., and P. Swansburg. 1984. *Strategic career development for nurses.* Rockville, MD: Aspen.

Thompson, J. 1967. *Organizations in action.* New York: McGraw-Hill.

Turkoski, B. 1988. Nursing diagnosis in print, 1950–1985. *Nursing outlook* 36(13): 142–144.

Vestal, K. 1984. Financial considerations for career ladder programs. *Nursing Administration Quarterly* 9: 1–8.

Von Glinow, M. 1988. *The new professionals.* Cambridge, MA: Ballinger.

Wadle, K., and D. Munns. 1983. A plea for a research-based curriculum. *Nursing and Health Care* 4: 261-264.

Williams, C., ed. 1983. *Image making in nursing.* St. Louis: American Academy of Nursing.

Wood, L. 1972. *Career model for nurse practitioners.* Los Angeles: UCLA Division of Vocational Education.

Yura, H., and M. Walsh. 1988. *The nursing process: assessing, planning, implementing, evaluating,* 5th Ed. Norwalk: CT: Appleton & Lange.

## *Appendix 2A*
## Nursing Defined

### Nursing

Nursing is the diagnosis and treatment of human responses to actual or potential health problems.

### Phenomena of Concern

The phenomena of concern to nurses are human responses to actual or potential health problems. Any observable manifestation, need, condition, concern, event, dilemma, difficulty, occurrence, or fact that can be described or scientifically explained and is within the target area of nursing practice is of interest to nurses.

### Human Responses

The following provides an illustrative list rather than a comprehensive taxonomy of human responses that are the focus for nursing intervention:

- Self-care limitations
- Impaired functioning in areas such as rest, sleep, ventilation, circulation, activity, nutrition, elimination, skin, sexuality, and the like
- Pain and discomfort
- Emotional problems related to illness and treatment, life-threatening events or daily experiences, such as anxiety, loss, loneliness and grief
- Distortion of symbolic functions, reflected in interpersonal and intellectual processes, such as hallucinations
- Deficiencies in decision-making and ability to make personal choices
- Self-image changes required by health status

- Dysfunctional perceptual orientations to health
- Strains related to life processes, such as birth, growth and development, and death
- Problematic affiliative relationships

(From *Nursing: A social policy statement*. American Nurses' Association, 1980. Reprinted with permission.)

## Appendix 2B
## Code for Nurses

1. The nurse provides services with respect for human dignity and the uniqueness of the client unrestricted by considerations of social or economic status, personal attributes, or the nature of health problems.

2. The nurse safeguards the client's right to privacy by judiciously protecting information of a confidential nature.

3. The nurse acts to safeguard the client and the public when health care and safety are affected by the incompetent, unethical, or illegal practice of any person.

4. The nurse assumes responsibility and accountability for individual nursing judgments and actions.

5. The nurse maintains competence in nursing.

6. The nurse exercises informed judgment and uses individual competence and qualifications as criteria in seeking consultation, accepting responsibilities, and delegating nursing activities to others.

7. The nurse participates in activities that contribute to the ongoing development of the profession's body of knowledge.

8. The nurse participates in the profession's efforts to implement and improve standards of nursing.

9. The nurse participates in the profession's efforts to establish and maintain conditions of employment conducive to high-quality nursing care.

10. The nurse participates in the profession's effort to protect the public from misinformation and misrepresentation and to maintain the integrity of nursing.

11. The nurse collaborates with members of the health professions and other citizens in promoting community and national efforts to meet the health needs of the public.

(*Code for Nurses, with Interpretive Statements.* American Nurses' Association. 1976. Reprinted with permission.)

## Appendix 2C
## Differentiated Competency Statements

### General Statement

The ADN cares for focal clients who are identified as individuals and members of a family. The level of responsibility of the ADN is for a specified work period and is consistent with identified goals of care. The ADN is prepared to function in structured health care settings. The structured settings are geographical and/or situational environments where the policies, procedures and protocols for provision of health care are established and there is recourse to assistance and support from the full scope of nursing expertise.

The BSN cares for focal clients who are identified as individuals, families, aggregates, and community groups. The level of responsibility of the BSN is from admission to post-discharge. The BSN is prepared to function in structured and unstructured health care settings. The unstructured setting is a geographical and/or situational environment which may not have established policies, procedures, and protocols and has the potential for variations requiring independent nursing decisions.

### Provision of Direct Care Competencies

The ADN provides direct care for the focal client with common, well-defined nursing diagnoses by:

The BSN provides direct care for the focal client with complex interactions of nursing diagnoses by:

A. collecting health pattern data from available resources using established assessment format to identify basic health care needs.

A. expanding the collection of data to identify complex care needs.

B. organizing and analyzing health pattern data in order to select nursing diagnoses from an established list.

B. organizing and analyzing complex health pattern data to develop nursing diagnoses.

C. establishing goals with the focal client for a specified work period that are consistent with the overall comprehensive nursing plan of care.

C. establishing goals with the focal client to develop a comprehensive nursing plan of care from admission to post-discharge.

D. developing and implementing an individualized nursing plan of care using established nursing diagnoses and protocols to promote, maintain, and restore health.

D. developing and implementing a comprehensive nursing plan of care based on nursing diagnoses for health promotion.

E. participating in the medical plan of care to promote an integrated health care plan.

E. interpreting the medical plan of care into nursing activities to formulate approaches to nursing care.

F. evaluating focal client responses to nursing interventions and altering the plan of care as necessary to meet client goals.

F. evaluating the nursing care delivery system and promoting goal-directed change to meet individualized client needs.

## Communication Competencies

The ADN uses basic communication skills with the focal client by:

The BSN uses complex communication skills with the focal client by:

A. developing and maintaining goal-directed interactions to encourage expressing of needs and support coping behaviors.

A. developing and maintaining goal-directed interactions to promote effective coping behaviors and facilitate change in behavior.

B. modifying and implementing a standard teaching plan in order to restore, maintain, and promote health.

B. designing and implementing a comprehensive teaching plan for health promotion.

The ADN coordinates focal client care with other health team members by:

A. documenting and communicating data for clients with common, well-defined nursing diagnoses to provide continuity of care.

B. using established channels of communication to implement an effective health care plan.

C. using interpreted nursing research findings for developing nursing care.

The BSN collaborates with other health team members by:

A. documenting and communicating comprehensive data for clients with complex interactions to provide continuity of care.

B. using established channels of communication to modify health care delivery.

C. incorporating research findings into practice and by consulting with nurse researchers regarding identified nursing problems in order to enhance nursing practice.

## Management Competencies

The ADN organizes those aspects of care for focal clients for whom s/he is accountable by:

A. prioritizing, planning, and organizing the delivery of standard nursing care in order to use time and resources effectively and efficiently.

B. delegating aspects of care to peers, LPNs, and ancillary nursing personnel, consistent with their levels of education and expertise, in order to meet client needs.

The BSN manages nursing care of focal clients by:

A. prioritizing, planning, and organizing the delivery of comprehensive nursing care in order to use time and resources effectively and efficiently.

B. delegating aspects of care to other nursing personnel, consistent with their levels of education and expertise, in order to meet client needs and to maximize staff performance.

C. maintaining accountability for own care and care delegated to others to assure adherence to ethical and legal standards.

C. maintaining accountability for own care and care delegated to others to assure adherence to ethical and legal standards.

D. recognizing the need for referral and conferring with appropriate nursing personnel for assistance to promote continuity of care.

D. initiating referral to appropriate departments and agencies to provide service and promote continuity of care.

E. working with other health care personnel within the organizational structure to manage client care.

E. assuming a leadership role in health care management to improve client care.

(Reprinted with permission from Primm, P. 1987. Entry into practice: Competency statements for BSNs and ADNs. *Journal of Professional Nursing* 3(4): 218–224.)

# Summary Section I

Section I establishes that:

1.  Career concepts provide a new paradigm for understanding the work patterns of registered nurses and redressing the imbalance of rewards available to transient and spiral nurses as contrasted with steady-state and linear nurses.

2.  Nursing is a heterogeneous occupation whose members are not united by a common educational experience, common tasks, or a shared social background.

3.  Licensure produces uniform entry competency requirements and discourages task differentiation related to education, while it promotes geographical mobility

4.  The wide range of nursing tasks and responsibilities requires nurses with different levels of preparation, experience, and pay (i.e., differentiation).

5.  Employers should use career concepts to develop disaggregated policies and strategies. This is possible because differentiated competency statements exist and managers have much discretion over task assignments and working conditions.

6.  Career structures can be formalized by state and local laws because nursing associations have experience in developing job-related examinations and model licensing statutes for all states when the employment system, which is dominated by hospitals, cooperates.

Hospital executives need to replace the disposable nurse syndrome, in which every nurse is treated alike, with a differentiated career strategy that attracts and retains the mix of nurses necessary for both short-term and long-

83

term survival of needed hospitals and the industry as a whole. For most hospitals and communities, this means formalizing the career structure for steady-state and linear nurses while deemphasizing the incentives for transient and spiral career orientations.

The new approach assumes that:

1. Nurses cannot be isolated from societal preferences about education, work, or careers.

2. Nurses have a strong commitment to work.

3. Work force experiences and opportunities are important influences on the amount of time worked and on personal investment in education to improve performance.

4. The caliber of new recruits, both men and women, ultimately depends on observation of the career patterns incumbents experience.

5. The locus of the career structure is within the hospitals, although the profession is encouraging career progression through the credentialing process.

This shift toward career-oriented management requires reexamination of current beliefs and management practices. Section II will synthesize relevant organizational research into areas where executives and managers have authority and responsibility:

• Organization culture and values

• Decision-making (governance and decentralization)

• Work specification (departmentation and staffing)

• Control systems, including the career system

• Reexamination of motivation, unions, and quality of work life projects.

Section III will present policy perspectives on the recurring cycle of nursing shortages and future alternatives.

*Section II*

# Management Issues

# Chapter 3

# Values: Organizational and Individual

---

Consideration of these questions over a period of years has led me to conclude that the fundamental questions of hospital management are not scientific.

(Griffith 1983, 27)

the...central challenge posed by the changing roles of nurses, the emergence of lay women managers and the ethical and professional dilemmas created by the new technologies is to the health care manager's value system.

(Shortell 1982, 20)

## Values in Organizations

Organization members share, to varying degrees, a set of values that, together with attitudes and beliefs, form a corporate culture. This shared value pattern is essential if workers are to take some things for granted and perform their specific jobs. When managers and workers share values, the organizational culture will be more homogeneous, consistent, and clear to the workers. del Bueno (1986) defines culture as the combination of symbols, language, assumptions, and behaviors that overtly manifest an organization's norms and values.

Organizations are not monolithic, however. Just like individuals, they subscribe to many values that vary in consistency, intensity, and direction. Where there is diversity, there may be more conflict, more tolerance for nonconformists, and a more diffuse strategy. Organizational values are not static but are modified by feedback from experience. In any organization there will be a constellation of important values that managers and workers share, but others that they do not. Although most people have a personal preference, it is unlikely that one can prove what is "best" for a given set of circumstances.

Before turning attention to the unique value dilemmas of hospitals, following is a brief summary of research about values that applies to all organizations.[1]

An organization's articulation of its mission includes a statement of both organizational philosophy and purpose. The philosophy establishes the values, beliefs, and guidelines for how the organization is going to conduct its business. Taken together, these values, beliefs, and guidelines form the culture of the organization. Certainly, organizational culture is not the sole determinant of organizational performance. However, potent ideologies and interconnected sets of values and beliefs that describe a preferred social system are important because they engender devotion and high spirits and add drama to everyday activities.

Executives can anticipate that values are more stable at the operational level than at the administrative level. Employees from a culture that emphasizes independence are more likely to be comfortable with structures and policies that enhance autonomy than with policies that stress conformity and authority. Employees who distrust the prevailing value system cannot be integrated without special effort. A characteristic of good management is its ability to make sound decisions in marginal cases where the unique subsystems are in substantial disagreement.

Prescriptions for employee motivation and control are affected by the leaders' views of the essential character of humanity—whether people are fundamentally good or evil. Thus, the values and beliefs of leaders, especially about the work ethic, help define supervisory behavior and preference for employee development activities.

Whatever their personal preferences, executives and managers cannot ignore the shared values of employees or potential employees. Workers are not captives. Although some workers have little or no choice about whether or where to work, this is not the case for most educated, skilled workers. Since employees tend to find their jobs in communities through a network of friends and acquaintances, employers depend on their reputation and on current workers' word-of-mouth recommendations for new applicants.

Consensus about values facilitates change. Values also set limits for ethical behavior—the extent to which one will accept or resist organizational goals or pressure; some things just are or are not allowed in an organization. The ideology pervades everyday experiences and limits employee options even when the employee is not being observed; this is an important consideration in hospitals, where patients frequently are dependent and unable to protect their own interests.

The flow of people into and out of the organization completes the circle of values: from culture to individual, from individual to organization, from organization to worker, and back to society. Employers may find it difficult to resist the momentum of this self-perpetuating cycle because change requires circular reasoning, which is more complex than simply separating work from life. But circular thinking is appropriate. It is nothing more than recognizing that people change in response to events and other people.

## Management Ideologies

The period from 1920 to 1970 has been described as the "era of management" (Reich 1983). Much management ideology is based on three principles: specialization of work through simplification, predetermined rules to coordinate tasks, and detailed performance monitoring. The result has been the splitting of thinkers from doers. The personal characteristics of workers have become more important than the personal character of executives and managers.

Within management, four ideologies have been identified: classical, human relations, structuralist, and systems; the last of these is a combination of the first three (Neugeboren 1985). Schools of administration tend to favor the first model, with its emphasis on economics. The human relations model has been closely linked with industrial psychology, and the structuralist model stems from organizational sociology. Within organizations, executives and managers tend to favor one ideology over another. These ideologies are not necessarily shared by other managers or workers.

The present era is characterized as one in which the market alone has failed to generate investments in human skills. As a result, many if not most workers lack a sense of shared purpose or believe that workers do not benefit from improved productivity. Yet as capital and management move to exploit entrepreneurial opportunities, workers are the only ones with a long-term stake in the organization.

## Organizational Values in Hospitals

Hospitals are a special subset of organizations, and their very purpose, saving lives, encourages shared values. At least one hospital proponent believes that hospitals should be bristling with enthusiasm, purpose, and mission (Kaiser 1983). Productivity and future survival depend, in his view, on *esprit de corps* and self-designing organizations. Managerial design of cultures, he predicts, will become much more prominent in the future.

Most researchers would agree that hospitals have a social purpose that cannot be captured by economic or technical analysis alone. The public places them in a different category from other businesses. Much of the concern shown by investor-owned hospitals about the cost and quality of care is rooted in competing values. Business strategies, however, do not necessarily dictate an expedient, profit-maximizing approach. An equally legitimate strategy is one of integrity and perpetuation with focus on long-term continuity and growth. In this case, worker welfare is not an optional luxury but the basis for achieving multiple goals of quality and cost-effectiveness (Hiller and Gorsky 1986).

The effect of hospital ownership on strategic behavior was studied in a sample of 164 multihospital system hospitals (Begun et al. 1987). Culture was measured by asking chief executive officers (CEOs) questions designed to elicit values regarding profit and public service. The findings were that hospitals in investor-owned chains claimed a higher preference for belief in profit making, whereas hospitals in Catholic systems held stronger beliefs in community service values and a less pervasive belief in the importance of making a profit. The Catholic hospitals showed a low level of internal conflict between individual hospitals and the corporate office, in spite of their being more decentralized; conflict was significantly higher in the investor-owned systems.

Hospital culture has also been connected to growth in social innovation (Nathanson and Morlock 1980). In obstetrical departments (12 in the same area) where decision-makers were committed to social change, innovations prospered. The authors concluded that the values of the elite represent a guiding force in the organization; these values are especially important to the introduction of change but of less significance to the determination of the means for accomplishing the desired ends. This confirms an earlier study, which found that values were more important than structure (complexity, centralization, and formalization) in understanding program innovation in health and welfare organizations (Hage and Dewar 1973).

Hospital workers are highly interdependent and are guided by informal norms of reciprocity, trust, and mutual helpfulness. Hospitals depend on the social power of peers as well as supervisors, more than on coercive or remunerative power, to control professional workers. Because the hospital is a service organization, the ultimate objectives of managers and providers coincide. The problem comes when immediate objectives conflict; in such cases the organization may sacrifice some interests to further those of the majority or of future patients.

Meyer's (1982) study of 19 hospitals suggested that, during tranquil periods, ideologies supplant elaborate control structures by fostering self-control. During crises, reservoirs of goodwill sanction unorthodox procedures. The risk is that ideologies themselves will become utopian or fanatical, as in the case of a hospital whose hyperactive entrepreneurial activity led to a stream of successes but produced an inefficient organization that was both unstable and expensive. Similarly, enthusiasm for short-term objectives without concern for long-term interests, such as the current tendency to reject the patient service ethic in favor of materialism and economic controls, may fuel a counterproductive cynicism among patients and employees.[2] Overemphasis on short-term objectives could backfire and lead to more restrictive reimbursement policies, entry-level restrictions, and regulations than now exist.

## Individual Values

### Nursing Values

The American Association of Colleges of Nursing, which is the professional association of four-year nursing colleges, recommends seven values as essential for a professional nurse to have. They are altruism, or a concern for the welfare of others; equality, or a belief that everyone should have the same rights, privileges, or status; esthetics, or an appreciation of the qualities of objects, events, and persons that provide satisfaction; freedom, or the capacity to exercise choice; human dignity, or the inherent worth and uniqueness of an individual; justice, or the upholding of moral and legal principles; and truth, or faithfulness to fact or reality (American Association of Colleges of Nursing 1986). The AACN gives examples of attitudes and professional qualities and of professional behaviors to assist in curriculum development.

Compared to 148 other occupations, nurses as a group have high vocational needs for achievement, security, and social service. Needs for activity, use of abilities, and advancement are moderate. Although their scores on authority and moral values are lower on the vocational need scale, only a few occupations score higher. As employees, nurses are an easy group to manipulate, given the low or moderate importance they give to company policies, recognition, working conditions, and human and technical supervision. Occupations with similar occupational patterns include cost accountants, dietitions, engineers (civil, mechanical, time study, highway), librarians, physical therapists, computer programmers, applied statisticians, and claims examiners (Rosen et al. 1972).

Nurses have been described as possessing an intrinsic value system (Zytowski 1978). As a group, nurses appear to hold strong religious and social service interests but low economic interest (Pietrofesa and Splete 1975). This may be changing, according to Meleis and Dagenals (1981), but a comparison of freshman college students who aspire to be nurses with other freshmen indicates that nurses still value "being well off financially" slightly less than the others. Would-be nurses also rated becoming an authority in their field, obtaining recognition from colleagues, and developing a meaningful philosophy of life lower than did their peers. Items that they valued more highly than their peers were raising a family, helping others in difficulty, and making a theoretical contribution to science.

Successful clinical nurses like working with people and are not achievement oriented in the sense of climbing educational or administrative career ladders (Dyer et al. 1975). Graduate nursing students have a personality profile that emphasizes artistic, intellectual, and sociability attributes. Those who have managerial interests score higher on characteristics traditionally attributed to managers but are not more masculine (Hanson and Chater 1982). In spite of the considerable research on nurse personality, however, none of the measures enables us to predict outcomes such as career development, performance, or turnover (Redfern 1977).

The literature fails to reach any firm conclusions about the characteristics of nurses who stay in the profession and do well (Lewis and Cooper 1976). Nurses are like all other women in this respect. If nurses differ from other women, it may be in ways other than commonly believed. More recent studies of nursing students, for example, dispel the myth that nursing students manifest more feminine characteristics than other college women (Meleis and Dagenals 1981).

Since values organize facts, information on education can be analyzed in two ways: (1) Individuals not predisposed toward higher education could argue that preference should be given to community college graduates and programs and that recruitment should focus on young women as well as mature women who are returning to the labor force; (2) individuals who value higher education could argue that the incentive system in hospitals should be restructured to retain bachelor's degree nurses in hospitals. They would also note that, although the system depends on new recruits, all programs need faculty with postgraduate education, and faculty supply ultimately is tied to the number and quality of nurses with bachelor's degrees. To threaten the supply of teachers and supervisors is equivalent to killing the goose that lays the golden eggs.

If one needs a rule of thumb for understanding nurses, it is best to consider that nurses will mirror the values of a cross section of women. The nursing occupation is heterogeneous, drawing recruits from all social classes. Over the last decade, nursing has become more attractive to the middle as opposed to the lower middle class. Now it is in jeopardy of losing upper-middle-class women, who have always comprised a minority of the nursing population, to higher status careers.

## Managerial Values

The mind of management is also an integral part of human relationships. Just as with workers in other professions, however, there is no proven association between values and effectiveness. Managers, as well as nurses, embrace a variety of contemporary values. For example, managers also experience reality shock—50% of college recruits leave within the first year of employment because of an inadequate progression plan (Lopez 1970).

Cross-cultural studies allow us to make some generalizations about American managers, to place comments about hospital managers into better perspective. Two hundred concepts were used to compare the personal value systems of American managers with those of managers from Japan, Korea, India, and Australia (England 1976). American managers had a large element of pragmatism, a strong need for achievement, and an orientation toward competence. In relation to the organization, American managers emphasized maximizing profit, efficiency, and productivity; that is, they had an organizational goal orientation that did not incorporate an egalitarian view. England (1976) also found that values did not change rapidly; they did influence solving problems and making decisions. Values also differed in varied contexts: In larger organizations there was more concern with productivity, profit, growth, and efficiency; not surprisingly, union leaders had different value systems. American managers were also found to have a high need for utilization of abilities, opportunities for advancement, creativity, recognition, responsibility, variety, and compensation (Gay et al. 1971).

Managers as a whole have been classified into four primary value orientation groups: pragmatic, moralist, affective, and mixed. A comparison of the two polar and largest groups shows that pragmatists hold higher positions, earn higher incomes, and have a higher achievement orientation than do moralists. The two groups differ in their perception of organizational goals, on most of the concepts associated with people, and on nearly half of the ideas related to personal goals. The moralists, although not as homogeneous, have a humanistic, bureaucratic orientation rather than the economic-organizational view of the pragmatists. This primary value framework links the manager's motivational behavior with the framework used to make decisions. Pragmatic managers look at consequences in terms of success and failure. The indices they use are easy to quantify and compare. The moralists seek the right answer, which of course is subjective rather than objective and difficult to evaluate. Fifty-seven percent of the American managers were classified as having a pragmatic orientation, and 30% as having a moralistic orientation (England 1976). Although the degree of pragmatism increased from small to large companies, it was not related to level in the organization, type of company, age of the manager, or level of job satisfaction.

When it comes to behaviors—such as designing incentive systems, changing strategies, or organizing management development programs—operative values are more important than intended values. Operative values, as expected, cluster around productivity, profit, and efficiency; ability, ambition, skill, cooperation, and competition are not just intended or adopted values to be used only when needed. The American managers resist organizational egalitarianism. Employee welfare is regarded only at a moderate level as an intended value, and social welfare is a very weakly held value. The humanistic orientation tends to be an intended orientation. As such, related behaviors will probably occur when they do not conflict with organizational goals or values related to achievement and competency.

Such generalizations serve as a reference but need refinement. There is evidence that public-sector managers—and by implication managers attracted to service organizations—may not have the same value profiles as managers in profit-oriented businesses (England, Dhingra, and Agarwal 1974; Warrier 1982; Gold 1982). Students in master's degree public administration programs had different value preferences for their professional and personal lives that were unaffected by their going to work (Edwards, Nalbandian, and Wedel 1981). Public administration students and alumni were more concerned with the public interest; business administration students and alumni were more concerned with efficiency. Although both groups had a similar commitment to professionalism, they defined it differently. These studies suggest that care should be taken when generalizing within broad occupational groupings.

One of the most troublesome considerations for executives and managers is determining to what degree businesspeople need to sacrifice personal values to succeed in their careers. Managers' careers, like those of other workers, involve a trade-off between security and risk, and between success and family life. Managers' rational behavior is directed at least partly by self-interests. Those managers who value power, income, and prestige are either climbers or conservers. Managers can be zealots seeking power for themselves and policies to which they are loyal, or advocates loyal to a broader set of functions, or statesmen loyal to society as a whole.

Research into differences among male and female managers is neither exhaustive nor definitive, but findings suggest that sex role stereotyping may have little basis in fact. Contrary to expectation, female managers placed a greater emphasis on their careers as opposed to family and home life than did male managers (Powell, Posner, and Schmidt 1984). This may be because a woman of the same age and education, receiving the same salary, and at the same managerial level as a man has had to make more sacrifices and make a greater commitment to a career than a man in the same position. Men were more likely to describe themselves as religious and more concerned about ethics in relation to other workers than were the female managers in the same study.

What about hospital managers who often straddle private-sector and public-sector management? A study revealed that, in Canadian teaching hospitals, middle managers' needs for security, independent thought and action, and opportunity to help people were met (Hurka 1980). In other areas such as social esteem, autonomy, and self-actualization, however, their needs were not met as well as those of top management. Positions in medium-sized hospitals provided less job security and need satisfaction than positions in large hospitals.

Research does not address the most fundamental concern, namely, the relationships between values and success in the organization or career. For now, the value profile and personality characteristics of hospital managers remain largely speculative. The evidence does not allow us to make generalizations about how values relate to social position, education, or work experience, since there has been much less interest in studying the motivation of hospital managers than in studying the motivation of nurses.

Intuitively, it would seem that executives and managers who gravitate to high-level positions in hospitals—where the authority of the medical staff limits administrative discretion, where outcomes are difficult to quantify, and where salaries are lower—must differ from traditional managers. In all probability, health care managers value service more highly than other managers but less than direct providers do.

Perhaps now that consultants to profit-oriented businesses are illustrating that corporate culture is essential for success, hospital managers will be more inclined to reassess their own values, attitudes, beliefs, and personalities before reshaping the hospital culture. Certainly, the current competitive environment is creating an interdependence between managers and employees, which should reinforce the trend toward a decrease in social distance occurring at work sites generally (Miles 1981). The need for mutual adjustment of managers and employees to each other has never been greater.

## Nurse Executives: Captives of Competing Values

History tells us that the director of nursing services influences both nursing education and hospital organization. Aspiring nurse executives do not lack models for influencing social policies, nursing education, nursing practice, and the development of professional organizations (Bullough and Bullough 1984; Fitzpatrick 1983; Dolan, Fitzpatrick, and Herrmann 1983).

Nursing administrators are described in opposite ways by historians and practitioners. Sometimes they are portrayed as subservient to physicians, as unable to meet the challenge of lay managers, or as generally inept, poorly educated, dogmatic women who have had, and continue to have, a secondary role. This portrayal can be explained as an extension of the problems faced by women in obtaining equal education and professional status. Suggested remedies usually include equalizing power by some combination of enhancing the status of nursing and decreasing the power of physicians and general administrators.

Others see nursing administrators as an extension of nursing superintendents (their original job title), women from the higher social classes with much organizational power who felt a responsibility to train genteel women. When forced to choose between upgraded education and cheap labor, they chose the latter. This accommodation to managerial preferences perpetuated social class differences by fragmenting work among aides and thus created the current "nursing disorder," the term used to convey the social class conflicts within nursing (Reverby 1982).

Most nursing administrators receive mixed messages emanating from these two myths: one conferring inordinate power, the other conveying pervasive ineptness, but both resulting from belonging to a certain class of female. To place these polar views in context, it helps to remember that hospitals were organized following the military and ecclesiastical models. Both are characterized by a hierarchical structure, a long history, and a strong, sustaining central direction. Subordination to duty, although exaggerated by the position of women in society, can also fairly be said to be influenced by these origins.

The literature on women in management has emphasized the problems of women in nontraditional occupations. Nursing service administrators are not usually seen or studied as female executives; this in itself is a revealing comment on the status of nursing service directors. Much of the available research on female leadership has a psychological thrust. For example, women have a more participative leadership style than men (Jago and Vroom 1982), and nurse managers are likely to perfect this style given worker preference and the prevailing negative evaluation of females who use an autocratic style.

Thus, female nurse leaders frequently end up in a "catch-22" situation. The more adeptly they embrace a participative management style, the more male managers and token nurse executives insinuate that their leadership is ineffectual and that they should "take charge" (i.e., adopt an autocratic style). However, any attempts at autocratic methods will also be evaluated negatively by those superiors who do not want "bossy" nurses. Female nurses who prefer a more autocratic style likewise have a tough time. Not only are they likely to encounter more situations in which nurses will not follow their leadership, but they will face rejection on the grounds that their behavior is not proper.

Psychological approaches such as this implicitly assume that the person is responsible for whatever differences or problems exist and that the remedy is to have women act like men (Riger and Galligan 1980). Yet sex is most likely a proxy for other attributes, such as education, job level, or work experience. Great caution should be taken when making generalizations about sex differences in attitudes and behaviors.

## Value Awareness

Because managers, physicians, and nurses choose occupations based on value preferences that are reinforced in college and at work, these important hospital workers define problems and acceptable behaviors differently. Being sensitive to existing perceptions is at least as necessary as having a keen analytical mind and knowledge of management solutions.

### Managers as Seen by Nurses

Nurses may not view positively the interconnected sets of values that determine managerial behavior. In a leading nursing administration textbook, a section introducing the topic of interpersonal relations portrays individuals as evolving through consecutive psychological levels that describe personal values and life styles (Graves 1970; Rowland and Rowland 1985). The level typical of business executives is characterized as manipulative or materialistic; they achieve their goals through manipulating the environment; they thrive on gamesmanship, politics, competition, and entrepreneurial effort; they measure success in terms of income and power and are apt to perceive workers as expense items rather than assets.

At a higher level are individuals who have high affiliation needs. Getting along with and receiving approval from important others are more highly valued than getting ahead or being recognized. At the highest level, the existential level, individuals have a high tolerance for ambiguity and for people with differing values; they like to do their jobs without the constraints of authority or bureaucracy; they are goal oriented but have a broader arena and a longer time perspective. These are the values that attract nursing students and receive reinforcement by nursing faculty and the norms of clinical practice. For many nurses, prescriptions for success that depend on "stepping on others," "creating a scene," "playing games," or "cozying up" are demeaning and demoralizing, not a "fact of life" or "common sense" as many executives and managers assume.

## Nurses as Seen by Managers

How do hospital managers view nurses? One method for clarifying the perceptions of hospital managers is to examine the case studies used in programs in health services administration. A review of several popular hospital casebooks suggests that aspiring managers have been taught to manage nurses (and other female workers) as secondary workers rather than develop them as professional workers. That is, the emphasis is on orienting young nurses, viewing pay as a short-term incentive, and controlling nurse employees by means of elaborate rules, procedures, and documentation of events. When nurses in casebooks are portrayed as powerful, they are threatening to undermine the administrator's job. Nurses do not have a significant role in cases about quality control, long-range planning, marketing, finance, or career structures.

Thirty cases from a recent book of case studies (with an accompanying instructor's manual) developed by leading educators provide a "comprehensive collection of fact situations" which are "rich in applied lessons" (Rakich, Longest, and Darr 1983). Sixteen of the cases refer to nurses, but only one case, in the human resource section, is centered on nursing. In the other cases, nurses and the nursing department are given a minor role or one secondary to the larger issue. Since cases are developed for problem-solving purposes, we do not expect to find idealized portraits or exemplary behavior. Yet taking all the cases together should illustrate how administrators are taught to anticipate behaviors and develop solutions.

In the key nursing case, the heading used to introduce the department is "The 'Leper Colony'," a term that reflects the propensity to view and therefore manage nursing as an isolated department.[3] In this case, the director of nursing services has a focal role but has serious operational difficulties with the other department heads. Her decision-making is described as intuitive. "I felt it was absolutely wrong, but I didn't know exactly why," is her way of describing her opposition to the personnel director doing nurse recruiting.

In the policy, planning, and marketing cases, nurse-related issues included:

1. Obtaining agreements from other hospitals not to hire any applicants from a hospital about to close.

2. Dealing with the concern that nurse supply would not keep up with growth should the hospital expand.

3. Involving the director of nurses in Career Week and listing the Future Nurses Club as potential users of the new education center.

Of the cases that portrayed governance, senior management, and medical staff problems, nursing played a minor role in only three. In one case, the director of nursing was portrayed as a "well-qualified professional nurse" who by nature was "very domineering," which apparently explained the high turnover of nurses, aides, and orderlies. In another, operating room nurses went with the physicians to a meeting of the board of trustees to argue for scheduling changes. In the third case, the instructor's guide suggested that the nursing staff should "increase communication," but nothing in the case suggests that problems in surgical scheduling and patient ward assignments were, in fact, related to the nursing department.

Although nurses appear in five of the financial management cases, none of the nurses are involved in budget or financial matters. Altogether, only once is the prescription given that nurses should have authority commensurate with their responsibility. Even here the authority does not relate to administrative matters. Instead, it is recommended that the nurses, rather than physicians, should control nurse staffing assignments—hardly an earthshaking recommendation. A supervisor in the public health setting is diagnosed as not having a power base, as the job is largely administrative. Lacking power, she is advised to cautiously implement a performance appraisal system for all employees and evade the issue of a problem nurse who has been disciplined poorly in the past.

The point is not that these cases are not well developed; the contrary is true. They are well chosen to illustrate important problems. The contextual material certainly feels right to persons familiar with the intended audience. That is, the material is culturally appropriate and it conforms to expectations. Prevailing culture is well portrayed. Nurses are often viewed as commodities. Communication is "in." Power is OK outside of hospitals. Executives have no responsibility for hiring educationally prepared nurse executives and managers or for developing managerial competence in them. Nurses function as technicians or controllers. Quality control is confined to utilization review and is a financial issue rather than a rallying point for organizing and monitoring the nursing and medical staffs. Possessing a bachelor's degree is equated with poor performance. Nurses are emotional and intuitive, even in management positions. The role of nurse specialists is ill defined.[4]

This book is not an exception. It continues a tradition among hospital teaching casebooks. In an important early casebook, explicit instructions were given on how to clear salary increases with other hospital administrators (Billington 1959). A later casebook detailed the reasoning behind assigning nurse anesthetists exempt employee status. If the hospital had conformed to the labor law and paid overtime, salary expense would have increased by 64%. The lesson here is that business necessity overrides the law (Coe 1970).

In the 1959 cases, personnel problems centered around "arrogant" nursing aides. Scheduling difficulties involved visiting hours and pressures brought by a board member and administrator on the nursing staff. Almost a decade later, nursing problems included smoking in a public area, reality shock experienced by new nurses, incident reports, and jurisdictional disputes about serving meal trays (Tappan 1968). More recently, a text gave aspiring managers an introduction to the role of the manager, organization design, control, professional integration, adaptation, and accountability (Kovner and Neuhauser 1981). Nursing seldom had a focal role. A patient's description of conscientious, busy, dedicated, inexperienced, beautiful young nurses under age 25 certainly could be a springboard for discussion about the lack of hospital-based careers and underrepresentation of mature women in nursing. More likely, students will recall the description of nursing attributed to the chief executive officer: that nursing is difficult; that morale is always a problem because young women must work evenings, nights, and weekends; that nursing is physically, emotionally, and administratively demanding.

What does this convey? By omission, the cases imply that nursing administrators have a marginal role in hospital life. The cases perpetuate a concern with the personality characteristics of nurses and thus trivialize serious dilemmas. The cases ignore the three major administrative problems related to nursing at the heart of hospital work: quality control (which requires physician involvement), nurse communication with the governing board, and organizational integration of the nursing department.

## Nurses: Victims or Masters?

Two polar constellations of beliefs exist about nurses. Since stereotypes based on these beliefs tend to persist over time and lead to poor judgments, it is advisable to delineate them. At one extreme, nurses are seen as an oppressed group (Roberts 1983). Individuals of this persuasion study nurses using the model that has been developed to understand blacks, Jews, and women in general. Their viewpoint is that the oppressed group is controlled by forces not within themselves, but by those who have greater prestige, power, and status. These forces act in mutually reinforcing ways to exploit the less powerful group. The evidence used to support the argument that nurses are oppressed includes the low and compacted salaries, the dependence on physicians to assume new tasks and responsibilities, the difficulty nurses have had in moving from apprenticeship to collegial education, and the divisiveness that exists among nurses.

Oppressed groups are characterized by some common behaviors (Roberts 1983). They internalize the expectations held by the dominant groups and aspire to join them. As individuals become assimilated, they are often alienated; they are on the fringes of both groups without identity in either. In the process of trying to become like the powerful group, which is the ideal, individuals experience self-hatred and low self-esteem, and reject the original group. When all behaviors are taken together, the upwardly mobile but blocked person exhibits what is labeled as a "submissive-aggressive" syndrome. This is characterized by chronic complaining against the high-status group, but with little direct expression of grievances. Since such behavior is ineffective in negotiations, frustration, failure, and even lower self-esteem result.

A direct consequence of this downward spiral is intergroup conflict, which is accompanied by a gradual loss of faith in one's own ability and responsibility. This divisiveness makes it difficult for the group as a whole to unite and overcome the oppression that they experience. Leaders in the affected groups are described as "queen bees" or "Aunt Janes," meaning that they are committed to maintaining the status quo and rejecting current feminist doctrine. Nursing service directors who side with management rather than advocate autonomous behavior are described as "selling out." Educating nurses to overcome reality shock rather than instituting an internship program is another example of a misplaced emphasis.

The contrary view is that nurses have extraordinary power that needs to be contained. This view is not as well verbalized in the management literature as oppression is in the nursing literature. Nevertheless, observers who listen carefully during management meetings and informal discussions hear a concern that nurses possess much power—maybe more than they know how to use properly. Objections to nurse involvement on high-level committees are often based on the fear that nurses would advocate unrealistic building programs or usurp medical authority. There is even a fear that nurses are seeking rewards and influence for destructive purposes, at the expense of other groups.

The belief that nursing power will be destructive stems from several factors. First, nurses dominate the hospital work force in terms of sheer numbers. Second, their close ties to physicians enable them to bend organizational rules. Third, their work cannot be supervised closely, since they perform tasks in private and their responsibilities are diffuse. Fourth, nursing careers are influenced by extraorganizational sanctions and rewards to a greater extent than are the careers of managers, since nurses are usually not so financially deprived that they must accept the dictates of a steady-state or linear career when such careers do not fit their personal aspirations. Those who are providing a second income often have more freedom to exit than do hard-pressed middle managers. Further, the financial rewards are not so high that nurses have a personal investment that causes them to want to remain. Finally, nurses in most areas have other employment alternatives, both in and out of hospitals. Taken together, nurses exhibit a relatively high independence of the organization, which managers often envy and fear. Although it is difficult for managers to acknowledge and recognize their discomfort with nursing career potential, managerial envy and distrust may well impede the organizational integration of nursing.

The existence of both of these constellations—that nurses lack power and that they possess inordinate power—perpetuates the development of an out-group, which when institutionalized constitutes a caste system. In such a system, there is social distance between nursing and other departments. There is considerable difficulty in merging nursing activities with other hospital activities, and this results in turf fights. Unless the work force is docile, there is likely to be tension around status issues and a high level of dissatisfaction among the workers.

Perhaps the reality lies between these extremes. Certainly, patterns can be explained differently. The lack of unity among nursing groups may be the direct consequence of their constituting a large, heterogeneous work force in our pluralist society. The changes that have occurred in state nursing practice acts throughout the country suggest that physician domination has its limits. The failure of nurses to achieve economic parity may reflect social class and value preferences about unions rather than employer collusion. Reality shock, as an organizational phenomenon, is not unique to nursing, nor are organizational socialization programs limited to female-dominated organizations. Among executives and managers, perceptions about the relative power of the work force vary throughout the industrial sector. There is no evidence that hospital management has a disproportionate representation of those who question the aspirations and motivation of the staff or hesitate to share power. Even though no conceptual synthesis of these competing views exists, it is fruitful to assume that workers are neither victims nor masters but that their actual status is between these two extremes.

## Practice Recommendations

The purpose of examining values is to develop a consciousness about the role values play in organizations and educational programs, since manipulation of organizational culture depends on respecting the values of managers and workers. Recommendations appropriate for organizations, management education, and nursing education follow.

### Organizational Implications

It has been predicted that the winners in the new, competitive hospital climate may not be those with the best data systems but those who understand the political and social structures of the hospital and the community (Lindner and Wagner 1983). The characteristics of high-performing health care organizations have been identified (Shortell 1985) as including a propensity to:

- Stretch themselves
- Maximize learning
- Exhibit transforming leadership
- Have a bias for action
- Manage ambiguity and uncertainty
- Exhibit loose coherence
- Develop a well-defined culture
- Embrace spirituality.

To become a high-performing organization, the objective is not to change the values of others. Little is known about how to change central values, and a rational attack on strongly held beliefs will only harden them (Rokeach 1979b).The most realistic goal is to understand how personal values and beliefs affect organizational policies and procedures. An increased sensitivity to the differing dimensions of values in the situation at hand has the best chance of leading to feasible solutions to organizational problems.

This sensitivity to values, which is called a value-critical approach, is applicable regardless of specific organizational strategies or prevailing management style. Even though the approach may be greeted with exasperation or indifference, in the long run it will make an enduring contribution (Rein 1978). A good case example of developing value awareness within a management team is offered by Timmel and Brozovich (1981).

Socialization of workers requires harmonizing divergent professional cultures. Even though there is a community culture, individual professions embrace different value systems. Because patient care depends on many professions, the management challenge is to construct an environment where the differences are not destructive. After all, except through selection processes, organizations have little direct control over the beliefs about work that individuals bring with them. Nor is it realistic to expect schools and colleges to indoctrinate graduates with a universal value set, as some employers believe to be possible.

The dangers to be avoided in managing cultural change are value-laden exhortations (propaganda), attempts at brainwashing, and manipulative interventions. Workers easily contrast the espoused value system with the one in operation by examining the career structure and opportunities. In situations where communication is necessary and the extent of value sharing is unknown, these ground rules of cross-cultural communication should be followed:

1. Communicate respect.
2. Be nonjudgmental.
3. Accept the relativity of one's own knowledge and perceptions.
4. Display empathy.
5. Be flexible.
6. Take turns.
7. Tolerate ambiguity (Ruben 1977).

There is much interest in developing a value management model for health care to promote the real quality of goods and services, differentiate their quality for purchasers, and promote productivity and reinvestment capital (Sisk and May 1986). Values and corresponding design philosophy statements are listed in Brozovich and Shortell (1984). Six steps executives must take to create a positive hospital culture have been identified (Deal, Kennedy, and Spiegal 1983):

1.  Consider seriously the mission of the hospital, aside from basic types of service, community needs, and other institutions.

2.  Trace these basic issues through to the departmental level where the work gets done.

3.  Build a consensus leading to a theme or rallying cry that captures the essence of the vision.

4.  Encourage subcultures through staff conferences, parties, and rewards, which foster a sense of mutual dependence and respect.

5.  Nurture heroes through certificates, awards, newsletters, personal congratulations, and assignment to highly visible task forces.

6.  To keep the various subcultures focused on organizational issues, create multifunctional task forces to work on major problems.

One expert suggests looking for rituals—ceremonies and occasions that bring people together—as an absence of rituals suggests a paucity of values (Zaleznik 1983). Another method appropriate for today's work force is to examine the career structures for each group of employees. After mapping cultural events, managers can assess which organizational practices have been responsible for both the strengths and the weaknesses they perceive. This assessment can be followed by an emphasis on employee development for managers as well as other workers.

Strategies for dealing with value impacts in organizations have been identified by Beyer (1981), who first presents her own biases: valuing ambiguity and change, emphasizing the limitation of intelligence, and assuming that environments cannot be manipulated very much. Given these biases, the options as she sees them are to nurture conflict, create similar ideologies and values, generalize to forge a synthesis, separate structurally, create a metasystem to override the existing ones, and uncouple ideologies from behaviors.

Changing career expectations and opportunities for women and the maturing of the work force require that executives and managers develop professional partnerships even when there are no presenting problems or budgeted vacancies. The fact that hospitals must import foreign-educated nurses suggests that hospitals are not offering the minimally acceptable value levels to potential workers. Managers are taught that recruitment and selection are management phenomena, but in reality workers make the first choice—the application—after assessing value compatibility. Once managers concur with the applicants' choice, managers can use knowledge of career paths, of acceptable reasons for certain kinds of career behavior, and of the criteria used to judge career success to decipher the culture of the organization (Schein 1984). Careers usually involve tradeoffs in many areas, such as between risk and security, success and failure, and work life and family life. Careers also reflect prevailing cultural values. Policies for motivating people will have different effects with different groups of employees.

## Professional Education

Implications for education are mentioned briefly here to acknowledge controversies about both nursing and management education. This discussion is not meant to shift responsibility to educators, who have a poor history of either changing the values of entering students or overcoming the incentives provided by employers and society to the graduates over a lifetime.

**Nurses.** Nursing schools are more likely than management schools to include a value component in the curriculum, and may even have modules on values clarification. Nursing students consider patient-oriented dilemmas such as informed consent and the right to die. Apart from modules designed to prepare nurses for the reality of work, the educational process is normative; a professional issues course with a rhetorical approach is common. Emphasis is on learning how to perform. The faculty seeks to instill in their students a sense of right and wrong and the importance of adhering to professional standards, to ensure that the neophyte will act properly when no one is available to monitor behavior or outcomes.

Considerably more attention needs to be given to the development of nurses with management potential. The issues are broader than the norms of the profession, the influence of the nursing schools, or bureaucratic requirements. Managers in the transition struggle with the tensions of competing values, of intended versus operating values, and of new values. The best an outsider can do is to acknowledge the struggle, show respect for the previous value set, and provide positive examples of integration. This acceptance, rather than denial and rejection of professional values, is the job of the astute senior management team.

**Managers.** For managers the educational process is less normative, since there are few clearly defined situations in which the behaviors can be prescribed. The study of values, if it is done at all, is limited to special units such as conflict resolution. Management education that caricatures clinicians as a class of naive, emotional, misguided, poorly educated, outdated, irrelevant do-gooders hardly provides a good base for future dialogue or accommodation.

Value clarity matters. In a recent matrix of managerial performance, the professional association for health care administrators rated the need for value clarity as high for mid- and top-level managers in organizations of all sizes (Jain and Files 1982). Medical group managers apparently need to hold values supportive of entrepreneurial medicine to be hired and to remain (Allison, Dowling, and Munson 1975).

Changes in professional education seem warranted. The type of management that flourished from 1920 to 1970 works best for the management of simple, repetitive tasks. Its three principles—work simplification, predetermined rules for coordination, and detailed performance monitoring—are not an appropriate basis for providing patient care. The emphasis on more rigid accounting methods and "paper entrepreneurialism" creates cleavage between fiscal responsibility and professional practice and retards rather than encourages productivity.

Executives and managers often advocate that nurses be taught cost awareness and inculcated with values of efficiency. Arguing against these obvious virtues may be heretical, but practical constraints and priorities exist. Nurses learn about the values of clients and professional practice in basic education. Time is too limited to spend much of it on teaching workers about values important to managers. Indeed, management's clients are the staff workers. Therefore, logic suggests that the management curriculum should include an appreciation of employee values, organizational culture, and the management of clinical work. Organizational efficiency and productivity become important when nurses become supervisors; they are properly part of a management development program. They cannot be the primary concern of basic nursing education.

Others have called for the reform of management education in areas related to values. One expert asserts that management education is attempting to train professionals in concepts that conflict with organizational values, in that the current emphasis on long-term relations, the viewpoint of the high-ranking officers, and the purely rational and emotionally neutral approach pervading management education are not compatible with the real world of business (Schein 1979). Another management observer argued in an essay on productivity that the culture of management and education must change to accommodate shifts in modal values and changes in family life and demographics and in the nature of authority (O'Toole 1981). The competency gap of managers, if there is one, is not in accounting or finance but in the ability to discuss fundamental issues. O'Toole states the issue succinctly: "If they cannot ask what ought to be, they cannot create a just and productive environment."

The recommendation of a values-oriented curriculum is easier to make than to implement. The objections fall into two categories: Such a curriculum is not feasible because of time constraints, and it is difficult to measure learning and impact. The first objection is easier to rebut. Faculty can continually examine their own biases, course materials, guest lecturers, and field placements to encourage value awareness and cultural differences among patients, providers, managers, and organizations. This does not require more courses or class hours.

The second objection is itself a value issue. If one believes that provision of personal care requires workers with a commitment to service who are sensitive to the values of patients, then it follows that managers must have the leadership skills and control strategies compatible with that mission as well as with financial success. To argue differently suggests that managers do not have an influence on the kind of workers they attract and retain or how they carry out their jobs. If this is so, then how do we justify the rest of the curriculum? It also suggests that the public will accept depersonalized and mechanical care offered by demoralized and angry workers. This denies the basic social legitimacy on which health services depend for survival.

**Research.** For the future, culture-specific research in organizations is needed. Top management should be concerned with value consensus along professional, social harmony, administrative, and rational dimensions rather than spiritual or esthetic dimensions. Such a prescription is pragmatic, as the latter are difficult for employers to address. Yet the prescription may be unnecessarily limiting for hospitals. The healing culture incorporates spirituality dimensions for both patients and workers. Fortunately, there are career measures that include the service component; therefore, hospitals interested in research can include this dimension as well as the others (DeLong 1982). The imbalance of research on the motivations of managers as contrasted with the motivations of nurses needs to be addressed. The copious literature on the personality and motivations of nurses and the paucity of literature critically examining managers reflects the premise of the prevailing management ethic, that the character of the workers is more important than that of the managers. Some balance is necessary.

## Summary

The corporate culture is the combination of the values, attitudes, and beliefs of its members, but the executives and managers set the tone for the organization. As there are many value systems in organizations, it is important for executives and managers to construct an environment where the differences are not destructive.

From 1920 to 1970, management ideology was based exclusively on specialization, rules, and performance monitoring. Four basic management ideologies have been identified. Schools of administration tend to emphasize a model based on economics; professional schools emphasize a model based on client service. These divergent emphases, along with outside pressures, have led to a situation where it is difficult to create a shared purpose.

Hospitals have unique cultures and purposes that differ from those of other organizations. One main reason for these differences is the intimate relationship that is often formed between hospital workers and patients. This bond acts to increase value consensus among workers. Even though there is more of a shared value system in hospitals than in commercial businesses, the dichotomy between labor and management in the hospital persists and will never be entirely removed.

Studies have explored the values of nurses in such areas as individual and vocational needs. Confusion arises because of differing general beliefs about nurses. They are seen by some as victims, by others as masters. The end result of this is the isolation of nursing from general management.

Compared to their counterparts in other countries, American managers exhibit a strong need to maximize profit, efficiency, and productivity. Managers can be classified into four value orientation groups. A difference is noted between the values of public administrators and those of business administrators. Little research has been conducted on hospital managers, who often straddle both public and private sectors.

Two polar views of nursing service administrators exist. One views them as being very powerful; the other sees them as inept and weak. Female nursing service administrators are often caught in no-win situations where they are condemned whether they adopt a participative management style or one that is autocratic.

In an era of competition and slower growth in funding, a commonsense approach is to manage cultural change to create a positive hospital culture. Some case studies misrepresent the roles of nurses in hospitals, suggesting that executives and managers are ill prepared to address major administrative problems that concern nursing.

Educational programs for nurses and managers vary in their treatment of values. The nursing curriculum includes some coursework about values, but the emphasis is on sensitivity to client values. Management students often have no coursework about values or else focus on biomedical rather than administrative ethics. As a result of differences in core values and education, nurses and managers frequently have conflicting views regarding the proper functioning of hospitals.

In the future, research is needed not only to look at organizational culture, but also to look at the motivations of executives and managers as well as nurses.

## Endnotes

1.  For a fuller discussion of values see Bhaget and McQuaid (1982), Dickson (1982), England (1967a, b), Fagin and Diers (1983), Goodstein (1983), Guth and Tagiuri (1965), Hofstede (1980), Kemelsor (1982), Kluckhohn (1951), Lincoln, Pressley, and Little (1982), Nord, Brief, Atieh et. al (1988), Pettigrew

(1979), Rokeach (1979a,b), Roy (1977), Ryan, Watson, and Williams (1981), Schein (1984, 1985), Smircich (1983), and Wilkins and Ouchi (1983).

2. For a full discussion of this see Batistella and Smith (1974). They note that with the decline of the family, the neighborhood, and the church, health is the only remaining social institution to which people can turn for comfort. Although the values of compassion, sympathy, understanding, charity, and individual dignity may sound anachronistic, they are vital features of civilized life and are intimately bound with delivery of health services. It is difficult to see how people will accept materialism over quality of life considerations as the motivating force for health professionals.

3. When I suggest that nursing is often treated as a ghetto department, managers chastise me for being unnecessarily emotional. The title of this case reaffirms my assessment.

4. As a check, the other cases were reviewed to check on presentation of other individuals. Here is how key actors in other cases were portrayed.

*Incompetent administrator:* "efficient," overly concerned with statistics

*Doctor:* admittedly seeking power

*Administrator:* of "old school," contrasted with the director of nursing, who is described as "domineering"

*Wife of doctor:* becomes inflamed, behaves belligerently (this case was not used to explain behavioral concepts)

*Doctor (male):* comes on strong and is soon involved in conflict (this doctor is depicted as crying out of compassion, not because of a weak ego as is asserted of nurses)

*Administrator:* appears worried, speaks tensely

*Board member:* a gentle man, never raises his voice, nice guy but no dummy

*Board member:* getting warmer, silently invited to calm down with an amused look

*Pharmacist:* had been defensive, is now helpful

*Administrator:* decisions becoming more autocratic, seemingly unrealistic, "most unprofessional"

*Doctor:* cried openly when patients died (a flamboyant doctor ended up as the hero of this case)

*Chief resident:* inflexible and ruthless (in this case the teaching guide presents an extensive development of different theories of motivation).

# References

Allison, R., W. Dowling, and F. Munson. 1975. The role of the health services administrator and implications for educators, in *Selected Papers of the Commission for Health Administration*, Vol. II. Ann Arbor, MI: Health Administration Press.

American Association of Colleges of Nursing. 1986. *Essentials of college and university education for professional nursing.* Washington, DC: American Association of Colleges of Nursing.

Battistella, R., and D. Smith. 1974. Toward a definition of health services management: a humanist orientation. *International Journal of Health Services* 4: 701–721.

Begun, J., R. Luke, T. Jensen, et al. 1987. Strategic behavior patterns of small multi-institutional health organizations. *Advances in Health Economics and Health Services Research* 7: 195–214.

Beyer, J. 1981. Ideologies, values and decision-making in organizations, in P. Nystrom and W. Starbuck, eds., *Handbook of Organizations*, Vol. 2. Oxford, England: Oxford University Press, pp. 166–202.

Bhagat, R., and S. McQuaid. 1982. Role of subjective culture in organizations: a review and directions for future research. *Journal of Applied Psychology* 67: 653–685.

Billington, G. 1959. *Cases in hospital administration.* New York: Columbia University Press.

Brozovich, J., and S. Shortell. 1984. How to create more humane and productive environments. *Health Care Management Review* 9(4): 43–53.

Bullough, B., and V. Bullough. 1984. *History, trends and politics of nursing.* New York: Appleton-Century-Crofts.

Coe, R. 1970. *Planned change in the hospital.* New York: Praeger.

Deal, T., A. Kennedy, and A. Spiegal. 1983. How to create an outstanding hospital culture. *Hospital Forum* 26(1): 21–34.

del Bueno, D. 1986. Organizational culture: how important is it? *Journal of Nursing Administration* 16(10): 15–20.

DeLong, T. 1982. Reexamining the career model. *Personnel* 59(3): 50–61.

Dickson, J. 1982. Top managers' beliefs and rationales for participation. *Human Relations* 35: 203–217.

Dolan, J., M. Fitzpatrick, and E. Herrmann, 1983. *Nursing in society: a historical perspective,* 15th Ed. Philadelphia: W. B. Saunders.

Dyer, E., M. Monson, and J. Van Drimmelen. 1975. What are the relationships of quality patient care to nurses' performance, biographical and personality variables. *Psychological Reports* 36: 255–266.

Edwards, J., J. Nalbandian, and K. Wedel, 1981. Individual values and professional education: implications for practice and education. *Administration and Society* 13: 123–143.

England, G. 1967a. Organizational goals and expected behavior of American managers. *Academy of Management Journal* 10: 108–117.

England, G. 1967b. Personal value systems of American managers. *Academy of Management Journal* 10: 53–68.

England, G. 1976. *The manager and his values: an international perspective.* Cambridge, MA: Ballinger.

England, G., O. Dhingra, and N. Agarwal. 1974. *The manager and the man.* Kent, OH: Kent State University Press.

Fagin, C., and D. Diers. 1983. Nursing as a metaphor. *New England Journal of Medicine* 309: 116–117.

Fitzpatrick, M. 1983. *Prologue to professionalism.* Bowie, MD: Robert Brady.

Gay, E., D. Weiss, D. Hendel, et al. 1971. *Manual for the Minnesota Importance Questionnaire.* (Minnesota Studies in Vocational Rehabilitation, no. 28). Minneapolis: University of Minnesota Department of Psychology.

Gold, K. 1982. Managing for success: a comparison of the private and public sectors. *Public Administration Review* 42: 568–575.

Goodstein, L. 1983. Managers, values, and organization development. *Group and Organization Studies* 8: 203–220.

Graves, C. 1970. Levels of existence: an open system theory of values. *Journal of Humanistic Psychology* 10: 131–155.

Griffith, J. 1983. The proper way to live: remarks on the teaching of hospital administration education. *Journal of Health Administration Education* 1: 27–36.

Guth, W., and R. Tagiuri. 1965. Personal values and corporate strategy. *Harvard Business Review* 42(5): 123–132.

Hage, J., and R. Dewar. 1973. Elite values versus organizational structure in predicting innovation. *Administrative Science Quarterly* 18: 279–290.

Hanson, H., and S. Chater. 1983. Role selection by nurses: managerial interests and personal attributes. *Nursing Research* 32: 49–52.

Hiller, M., and R. Gorsky. 1986. Shifting priorities and values: a challenge to the hospital's mission, in G. Agich and C. Begley, eds., *The price of health.* Boston: D. Reidel.

Hofstede, F. 1980. *Culture's consequences: international differences in work related values.* Beverly Hills, CA: Sage.

Hurka, S. 1980. Need satisfaction among health care managers. *Hospital and Health Services Administration* 25(3): 43–54.

Jago, A., and V. Vroom. 1982. Sex differences in the incidence and evaluation of participative leader behavior. *Journal of Applied Psychology* 67: 776–783.

Jain, S., and L. Files. 1982. A concept of health administration: implications for education and quality control. *AUPHA Program Notes* (Fall): 1–8.

Kaiser, L. 1983. Survival strategies for not-for-profit hospitals. *Hospital Progress* 64: 40–46.

Kemelsor, B. 1982. Job satisfaction as mediated by the value congruity of supervisors and their subordinates. *Journal of Occupational Behavior* 3: 147–160.

Kluckhohn, C. 1951. Values and value orientation, in T. Parsons and E. Shils, eds., *The theory of action.* Cambridge, MA: Harvard University Press, pp. 395–425.

Kovner, A., and D. Neuhauser. 1981. *Health services management: a book of cases.* Ann Arbor, MI: AUPHA Press.

Lewis, B., and C. Cooper. 1976. Personality measurement among nurses—a review. *International Journal of Nursing Studies* 13: 209–229.

Lincoln, D., M. Pressley, and T. Little. 1982. Ethical beliefs and personal values of top level executives. *Journal of Business Research* 4: 475–487.

Lindner, J., and D. Wagner. 1983. DRGs spur management related groups. *Modern Healthcare* 13: 160–161.

Lopez, F. 1970. *Making of a manager.* New York: American Management Association.

Meleis, A., and F. Dagenals. 1981. Sex role identity and perception of professional self in graduates of three nursing programs. *Nursing Research* 30: 162–167.

Meyer, A. 1982. How ideologies supplant formal structure and shape responses to environments. *Journal of Management Studies* 19: 45–61.

Miles, R. 1981. Governance of organizations: leader-led roles, in G. England, A. Negandi, and B. Welpert, eds., *The functioning of complex organizations.* Cambridge, MA: Oelgeschlager, Gunn & Hain, pp. 173–202.

Nathanson, C., and L. Morlock. 1980. Control structures, values, and innovation: a comparative study of hospitals. *Journal of Health and Social Behavior* 21: 315–333.

Neugeboren, B. 1985. *Organization, policy, and practice in the human services.* New York: Longman.

Nord, W., A. Brief, J. Atieh et al. 1988. Work values and the conduct of organizational behavior. In *Research In Organizational Behavior.* 10: 1-42.

O'Toole, J. 1981. *Making America work: productivity and responsibility.* New York: Continuum.

Pettigrew, A. 1979. On studying organizational cultures. *Administrative Science Quarterly* 24: 570–581.

Pietrofesa, J., and H. Splete. 1975. *Career development: theory and research.* New York: Grune & Stratton.

Powell, G., B. Posner, and W. Schmidt. 1984. Sex effects on managerial value systems. *Human Relations* 11: 909–921.

Rakich, J., B. Longest, and K. Darr. 1983. *Cases in health services management.* Philadelphia: W. B. Saunders.

Redfern, S. 1977. Absence and wastage in trained nurses: a selective review of the literature. *Journal of Advanced Nursing* 3: 231.

Reich, R. 1983. The next American frontier. New York: Times Books.

Rein, M. 1978. *Social science and public policy.* New York: Penguin.

Reverby, S. 1982. *The nursing disorder: a critical history of the hospital nursing relationship 1860–1945.* Unpublished doctoral dissertation, Boston University.

Riger, S., and P. Galligan, 1980. Women in management. *American Psychologist* 35: 902–908.

Roberts, S. 1983. Oppressed group behavior: implications for nursing. *Advances in Nursing Science* 5(4): 2–30.

Rokeach, M., ed. 1979a. *Understanding human values.* New York: The Free Press.

Rokeach, M. 1979b. *Beliefs, attitudes and values: a theory of organization change.* San Francisco: Jossey-Bass.

Rosen, S., D. Hendel, D. Weiss, et al. 1972. *Occupational reinforcer patterns: II.* Minneapolis: University of Minnesota Department of Psychology.

Rowland, H., and B. Rowland, 1985. *Nursing administration handbook.* Germantown, MD: Aspen, pp. 337–342.

Roy, R. 1977. *The cultures of management.* Baltimore: Johns Hopkins Press.

Ruben, B. 1977. Guidelines for cross-cultural communication effectiveness. *Group and Organization Studies* 2: 470–479.

Ryan, W., J. Watson, and J. Williams. 1981. The relationship between managerial values and managerial success of female and male managers. *Journal of Psychology* 108: 67–72.

Schein, E. 1979. Organizational socialization and the profession of management, in D. Kolb, I. Rubin, and J. McIntyre, eds., *Organizational Psychology,* 3rd Ed. Englewood Cliffs, NJ: Prentice-Hall, pp. 19–23.

Schein, E. 1984. Culture as an environmental context for careers. *Journal of Occupational Behavior* 5: 71–81.

Schein, E. 1985. *Organizational culture and leadership.* San Francisco: Jossey-Bass.

Shortell, S. 1982. Theory Z implications and relevance for health care management. *Health Care Management Review* 7: 20.

Shortell, S. 1985. High-performing healthcare organizations: guidelines for the pursuit of excellence. *Hospital and Health Services Administration* 30: 35.

Sisk, F., and J. May. 1986. Moving forward toward value: a new era in health care. *Healthcare Financial Management* 40(11): 56–60.

Smircich, L. 1983. Concepts of culture and organizational analysis. *Administrative Science Quarterly* 28: 339–358.

Tappan, F. 1968. *Toward understanding administrators in the medical environment.* New York: Macmillan.

Timmel, N., and J. Brozovich. 1981. Managing through values. *Hospital Forum* 24(3): 31–39.

Warrier, S. 1982. Values of successful managers: implications for managerial success. *Management and Labour Studies* 8: 7–15.

Wilkens, A., and W. Ouchi. 1983. Efficient cultures: exploring the relationship between culture and organizational performance. *Administrative Science Quarterly* 28: 468–481.

Zaleznick, A. 1983. An introduction to work in the 21st century. *Personnel Administrator* 28(12): 28–31.

Zytowski, D. 1978. Vocational behavior in career development, 1977: a review. *Journal of Vocational Behavior* 13: 141–162.

## Chapter 4

# Decision-Making: Governance and Centralization

...considering the current problems of the system, it is likely that the general hospital eventually will require a self-governing structure which could give every professional and occupational group the opportunity to participate meaningfully in the decision making processes of the organization.

(Georgopoulos 1972, 43)

## Effectiveness and Efficiency

Discussions of governance, decision-making, and structure rest on the assumption that improvements in these areas will enhance organizational effectiveness. Numerous hospital studies suggest that efficiency and effectiveness occur together (Scott and Shortell 1984; Neuhauser 1971; Longest 1978; Flood et al. 1979; Shortell 1983). Overall, hospitals that are more efficient at cost containment are also more effective in terms of quality of care provided. Although the cost-quality relationship is a complex one, and not fully understood by researchers, well-managed hospitals are concerned with both financial and product outcomes, that is, with the value generated. The guiding principles are that initiatives to improve profitability are not inherently incompatible with either quality of care or professional prefer-

117

ences; and, conversely, that meeting financial objectives without consideration of quality of care or worker needs is self-defeating in the long run.

The lesson from the commercial sector, which the health care industry is emulating, seems to be that strong emphasis on profitability does not necessarily come at the expense of worker involvement. In service industries, most high-performing organizations emphasize value and quality of service, not cost (Peters and Waterman 1982).

## Decision-Making: Governance

Theorists have observed that a board of trustees that does not represent the political and social interests of the community or does not co-opt significant financial and political elites is not likely to survive (Pfeffer and Salancik 1978). The survival of a not-for-profit hospital also depends on the influence of the chief executive officer (CEO) on the governing board (Provan 1987). Because of recent revenue and cost pressures there has been an increased interest in hospital governance and strategic management (Jaeger 1988; Files 1988). In general, hospitals follow the same trends as other organizations. Therefore, we can expect that emphasis on the rights of ownership will be tempered by a growth in concern for the rights of other stakeholders, including employees (Quintana, Duncan, and Houser 1985).

A good overview of the evolution of hospital governance from the board of trustees perspective is presented by Prybil (1980). He noted that governing boards establish overall goals and policies. Legally and morally, the governing board is responsible for the institution and the services it provides. This responsibility, along with the fiduciary responsibility, cannot be delegated. Major board functions are to (1) formulate objectives, (2) approve plans, (3) appoint the CEO, (4) assess system performance, and (5) see that action is being taken to ensure quality of care. The Joint Commission on Accreditation of Health Organizations (JCAHO) has introduced new requirements for board assessment and more effective decision-making in community hospitals.

The role of community not-for-profit hospital boards does not have to be understood in terms of the traditional corporate model, despite the fact that that model is enshrined in accreditation standards and state hospital leaders. Starkweather (1988) argues that several economic and sociological approaches are more explanatory of hospital board power because they include concepts of unified versus competing power groups, resource dependency and coalitions, paid directors, conflictive equilibrium, and directors as tools rather than driving agents of the hospital.

However, Starkweather's preferred theory is that three major elements of the hospital—medical staff, management, and governing board—maintain an agreeable fiction, whereby the medical staff and management ostensibly submit themselves to board control while at the same time understanding that the board can do little. The advantage for management is that they increase their own influence over physicians by invoking the power of the board, while arranging to control the board through appointments, agenda-setting, and information flow. Physicians benefit from the fiction by enhancing their own power and thus maintaining autonomy over their practice. They are able to do this because board members must depend on the amount and type of expert information the physicians supply in approving and enforcing medical staff bylaws and rules. The trustees are amenable to this arrangement because the myth enables them to enjoy the social status and trappings of power.

This system, made possible by a benign environment, is being challenged by a more competitive environment and stricter payment methods. Starkweather concludes that, fundamentally, the amount and nature of board power are a function of the organization's relation to its environment. If this is true, it follows that there will be a realignment of the hospital away from its legitimacy as a social and community agency where the hospital is the doctors' workshop, toward a new legitimacy as a business enterprise.

A comparison of hospitals with parallel industries suggests that health care boards tend to be too large to make effective strategic policy decisions in a competitive market (Delbecq and Gill 1988). As a result there will be a trend for boards to have more paid members who possess greater expertise but serve shorter terms. In the future CEOs are more likely to have full voting rights and employment contracts that encourage risk-taking. Comparison of freestanding hospitals with system hospitals suggests that CEOs in multihospital systems have had more formal influence in decision-making and were held more accountable for performance than CEOs in independent hospitals (Morlock, Alexander, and Hunter 1985). Physicians in system hospitals, however, had less formal involvement in decision-making than their counterparts in freestanding hospitals did.

Although they should be, board policies and plans are not necessarily translated into operational decisions (Thakur 1985). Even though this deficiency is not unique to hospitals, it is counterproductive when administrators and department heads diverge in their perceptions of organizational direction.

There has been a heightened interest in governance among nurses. The term "governance," however, is used in different ways. A formal definition of governance in a nursing context is "the development of decision-making groups functioning in an orderly fashion; groups that are instrumental in the exercise of authority and control" (Camiller 1981). This definition may intimidate administrators who assume that nurses plan to usurp authority in strategic planning, tangle with the medical staff, and dominate the board of trustees. Common usage among nurses, however, suggests that for them governance means active participation on nursing, hospital, and medical committees (American Academy of Nursing 1983).

Nursing associations believe in a professional practice model and therefore have been active in supporting governance changes that lead to greater professional autonomy. In 1978, the American Nurses' Association listed shared governance as the first characteristic of a professional climate of administration and practice. By this was meant that there should be either contracted agreements or officially approved bylaws, rules, and regulations *within the nursing department* to provide means for accountability to the governing body of the institution and to the patient/client.[1] The Tennessee Nurses' Association has developed guidelines for establishing nursing staff bylaws (Holle and Blatchley 1982). Suggested nurse committees include those for credentials and appointments, professional practice, research, audit and peer review, evaluation, grievance, professional liaison, policy, continuing education, and bylaws. The 1,500 nurses at Strong Memorial Hospital in Rochester, New York, have had a participative management program since 1977. In March 1986 they began developing a professional nursing organization with bylaws (Ortiz, Gehring, and Sovie 1987). They are now focusing on needed nursing budget changes and JCAHO accreditation reports.

The National Commission on Nursing (1983) has recommended that physicians, administrators, trustees, and nurses ensure that the top nurse administrator is part of the institution's executive management. The commission stated further that nurses should have the authority to work with medical leaders to evaluate and improve patient care. These recommendations carry considerable weight because the committee was composed of leaders from all the major constituencies: nursing education and administration, physicians, boards of trustees, administrators, insurance companies, foundations, the government, and the American Hospital Association. It is no longer uncommon for nurses to participate on hospital and medical committees, but fewer than 4% of directors of nursing service vote on the hospital governing board, and only 8% vote on the medical executive committee (Aydelotte 1984).

The increased interest in having nurses actively participate in meetings of the executive committees of the medical board and boards of trustees stems from the belief that nursing participation in governance will yield the same positive benefits that accompany physician and trustee involvement. For example, one study (Scott and Shortell 1984) indicated that physician representation on the governing board was correlated with higher quality of care and lower costs per admission and patient-day. Another study indicated that there is a strong relationship between hospital trustee involvement in decision-making and quality of care (Morlock et al. 1979).

Analysts who view hospitals as traditional businesses disagree with this reasoning. They argue that nurses are merely employees. Therefore, it is appropriate for administrative superiors to speak to the board in a single voice after consulting with those who can make a contribution. The solution to this dilemma is to establish limitations in sensitive areas. It is not uncommon for boards to meet in executive session when personnel actions are under consideration, for example.

In any event, the multiplicity of models will continue. However, the trends that are encouraging management concern with integration of services will mean a greater nursing presence at all levels.

## Decision-Making: Decentralization

Decentralization is a dimension of decision-making that invariably involves beliefs about distribution of power and participation. Although many assume that workers in decentralized organizations have more participation in decision-making than workers in highly centralized organizations, this is not necessarily true. It is possible for an organization to be decentralized and yet have a low level of participation by the members in the organization. The opposite is also true. Essentially, no single approach, whether autocratic, consultative, or totally participative, can be used effectively in all situations (Schweiger and Leana 1986).

Workers' and managers' expectations about delegation are important. The behavior of top management has much influence on subordinate managers. The opportunity for participation may be as important as the actual fact of participation. Not all decisions are delegated even in decentralized organizations. Generally, strategic decisions are made by an inner circle, and the less important ones are delegated (Hage 1984).

Decentralization is neither a new nor an isolated idea. Scales for measuring decentralization have been used widely and challenged frequently (Dewar, Whetten, and Boje 1980). Other researchers believe that there is no necessary relationship between the degree of centralization of decision-making and effectiveness. There are two major explanations for the absence of a cause-and-effect relationship: (1) Decentralization is confused with participation, and (2) improved goal-setting and training, which occur along with decentralization, may be the real reason why positive changes follow efforts to decentralize (Kanter and Brinkerhoff 1981).

Several hospital analysts have argued for decentralization in large hospitals or have described decentralization programs in nursing and other departments (Starkweather 1978; Linville and Hudson 1963). A nurse theorist described the decentralization model as a practical way for making work more humane and democratic (Fine 1982). The current emphasis is not on participatory management models but on an accountability-based system for professional workers (Porter-O'Grady 1987; Allen, Calkin, and Peterson 1988).

In spite of much research, the relationship among decentralization, participation, and effectiveness remains poorly understood (Jennergren 1981). In a direct test of the effect of increased staff nurse participation on nursing units, it appears that satisfaction with supervision and co-workers will increase if enough time elapses (Counte, Barhyte, and Christman 1987).

The following case examples illustrate the complex effects of decentralization in health care organizations.

## Example 1

A recent study of the impact of prospective reimbursement on New Jersey hospitals showed that, in order to implement this system, hospitals took steps that were compatible with self-governing structures and professional participation in decision-making (Boerma 1983). Prospective reimbursement based on diagnosis-related groups (DRGs) led to:

1. Decentralization of hospital departments
2. Department heads having more authority

3. A more interactive work mode

4. More communication

5. A higher level of formalization of interdepartmental and management relationships.

The changes among departments were most dramatic between the medical and nursing staffs, primarily because nursing controls the flow of information between medical records (a key department) and the medical staff.

Two of the effects—moving power down the hierarchy while simultaneously increasing bureaucracy—seem contradictory on the surface. However, the potential loss of top management control was balanced by the use of quantitative performance standards. The adjustments made by the New Jersey hospitals served three functions: First, decentralization helped the organization when the departments had to be depended upon to adjust their practice patterns. Second, the tightening up at the top helped management cope with what was perceived as a hostile environment. Third, the tight-loose method enabled managers to buffer the professional core from environmental pressures without directly interfering with activities in the individual departments.

## Example 2

One well-documented case of decentralization, written by the nurses involved, is entitled *Nursing Decentralization: The El Camino Experience* (Althaus et al. 1981; Althaus, Hardyck, and Pierce 1982). This report, plus the research on organizational impacts published by outside evaluators, provides a unique opportunity to study both process and the related finances (Department of Health, Education, and Welfare 1980; Battelle Memorial Institute 1973; Norwood et al. 1976). The purpose here is not to argue for or against decentralization, nor is it possible to generalize one hospital's cost experience to other hospitals. Instead, we can attempt to understand what the nurses in this case meant by decentralization, identify design elements, consider the outside evaluations, and relate these to current theories of organizational design.

El Camino Hospital, a district hospital located in a suburb of San Francisco, had 453 beds during the early 1970s when a hospital information system with strong support from management (medical information system or MIS) and a decentralized nursing structure were implemented. The medical staff was comprised of 340 physicians in private practice, plus 173 courtesy staff. Although the hospital was classified as a tertiary hospital, some analysts considered it to be only a large hospital serving complex cases, since it did not have the characteristics of a university teaching hospital. The average occupancy rate was 77.7%, and the average length of stay was 5.4 days. The nursing staff consisted of 400 full-time equivalents, of whom 60% were registered nurses; the educational mix was not known. Nurses had a low turnover rate (13% to 14% per year, as contrasted with a 20% average in the county), suggesting that labor relations were probably not a serious problem. Nurses' salaries were competitive with salaries in the region and tended to be a little higher than those paid by hospitals to the south but not as high as those paid at the university medical center to the north. There has been no serious union activity either before or since the change.[2] For the first quarter of 1985, the total cost per patient discharge for nearby hospitals in Santa Clara County was 62% higher than El Camino's costs (Sandrick 1985).

The purpose of the MIS was to develop an integrated patient information system rather than to generate management information reports. Many departments besides nursing were involved: admitting, dietary, medical records, laboratory, central supply, x-ray, and billing. The MIS served as a catalyst for restructuring (i.e., decentralizing) the nursing staff. Two detailed reports, one on nursing decentralization and one on the evaluation of the MIS, provide a unique opportunity to illustrate the complexity of organization design and the difficulties in determining cause and effect.

**Through the Nurses' Eyes.** In a complete report on the decentralization of the nursing department, the nurses described decentralization in positive terms, although no financial data were presented, nor did the nurses address interdepartmental or technical issues. The nurses believed that the MIS system, which preceded decentralization by a few years, enhanced communication and documentation, which in turn led to more nurses' time at the patients' bedside. They did not, however, believe that an MIS system was an essential component of decentralization. To the nurses, decentralization meant that the nursing service existed to support the patient and the bedside nurse. Nurse supervisors, even on evening and night shifts, were eliminated as line managers. Instead, staff nurses and head nurses had line authority and responsibility. They used the support staff and peers to make "... important decisions that keep the hospital running" (Althaus et al.

1981, 14). The patient was portrayed as being at the top of the organizational chart; nurses operated as independent practitioners with autonomy, authority, and accountability for patient care. In this instance, the key to decentralization was the philosophy of primary care nursing, even though the conversion was not total.

Moving down the organizational chart, assistant head nurses performed several functions in addition to maintaining leadership when the head nurse was absent. These functions included coaching personnel, staffing and scheduling, monitoring patient acuity, overseeing quality of care, interacting with patients' families, and communicating with other departments. Head nurses had around-the-clock responsibility for the unit and reported to the director of nursing. The functions of the first line supervisor were clinical, supervisory, and inspirational. As a patient care advocate, the head nurse acted as the clinical resource on the unit, intervened in crises, and participated in patient care. As a manager, the head nurse hired and terminated nurses (within the unit), obtained in-service education, delegated responsibilities, and prepared the unit budget. The ultimate objective of these activities was to provide a constant reminder that the patient is the consumer of nursing services.

The director of nursing, who served as the chief executive officer of nursing services, assumed new responsibilities for involving nursing in organizational decision-making and increasing the rapport among nursing groups. Within the nursing department, this was accomplished by monthly meetings with head nurses from each of the major specialty areas, an "open-door" policy for staff nurses, and the use of support groups for discharge planning, infection control, staff development, and management. Although the management support group reported to the director of nursing, responsibility could also be delegated to these nurses by the hospital administrator and head nurses. The management complement was two full-time nurses and three nurses at 80%-time for the evening and night shifts. There was also an 80%-time position for interdepartmental coordination. There were three full-time coordinators, one each for nurse recruitment, quality assurance, and budget and staffing.

Complex captain positions were developed to assume coordination of administration and budget and staffing responsibilities of multiple units (called complexes) serving similar medical diagnoses (maternal-child health, critical care, and medical-surgical). Head nurses served as complex captains on a rotating basis with specific assignments; their recommendations were seen by staff nurses as advisory, not supervisory. Their responsibilities, which were rotated, varied somewhat by specialty. For example, the maternal-child health captain served as a member of the executive advisory committee; the critical care captain was responsible for coordination of all staffing. The common functions of the complex captains were to (1) hire, orient, and make final decisions concerning the utilization of float nurses; (2) provide information about the complex to other department heads and organizational support personnel; and (3) set the agenda for, chair, and carry out actions recommended at the weekly complex meetings.

Staff nurses from all shifts and complexes participated in six standing committees that provided formal communication and group decision-making. The nurses' time on these committees was paid for out of the unit budgets. The management council was the decision-making body of the nursing service. Its membership consisted of one elected staff nurse, two members elected by the management support group, one member elected by staff development, and all the head nurses, as well as the director, who retained final approval rights. The other key committees were executive, nurse practice, nursing-care planning, product evaluation, and MIS nursing. The executive committee was a broadly representative committee with a short-term project orientation rather than a policy orientation. The MIS nursing committee was chaired by the quality assurance coordinator to record problems, identify accountable persons, propose solutions, and monitor progress in the MIS system. One effect of this system of formal communication was that nurses spent more time than before in meetings.

New staffing policies were formulated by a special task force. Staffing became the responsibility of the head nurse and was related to five budget planning steps. First, the director of nursing services and the head nurse established a productivity goal for the upcoming year. Second, the number of patient-days was forecast. Third, the number of nursing hours to be used in patient care was forecast. Fourth, a model staffing schedule organized by shift and day of the week was developed. Fifth, planned nonproductive hours (e.g., vacation, holidays, sick leave, education leave) were budgeted. Productive time included not only direct patient care but also unit administration, conferences, educational activities, and orientation. These changes were facilitated by a feedback system that provided patient dependency information, labor analysis (productive time, nonproductive time, and overtime), labor performance (by period and year to date), and labor distribution (by name).

Before assuming that these activities explain the enthusiasm demonstrated by the nurses or relate to the successful outcomes attributed to the

MIS, one should know that other changes occurred simultaneously. The major ones were changes in budget rules, educational programs, use of time, hiring and orientation, in-service education, patient admitting policies, pharmacy support, and cost allocation. Some specific examples follow.

*Hiring and orientation.* New nurses were asked to give a one-year work commitment. They received a two-week orientation on the day shift; evening and night nurses received an extra week of orientation on the appropriate shift. During this period, they spent 30 hours with a preceptor (mentor) and participated in a one-day workshop. Recent graduates got two months of orientation on the day shift. Nurses, both new and incumbent, self-selected themselves out of the hospital if they did not like the system. Altogether, fewer float nurses were needed.

*In-service education.* The hospital instituted clinical competency courses for all shifts of each complex. The courses consisted of a core curriculum and clinical skill validation.

*Budget.* In addition to the staffing and budgeting process described above, head nurses budgeted for each item costing over $250 that they planned to purchase within the next three years. Also, time cards were used to ascertain the number of hours worked in patient care, administration, education, and training of new employees by nursing unit (cost center). Four cost centers per unit were established: administration, new training, education, and patient care. These reports were used by the head nurse, who worked closely with the budget coordinator.

*Admitting.* Each Friday a forecasting committee reviewed admitting projections for the coming three weeks. Committee members were the director of nursing, the operating room scheduling nurse, a head nurse, a staffing coordinator, a management engineer, and three hospital administrators.

*Pharmacy support.* A unit dose system was initiated.

Other information about the case would be helpful but is not available from the case history. Physician involvement or resistance was not discussed. No mention was made of part-time or temporary nurses. Nor is there information about pay adjustments for nurses who assumed more responsibility or received more education.

Determining the change in the amount of time that nurses spent at the patients' bedside is difficult. Even more difficult to determine is the cause of the changes that occurred, since there were so many offsetting factors. On some units, there was an increase in the patient-to-staff ratio, which automatically decreased the available time per patient. Conversely, the new pharmacy unit dose system acted to decrease the amount of time nurses spent on medication activity and increase the time available for patient care. The MIS system, which was expected to reduce clerical time and increase patient care time, had little or the opposite effect. More time was spent, especially by nursing aides and ward clerks, at the nursing station and the computer terminal. Overall, a decrease in patient care minutes occurred in the early phases of the project (Battelle Memorial Institute 1973).

The following problems were identified: (1) Staff nurses resisted attempts to remedy deficiencies exposed in the core curriculum; (2) there was less slack time to review charts; and (3) nursing care plans were not of uniformly high quality. There was also a need to increase opportunities for lateral promotion based on enhanced clinical competency or willingness to learn new specialties. In sum, the source of nursing discontent after the change was related to clinical competence issues, not role-related concerns. This outcome can be seen as desirable. A design that frees practitioners to worry about clinical practice rather than working conditions or administrative trivia certainly meets one criterion of success for nurses.

The concluding "future fantasies" section of the book revealed the concern of nurses about their status. This is expressed by, for example, their desire to wear street clothes instead of a uniform, to hire some male unit secretaries, and to have equal status (and education) with physicians. The medical model for staff organization with monthly meetings was the nurses' ideal. They also hoped for more predictable staffing and better pay for nurses who completed the core curriculum. The example indicated that nurses did not fantasize about higher pay but instead about income varying with skill and energy. Overall, the reporting nurses were enthusiastic advocates of the decentralized organization.

**Through the Evaluators' Eyes.** Administrators wanted to know the impact of these changes on costs, turnover, and quality of care. Unfortunately, an independent outside evaluation of decentralization itself is not available. However, since the comprehensive information system was evaluated rigorously for several years by outside evaluators, it is possible to obtain some insights about the combined effects of a technologically advanced communication system and a decentralized nursing department.

The outside evaluators' reports analyzed costs, utilization, and acceptance. After two years of operation, 94% of the nurses favored the MIS, 78% of the physicians used it, and there were fewer pharmacy-related errors than prior to implementation (Norwood et al. 1976). There was no change in physician admitting patterns, although the doctors became slightly more negative. Ward clerks were able to handle more routine work, since data handling was defined more clearly (Battelle Memorial Institute 1973).

The comprehensive evaluation, which analyzed costs, utilization, and acceptance, spanned a six-year period and included four other area hospitals for comparison (Department of Health, Education, and Welfare 1980). The researchers conceded that they could not match hospitals precisely, but they did make data comparable and accounted for case mix, demand, labor expense rates, inflation, and trends in care. They did not review charts for patient care errors or adequacy. Instead, they restricted themselves to nonclinical measures of effectiveness, utilization, and cost. The cost of operating the MIS, which was covered by the grant, was not included. The financial measures studied were cost per patient, which is the social cost; cost per patient-day, which is important for reimbursement; and cost per month, which best reflects the overall hospital cost.

The comparative cost findings for the hospital that implemented the MIS and the concurrent decentralization were as follows:

*Nursing staff.* Nursing staff costs were reduced 5%.

*Cost per patient-day.* Neither nursing nor ancillary costs per patient-day changed. Support costs increased. Apparently, the same treatments were given in less time.

*Cost per month.* The hospital was described as more efficient, since admissions increased but occupancy remained the same.

*Cost per patient.* Turnaround time for tests was faster, and length of stay shorter. Ancillary costs were not affected. Overall, there was an inexplicable increase in support costs that offset the reduction in nursing costs. (Support costs included administration, industrial engineering, pharmacy, business office, admitting, central supplies, dietary, medical staff, and medical records) The increase was not explained by the medical records department.

*Costs attributed to MIS.* There is some disagreement about the findings with regard to MIS costs. The analysis indicated that the hospital recouped the cost of the system and saved $4.00 per patient-day. The outside evaluator developed three models: The first indicated high costs; the second indicated high savings; the published model found a 0% to 1.7% increase in cost that was not statistically significant. The evaluator acknowledged that this increase could have a large impact on the operating budget in spite of the fact that it was not statistically significant. The summary analysis is that it is exceedingly difficult to reach a reliable conclusion about the overall impact of the information system on total direct expenses per patient (Department of Health, Education, and Welfare 1980). In general, cost savings from MIS have been overstated because of unrealistic labor savings projections, inclusion of better revenue recovery, and understated system costs (Department of Health and Human Services 1981).

**Reflections on the Case.** Does this case exemplify decentralization? The answer is that it does not if "decentralization" means a federal form of decentralization, in which autonomous small units are responsible for their own performance, results, and contributions to the organization. Since the head nurse had limited ability to affect net income or bill for nursing services, the example is closer to the simulated decentralization model described by Drucker (1974). In the simulated model, the units are given a simulation of profit and loss, but performance is determined by internal management processes and external cost reimbursement policies (in this case, staffing standards, fixed salaries, and a capped expenditure budget). Generically, the limitations of simulated decentralization are that roles tend to be unclear, communication channels are overloaded, and the scope of control is limited. If there are too few supervisors, problems may be brushed off.

The evolution of the complex captains and the management support group could have been predicted to provide necessary vertical information systems and lateral relations adaptations (Galbraith 1977). For either type of decentralization, departmental administration must be large enough to support an adequate top management team, but not so large that it becomes an empire that serves itself at the expense of the larger organization.

The example illustrates the paradox of decentralization. To succeed, initiating support at the top management level is required. More formalized and centralized control systems become necessary. Thus, decentralization seems to be an outgrowth of a good climate rather than a cure for a poor climate. Ironically, staffs most in need of the benefits attributed to decentralization are most likely to be found in the very organizations unable to implement it.

How does this decentralization model conform to an established model for salaried professional practice? Mintzberg's (1979, 1981, 1983) formulation is useful. His premise states that effective organizations choose design elements to achieve internally consistent groupings that are consistent with their environments and technology. He identified four major configurations, in addition to professional bureaucracy: simple structure, machine bureaucracy, divisionalized form, and adhocracy.

Five forces pull organizations in different directions, according to Mintzberg (1983). These forces reflect the five configurational forms of organization: (1) Forces continually work to simplify the design and revert to a simple structure with highly centralized management and direct supervision. (2) Other forces seek to coordinate by standardizing the work processes and to achieve the advantages of machine bureaucracy. (3) Workers take initiatives to become professionals and thus maximize their autonomy in order to structure the organization as a professional bureaucracy. (4) The tendency for middle managers to create autonomous departments provides the pull toward the divisionalized form. Here the emphasis is on standardization of outputs. (5) Support staff and some core workers exert a pull toward the form called "adhocracy." These individuals seek involvement in decision-making and control by mutual adjustment rather than rules, output measurement, or peer review.

Professional bureaucracies such as hospitals, accounting firms, and universities cannot rely on work processes or outputs to coordinate workers' activities. Instead, they must depend on standardization of skills for such coordination. In such settings, professionals, who are selected and trained outside the institution, are responsible for performing primary tasks. Professionals are given considerable control over their own work. Few supervisors are required, and professionals do little direct supervision.[3] Instead, supervisors spend much of their time linking to the broader environment, especially in seeking adequate financing. Distinguishing characteristics of professional bureaucracies include:

1. An operating core rather than management or support staff as the key part of the organization

2. Much horizontal specialization

3. Much training and indoctrination

4. Little bureaucratic formalization

5. Large unit size at the bottom, small elsewhere

6. Little planning and control

7. Liaison devices in administration

8. Horizontal and vertical decentralization

9. Presence of both functional and market groupings.

Managers need the active involvement of the professionals who make up the operating core to help minimize costs by using supplies wisely, arranging work productively, and minimizing absenteeism and turnover. Organization designs, therefore, should foster integration of workers into the organization and reject the belief that professional and organizational needs are inherently in conflict. The cooperative organizational form has the advantage of avoiding the costs that accompany conflict.

Service managers, as contrasted to manufacturing managers, cannot design work standards and expect line managers to enforce them. Neither can they directly measure output or supervise workers. There is little middle management responsibility for planning and formalizing work. Support staff focus on serving the core operations, since professionals are expensive and often scarce.

This theory for managing professional employees suggests that:

1. A decentralized structure at the operational level is appropriate.

2. Professionals seek collective control of decisions that affect them (e.g., hiring, promotion, and distribution of resources). This means staffing the middle with their own.

3. Heavy reliance on committees is necessary, since the structure relies on mutual adjustment.

4. The professional administrator's job is to mediate jurisdictional disputes and buffer the workers from external pressures.

5. Managers can expect to spend time coordinating activities or "handling disturbances" to overcome departmental tendencies to act independently (Mintzberg 1979).

6. The interaction between the technical support system and the nursing structure is significant. Specifically, Shukla (1983) argues that the optimal utilization occurs when nurses use the primary nursing method of care (discussed in detail in Chapter 5) and a decentralized technical support system.

These propositions hold in the El Camino case. Decentralization allowed for more bottom-up influence as the head nurses assumed more management responsibility and the staff nurses received more clinical consultation, but it did not undermine the prerogative of management. It did change how managers worked. Probably, at El Camino Hospital the intermediate managers had their duties realigned to be more relevant to the task structure. The result was that top management ceased to perceive the middle managers as a barrier between themselves and subordinates and vice versa.

The El Camino example highlights an aspect of decentralization that often puzzles inexperienced advocates, namely, how to manage without supervisors. The nurses at El Camino were not unique in finding that the functions provided by supervisors could not be abolished. The need to adjust staffing and coordinate with other departments required substitutes. The nurses wanted other nurses whom they could view as colleagues rather than agents of a distant authority. However, these nurses, who had only informal power, did not meet the need for organizational accountability, quality assurance, budgeting and staffing, interdepartmental liaison, or handling "officer of the day" problems. These functions were handled by developing a management support group, which reported to the assistant administrator for nursing issues but also received assignments from head nurses and general management. The challenge in such cases is to solve the coordination difficulties at the top that predictably occur when bureaucracies are internalized (Meyer 1972).

It is impossible to determine how much decentralization contributed to the increase in nurse satisfaction. For example, successful admission schedules such as those used at El Camino enable a hospital to operate with less organizational stress by resolving the inherent conflicts among patient care providers: physicians who want to admit patients at will, nurses who want to staff appropriately, administrators who want to have optimum occupancy, and controllers who want to relate nursing hours to patient census. Also at El Camino, the potential for increased turnover was minimized by making organizational expectations clear,  investing in mentors, and relating work load to competence, especially for new nurses. Staffing goals based on an extensive job analysis made work schedules more predictable. In addition, a discretionary budget enabled nurses to easily obtain needed supplies and services. These were all managerial initiatives that did not require an information system. This example illustrates that successful change occurs when practitioners and managers are ready for change and the resources for precipitating change exist.

The finding that nursing staff can be reduced without affecting total cost per patient (the social cost) has important implications. Where did the "savings" go? A cynic might even argue that the introduction of technology along with decentralization is either a method of increasing productivity without sharing the benefits with those affected, or a way of shifting resources to departments that share management's rational management philosophy. At a minimum, the example suggests that MIS and decentralization should be defended on grounds other than economy.

A follow-up conversation in 1988 with the assistant administrator for nursing at El Camino allays a fear expressed by Mintzberg that a professional bureaucracy would be unwieldy and unresponsive to change. The administrator, who was involved in the implementation process as a supervisor and staff consultant, believed that the reorganization enabled the nursing department to adjust to reimbursement changes more effectively than they could have under the previous system. Whether the results would apply to all hospitals is an open question. At a minimum, it seems fair to infer that in an organization where the nurses perceive themselves as professionals, they act in ways that theory predicts. Managers will continually question how far they can go in the direction of decentralization without losing control.

## Product Line Management

Product line management (PLM), as practiced in health care services, is a form of management in which the organizational structure, management control systems, and delivery strategies are structured around clinical case types or major clinical lines rather than functional lines (Nackel and Kues 1986). Hospitals begin by distinguishing their core product lines from their convenience or feeder businesses. These core products can be organized in a variety of ways: by patient demographics, by physician specialty groups, or by specific procedures (Yaho-Fong 1988). So far, except in a few medical centers, the emphasis has been on new, discrete services, with the expectation that product diversification will increase profitability and reduce financial risk. However, early evidence from California suggests that neither outcome occurs (Clement 1987).

Prospective payment based on DRGs, which link clinical diagnosis to payment, gives hospitals an output measure for professional activities (Fetter and Freeman 1984). This, in turn, encourages managers to relate clusters of activities (product lines) to markets and revenues. When PLM is introduced in a hospital, it encourages analysis of relationships of the service mix to the marketplace, competitive pricing strategies, and the relationship between the service mix and the medical and nursing staff.

Therefore, PLM offers a unique opportunity for many disciplines to coalesce around clinical care and resource use in a way that places the patient at the center.

Managing by product line frequently requires a team organization that will overlay the functional organization (e.g., a matrix design). Hospitals could add extra staff to become product line managers. Alternatively, they could provide training and added responsibility to front-line managers.

When PLM is adopted, information systems play a key role to:

1. Identify and define the costs of individual services and case types

2. Measure profitability and contribution margin of services and case types

3. Evaluate the impact of changes in operating procedures and technology on costs of services and case types.

Such data will automatically change the control system and professional responsibilities. The successful use of product line philosophy requires not only physician support but also integrated administrative and clinical management. In this configuration, staff members in finance, personnel, and information systems work closely with departments but report to the CEO.

The disadvantages of PLM are that it creates stress for traditional managers, a narrow product focus at the expense of the overall organization, administrative accountability without line authority, questionable cost-benefit results, and internal competition where departmental and professional conflicts are already a problem. Further, matrix management is often difficult to implement and the transition period is long.

## Quality of Care

Few studies address the impact of various organization designs on quality of care. In a longitudinal study of family planning agencies (Weisman and Nathanson 1985), the job satisfaction of the nursing staff was the strongest determinant of aggregate satisfaction of the clients, which in turn predicted the rate of subsequent compliance with prescribed routines. Compliance was also affected by variations in the levels of hierarchy of the organization—the more levels there were, the less compliance was obtained. The ability of staff members to make autonomous work decisions, which would presumably be linked with decentralization and less bureaucratization, was the only internal organizational attribute that independently increased client satisfaction with humaneness of service in a study of 11 human service organizations (Greenley and Schoenherr 1981).

## Summary

The themes of this chapter are decision-making and governance in the hospital setting. Contrary to generally held beliefs, financial effectiveness and product outcomes (e.g., quality patient care and fulfillment of professional preferences) are not necessarily incompatible. Lessons to this effect can be learned from the private sector, where high-performing organizations emphasize value and quality of service as well as financial performance.

There are many differing opinions about the optimal governance of hospitals, and many models exist. For instance, hospitals have different policies about the roles of boards of directors, CEOs, and nurses (including the roles nurses should have in administration). The nursing literature suggests that nurses believe the top nursing administrator should be part of executive management, not to determine the strategic plans of the entire organization, but to exert more authority over practice issues. Because of the diversity among hospitals and in the qualifications of nursing service administrators, many models for nursing administration exist.

Decentralization does not imply a lack of central direction. Indeed, effective decentralization rests on strong executive vision, commitment, and ongoing support. This chapter discussed two case examples that illustrate the changes that can occur with different decentralization efforts. In the first example, the effects of prospective payment based on DRGs in New Jersey were that (1) hospital departments were decentralized, (2) department heads had more authority, (3) a more interactive work mode developed, (4) communications improved, and (5) interdepartmental and management interactions became more structured. In the second example, decentralization of the nursing department in a community hospital took effect simultaneously with installation of a medical information system using clinical as well as financial data. Although it is difficult to tease out the causes, nursing turnover was reduced as nursing satisfaction increased, nursing costs declined, overall costs remained the same, physicians accepted the changes, and quality of care as measured internally improved.

Overall, the two examples support the Mintzberg model of a professional bureaucracy. That is, professionals require goal-directed top management and a limited middle management. There should be many opportunities for professional self-management (governance) through the use of peer review processes for credentialing, promotion, training, staffing, and termination. This professional structure of governance and decision-making is also compatible with the current emphasis on product line management.

## Endnotes

1. Refer to Nyberg and Simler (1979) and the appendices in Hayne and Bailey (1982) for case examples and forms.

2. In conversations with members of the El Camino administrative and nursing staff who participated in the process, the author learned that the decentralization of the nursing department and the MIS continues. These individuals believe that the experiment was successful. They agree that technology was a catalyst for needed change, but state that there is no consensus about whether the information system was essential.

   Physicians are described as conservative case managers who always used tests, therapies, and medications judiciously. In the beginning, physicians had difficulty accepting that a head nurse was not available to give reports at their convenience; most of them soon learned that the assigned nurse provided better information. However, some still yearned for the single contact person. Physicians in obstetrics and gynecology supported the change first, followed by surgeons and internists. The nurse responsible for implementing the MIS system is credited by an administrative analyst with changing the attitudes of physicians.

   One of the supervisors who became a generalist staff consultant is now the assistant administrator responsible for nursing. (The new title for the director of nursing reflects the change in responsibilities.) She attends board meetings, presents formal reports to the board and answers their questions, votes on the Long-Range Planning Subcommittee of the board, and sits on the Executive Committee of the Medical Staff. She stated that the interdepartmental coordinator position is a full-time rather than an 80%-time position. She agreed that nursing morale is high. Many part-time nurses are used.

Current cost comparisons show that the nursing department has a lower fixed overhead-to-variable cost ratio than the other departments. California Office of Statewide Health Planning reports show that El Camino charges are 25% lower than those of the other 13 hospitals in the county. Pay for nurses is negotiated internally between a committee of staff nurses and a management coordinator, head nurses, and the personnel director. The assistant administrator for nursing has no formal role in the process but works informally with the personnel director on a regular basis.

The hospital enjoys a good reputation in the community. There is no definitive proof that quality of care was enhanced, since there were no quality measures in place before the initiative. However, concurrent audit scores have improved each year since the change, according to the assistant administrator. According to the Los Angeles Times (1988), data from the California Office of Statewide Planning and Development indicate that, among California hospitals performing coronary bypass surgery, El Camino was one of the eight hospitals with the lowest mortality rates and one of the ten hospitals with the lowest median charges ($18,466). El Camino performed 171 such operations in 1986.

I appreciate the time given by Mary Smithwick in reading an early draft of this case example. Any remaining errors are mine, not hers.

3.  The hypothesized effects of professional organization on middle management size differ, although this may be a matter more of definition and refinement than real disagreement. Heteronomous professional organizations, in which professional participants are clearly subordinated to an administrative framework, have a high proportion of administrators and supervisors (Scott 1982). Their function is to improve the transmission of information and improve decision-making rather than provide direct supervision. They are members of the profession. The unanswered question concerns the relationship between gen-

eral management size and productivity. Low costs and labor hours were not achieved by increasing the managerial component; inefficient hospitals had a higher proportion of managers in an early study (Neuhauser 1971).

# References

Allen, D., J. Calkin, and M. Peterson. 1988. Making shared governance work. *Journal of Nursing Administration* 18(1): 37–43.

Althaus, J., N. Hardyck, P. Pierce, et al. 1981. Nursing decentralization: The El Camino experience. Wakefield, MA: Nursing Resources.

Althaus, J., N. Hardyck, and P. Pierce, 1982. Decentralized budgeting: holding the purse strings: part I. *Journal of Nursing Administration* 12(5): 15–20.

American Academy of Nursing. 1983. *Magnet hospitals.* Kansas City, MO: American Academy of Nursing, American Nurses' Association.

Aydelotte, M. 1984. A survey of nursing administrators—part 2. *Hospitals* 58(12): 79–80.

Battelle Memorial Institute. 1973. *Evaluation of the implementation of a medical information system in a general community hospital,* vol. 1. Columbus, OH: Battelle Memorial Institute.

Boerma, H. 1983. *DRG evaluation: Vol. IV B: the organizational impact of DRG's.* Princeton, NJ: Health Research and Educational Trust of New Jersey.

Camiller, D. 1981. Governance, in J. McCloskey and H. Grace, eds., *Current issues in nursing.* Boston: Blackwell, p. 402.

Clement, J. 1987. Does hospital diversification improve financial outcomes? *Medical Care* 25: 988–1001.

Counte, M., D. Barhyte, and L. Christman. 1987. Participative management among staff nurses. *Hospital and Health Services Administration* 32(1): 97–108.

Delbecq, A., and S. Gill. 1988. Developing strategic direction for governing boards. *Hospital and Health Services Administration* 33(1): 25–36.

Department of Health, Education, and Welfare. 1980. *How a medical information system affects hospital costs: the El Camino Hospital Experience.* Washington, DC: National Center for Health Services Research.

Department of Health and Human Services. 1981. *Methods for evaluating costs of automated hospital information systems.* Washington, DC: National Center for Health Services Research.

Dewar, R., D. Whetten, and D. Boje, 1980. An examination and validity of the Aiken and Hage scales of centralization, formalization, and task routineness. *Administrative Science Quarterly* 25: 120–128.

Drucker, P. 1974. *Management: task, responsibilities, practices.* New York: Harper and Row.

Fetter, R., and J. Freeman. 1984. A product approach to productivity improvements in health care, in John Virgo, ed., *Health care: an international perspective.* Edwardsville, IL: Southern Illinois University at Edwardsville, pp. 149–173.

Files, L. 1988. Strategy formulation in hospitals. *Health Care Management Review* 13(1): 9–16.

Fine, R. 1982. Creating a workplace for the professional nurse, in A. Marriner, ed., *Contemporary nursing management.* St. Louis: C.V. Mosby, pp. 96–109.

Flood, A., W. Ewy, W. Scott, et al. 1979. The relationship between intensity and duration of medical services and outcomes for hospitalized patients. *Medical Care* 17: 1088–1102.

Galbraith, J. 1977. *Organization design.* Reading, MA: Addison-Wesley.

Georgopoulos, B. 1972. *Organization research on health institutions.* Ann Arbor, MI: Institute for Social Research, University of Michigan.

Greenley, J., and R. Schoenherr. 1981. Organization effects on client satisfaction with humaneness of service. *Journal of Health and Social Behavior* 22: 2–18.

Hage, J. 1984. Communication and coordination, in S. Shortell and A. Kaluzny, eds., *Health care management.* New York: Wiley, pp. 224–249.

Hayne, A., and Z. Bailey. 1982. *Nursing administration of critical care.* Rockville, MD: Aspen.

Holle, M., and M. Blatchley. 1982. *Introduction to leadership and management in nursing.* Monterey, CA: Wadsworth.

Jaeger, B., ed. 1988. *Hospital management and governance in the new era.* Durham, NC: Duke University.

Jennergren, L. 1981. Decentralization in organizations, in P. Nystrom and W. Starbuck, eds., *Handbook of Organizational Design,* Vol. 2. Oxford, England: Oxford University Press, pp. 39–59.

Kanter, R., and D. Brinkerhoff. 1981. Organizational performance: recent developments in measurement. *Annual Review of Sociology* 7: 321–349.

Linville, C., and W. Hudson. 1963. We taught our nurses how to become managers. *Modern Hospital* 100(4): 96.

Longest, B. 1978. An empirical analysis of the quality-cost relationship. *Hospital and Health Services Administration* 23: 20–35.

Los Angeles Times. 1988. Heart surgery death rates found high in 1 in 6 hospitals. *Los Angeles Times* July 24, pp. 3, 32.

Meyer, M. 1972. *Bureaucratic structure and authority.* New York: Harper and Row.

Mintzberg, H. 1979. *Structuring of organizations.* Englewood Cliffs, NJ: Prentice Hall.

Mintzberg, H. 1981. Organization design: fashion or fit? *Harvard Business Review* 59(1): 103–116.

Mintzberg, H. 1983. *Structure in fives: designing effective organizations.* Englewood Cliffs, NJ: Prentice Hall.

Morlock, L., J. Alexander, and H. Hunter. 1985. Formal relationships among governing boards. *Medical Care* 23 (10): 1193–1213.

Morlock, L., L. Nathanson, D. Schumacher, et al. 1979. *Decision making patterns and hospital performance: relationships between case mix adjusted mortality rates and the influence of trustees, administrators, and medical staff in 17 acute care general hospitals.* Paper presented at the Association of University Programs in Health Administration meeting, Toronto, Canada, May 7–8.

Nackel, J., and I. Kues. 1986. Product line management: systems and strategies. *Hospital and Health Services Administration* 31: 109–123.

National Commission on Nursing. 1983. *Summary report and recommendations.* Chicago: Hospital Research and Educational Trust.

Neuhauser, D. 1971. *The relationship between administrative activities and hospital performance* (University Research Series no. 28). Chicago: Center for Administrative Studies, University of Chicago.

Norwood, D., R. Hawkins, J. Gall, et al. 1976. Information system benefits improves patient care. *Hospitals* 50 (18): 79–83.

Nyberg, J., and M. Simler. 1979. Developing a framework for an integrated nursing department. *Journal of Nursing Administration Quarterly* 9(11): 9–15.

Ortiz, M., P. Gehring, and M. Sovie, 1987. Moving to shared governance. *American Journal of Nursing* 87(3): 33–36.

Peters, T., and R. Waterman. 1982. *In search of excellence*. New York: Harper and Row.

Pfeffer, J., and G. Salancik. 1978. *The external control of organizations*. New York: Harper and Row.

Porter-O'Grady, T. 1987. Shared governance and new organizational models. *Nursing Economics* 5(6): 281–286.

Provan, K. 1987. Environmental and organizational predictors of adoption of cost containment policies in hospitals. *Academy of Management Journal* 30: 219–239.

Prybil, L. 1980. The Evaluation of Hospital Governance, in S. Levey and T. McCarthy, eds., *Health management for tomorrow*. Philadelphia: J. B. Lippincott, pp. 76–90.

Quintana, J., W. Duncan, and H. Houser. 1985. Hospital governance and the corporate revolution. *Health Care Management Review* 10(3): 63–71.

Sandrick, K. 1985. Pricing nursing services. *Hospitals* 59(21): 75–78.

Schweiger, D., and C. Leana. 1986. Participation in decision making, in E. Locke, ed., *Generalizing from laboratory to field settings*. Lexington, MA: Lexington Books, pp. 147–166.

Scott, W. 1982. Managing professional work: three models of control for health organizations. *Health Services Research* 17: 213–240.

Scott, W., and S. Shortell. 1984. Organization performance: managing for efficiency and effectiveness, in S. Shortell and A. Kaluzny, eds. *Health care management*. New York: Wiley, pp. 418–455.

Shortell, S. 1983. Physician involvement in hospital decision making, in B. Gray, ed., *The new health care for profit*. Washington, DC: National Academy Press, pp. 73–101.

Shukla, R. 1983. Technical and structural systems and nurse utilization: systems model. *Inquiry* 20: 381–389.

Starkweather, D. 1978. The rationale for decentralization in large hospitals, in K. Anthony and N. Duncan, eds., *Health services management*. Ann Arbor, MI: Hospital Administration Press, pp. 179–205.

Starkweather, D. 1988. Hospital board power. *Health Services Management Research* 1(2): 74–86.

Thakur, M. 1985. Planning for hospitals: no focus, no strategy. *Long Range Planning* 18(6): 77–83.

Weisman, C., and C. Nathanson. 1985. Professional satisfaction and client outcomes. *Medical Care* 23: 1179–1192.

Yaho-Fong, B. 1988. Advantages and disadvantages of product-line management. *Nursing Management* 19(5): 27–31.

*Chapter 5*

# Work Specification
# and Departmentation

---

All echelons of the staff will coordinate the configuration of the plans with the requisite tailoring of the overview in order to expedite the functional objective.

(Capt. Scarrett Adams, USN, in Kent 1985, 282)

## Departmentation

### Overview

Departmentation or the grouping of managers, workers, and technology, sets the parameters for defining the power, responsibility, authority, and discretion of persons in an organization. Nursing departments are typically a mixture of process, territorial, and product organization.[1] For example, the operating room is a process department, the obstetrical service is a product-line department, and medical-surgical wards are often specified territories (e.g., "Four South").

Generally three forms of nursing department organization have been identified: (1) the functional form, (2) the divisionalized structure, and (3) the matrix design. Departments based on process are surgery, delivery, and emergency care, where there is an emphasis on particular human-machine

143

relationships. Nursing units (wards, stations) where patients are admitted for care are a form of territorial organization (e.g., second floor, east wing). Since these spaces are usually reserved for patients with certain medical, surgical, obstetrical, pediatric, or specialty diagnoses, these units can also be classified as product departments. The advantage of grouping patients in this way, aside from physician convenience, is that it is easier for the nursing staff to become experts in caring for patients with specific conditions. The disadvantages are that there is less flexibility in the use of beds and that patients with similar nursing problems (as contrasted with medical problems) are not necessarily grouped together. This makes it more difficult to view the patient as a whole and the family as a unit—two key tenets of nursing practice.

The functional form rather than the decentralized product line forms discussed earlier predominates in the organization of nursing departments. The functional form adopts the pyramidal shape derived from classical management theory, which emphasizes unity of command, a scalar chain of command, lines of authority, and accountability of subordinates to their immediate superiors. Even though it may be efficient, the functional form lacks both lateral links with other departments and professional credentialing mechanisms. Too much of the necessary coordination of activities may depend on interest or friendship groups. As a result, problems are defined as personality problems or leadership style defects rather than design problems.

The divisional structure is seldom used but is found in some large teaching hospitals when the environment is complex and changing rapidly. (Traditionally, nurses in teaching hospitals have had more discretion over the work performed at lower levels than in other hospitals.) In this design, the clinical divisions have their own clinical and administrative support services. The divisional structure works best when there are abundant resources. Nursing acceptance of this structure is related directly to the degree of autonomy over nursing decisions and participation in decision-making (Kimberly, Leatt, and Shortell 1984). The divisional structure is unlikely to increase in prevalence in the future (Burns 1985).

The matrix design is a combination of a project structure superimposed on a functional or traditional vertical design. It is most likely to be found in medical centers. Separate task forces are formed to work on defined problems such as accreditation preparedness or standardization of regimes for care. Since staff members report to both a line manager and a project manager, it is sometimes necessary to assign a top administrative person to coordinate task forces and mediate conflict. These managers must be well-educated, fairly sophisticated, and experienced. This form may be most appropriate when a complex and dynamic environment requires much processing of information.

## Unit Managers

Matrix management in hospitals is usually associated with the presence of administrative managers on nursing units (Wieland and Ullrich 1981). The managerial hierarchy extends down from the hospital administrator or nursing director to a director of unit management. Technical and support services are centralized and controlled, as usual, by operating department heads. The lower-level managers facilitate the work of personnel from these other departments who work in patient care departments.

The trend toward matrix management continues, although less rapidly than in the past. The dissemination has been from large teaching hospitals to smaller facilities. Some hospitals have discontinued experiments in this area, for reasons that include lack of cost effectiveness, inability to retain good unit managers, and conflict between providers and unit managers (Burns 1982).

One early researcher observed that emancipating the nurse from unit management will not be sufficient to bring about desired changes, because those who are responsible for coordination need managerial authority, not just informational power (Mauksch 1966). Further, the individual must have the symbolic authority to bridge the discontinuity of responsibility and authority caused by the usually absent physician. Communication between physicians and nurses is essential. Nonnurse managers may fail because they lack either managerial power or symbolic authority over nurses and physicians, or because they impede communication among nurses and physicians.

A recent examination of the diffusion of matrix management in 277 hospitals confirms the Mauksch's prediction. The prevalence of nursing control over inpatient areas and unit management programs has halted the elaboration of these designs along administrative lines. This has happened because "political conflicts with nursing necessitated compromises in program structure" (Burns 1985, 20).

## Subunit Design

The nursing delivery system has unique subunit design aspects. The four main alternatives are the case method, the functional method, team nursing, and primary nursing. Currently several innovative models are being evaluated.

**Case Method.** Private-duty nursing, in which one nurse provides all care for one patient exclusively during a shift for the entire hospital stay, is the pure form of the case method. This method and its modification, one nurse for each of three eight-hour shifts, has all but disappeared except on burn or other critical care units. It is economical only when there is a high degree of task diversification and a high degree of uncertainty. In such situations, the nurse can work in an organic rather than a mechanistic way, handling emergencies, collaborating with others, and innovating to achieve results.

**Functional Design.** The functional design organizes work by functions or specialties. Most large nursing divisions are organized by clinical specialty (medical/surgical, obstetrics, critical care, etc). Within the units, the head nurse delegates tasks to nurses according to their level and competency. Registered nurses (RNs) give medications, administer intravenous medications, perform sterile and complex treatments, and monitor the critically ill. Licensed practical nurses (LPNs) perform in the broad middle range. Aides handle bedpans, make beds, and assist in bathing less critically ill patients. Volunteers give water and juice. An example of successful limited use of this method in large hospitals is having a team of nurses start all intravenous infusions, monitor the patients' intravenous sites daily for adverse effects, and rotate sites every three days to prevent infection.

The advantages of the functional design are increased technical expertise, clarity of roles, organizational stability, enhanced communication, and enhanced productivity on units that have low task diversification. The drawbacks are that workers tend to defend their own specialization at the expense of departmental and organizational needs, and that potential leaders do not get an opportunity to grow and develop. Thus, short-term efficiencies may sow the seeds of future problems. The Hospital Nursing Personnel Survey conducted by the American Hospital Association (1987a) found that fewer than 16.7% of hospitals reported any use of functional nursing.

**Team Nursing.** Team nursing attempts to remedy the problems of fragmented care and overload of experienced head nurses (Kron and Durbin 1981). The American Hospital Association (1987a) Hospital Nursing Personnel Survey found that team nursing was used most frequently by smaller, government, and rural hospitals.

Following the principle of democracy, members of the nursing team share the care of a number of patients. The head nurse assigns a group of patients and patient care team members to a team leader who is an RN. Assignments are carried out under the guidance of the team leader, who uses leadership skills to match patient needs with worker interests and abilities. The patient care plan is developed and modified in team conferences. Unfortunately, team nursing is often poorly understood and implemented. Among the common misconceptions are that team nursing is:

- Practiced only on the day shift or when students are present
- Any method that requires cooperation and mutual adjustment
- Assigning patients to a team on the basis of location (far end of the corridor, east side of the hall, etc.)
- Assigning duties and patients equally to various workers.

There are several advantages to team nursing when it is the enactment of a philosophy rather than a mechanical method of assignment. It was devised to provide better patient care with available staff; it provides flexibility in assignments and favors innovation. In addition, the head nurse has a smaller span of control and has more time for management and clinical consultation.

The disadvantages of team nursing are that it decreases organizational stability unless there is a strong team leader to clarify roles, explain the overall strategy, and fill communication gaps; increased coordination and communication demands decrease its utility; patient care is more fragmented, and patients often complain that they are confused about who does what; it favors a narrow perspective and does not develop nurses for management positions; it (like functional nursing) reinforces "class" differences and conflicts, since the lowest order tasks usually go the lowest class of nurses.

Hospitals with a rigid and caste-like organization tend to provide ritualized patient care and discourage the feedback necessary for making adjustments. Therefore, when the team form is used, procedures to encourage full participation by all members and structural arrangements to reduce stratification are important (Christman and Counte 1981).

Given the nature of hospital staffing, the word "team" is frequently used inappropriately. Teams depend on stable relationships and adequate staffing for conferences, prerequisites that often do not exist. Rotating shifts, off-duty days, variable staffing practices, turnover, absenteeism, emergencies, and staff shortages (plus nonparticipation by a few nurses) frequently make teamwork impossible at the patient care level. Another problem is that team nursing is sometimes confused with the organizational development process labeled "team building." This is not harmful for those who have had a successful experience with either one or both. However, among nurses who have experienced team building when it was a euphemism for getting them to accede to decisions already made by administrators or physicians, the term itself causes a negative reaction.

Some theorists believe, however, that the team approach is the preferred design for enhancing top management and innovative work. A variation of team nursing is to organize a project team around each patient, with representatives from various services involved. This is most appropriate in hospitals or units where both staff and patients are stable (e.g., rehabilitation or research units). To succeed, members need mutual respect so that the ambiguity does not become dysfunctional. In this case, the team manager may be a physician, nurse, or administrator.

**Modular Nursing.** Modular nursing is a modification of team nursing in which 8 to 10 patients receive their care from an RN and an assigned LPN or aide. The number of patients is adjusted depending on patient acuity and shift.

**Primary Nursing.** Primary nursing is the approach most frequently discussed. It incorporates the concept of assigning total care for one patient to a single nurse throughout the entire care episode.[2] The Hospital Nursing Personnel Survey reported that primary nursing was used often in very large to medium-sized hospitals (200 to 500 beds), although these hospitals frequently combined primary nursing with total patient care or modular nursing.

In its ideal form, the head nurse assigns patients to RNs who write, monitor, and implement the care plan throughout the patient's stay with 24-hour responsibility. When the nurse is not there, associate nurses care for the patient and transmit the information. Primary nursing in its pure form requires an all-RN staff. In practice, when LPNs and aides are used, the head nurse assigns them to assist with specific tasks.

Primary nursing offers the best answer to the problem of continuity for both patient and personnel. Advocates of this method see it as a first step that will lead to joint practice models between nurses and physicians as well as between staff nurses and nurse educators (Spitzer 1981). In all likelihood, when nurses realize that the real virtue lies in care planning, not delivery, primary care will have the flexibility to be combined with any delivery model and respond to nurse shortage situations.

Advocates of primary nursing usually also want changes in nursing governance, because of the interdependencies the method implies. Primary practice is based on the principles of autonomy and accountability, which then require:

- Controlling access to staff and practice privileges
- Confirming educational background and certification
- Assessing practice shortfalls and remedies
- Delimiting practice privileges
- Developing quality assurance and continuing education standards
- Participating in the education of students
- Conducting research (Christman 1976).

The prevailing medical care perspective influences nursing practice. The continuum for medical care concepts is anchored at one end by the diagnosis-and-cure approach and at the other end by the wellness-illness prevention approach. In the former, the physician is the captain of the team, and prescribes on the basis of personal judgment what both patients and nurses should do; in the latter, the physician serves as a consultant to the patient and is open to the judgments of other providers about the therapeutic regimen. It is hypothesized that (1) primary nursing flourishes when the wellness paradigm and a facilitative management style predominate, and (2) primary care and decentralization face more difficulty in organizations or units where physicians are more traditional and management is more authoritarian.

It is impossible to establish primary nursing care without changing relationships among physicians, nurses, and other providers. Therefore, it requires organizational readiness and increased participation on administrative and clinical committees. Hospitals that use functional, team, or modular nursing may also have the characteristics associated with primary nursing: decentralized decision-making, few subordinates, a high degree of professional autonomy and accountability, high performance standards and knowledge, and comprehensive, continuous peer review. That is, the subunit design relates to governance, but neither one wholly determines the other.

The disadvantages of primary nursing relate to its implementation. Primary nursing demands increased independence and accountability, and the ability to make nursing assessments and to plan accordingly. Nurses without a professional career orientation may not want this responsibility. Coordinating the activities of at least six nurses (three nurses to cover three eight-hour shifts in a day and another three to substitute for them on days off) is a challenging responsibility. Many nurses need more education or mentoring to perform these new functions well. In addition, many ancillary personnel resent losing their role as caregivers and have less opportunity for upward career mobility than under the team method. In hospitals where employers rely on transient or part-time workers it is difficult to have 24-hour accountability.

**Comparisons Among Methods.** Evaluators of these models address the question of how costs, nurse satisfaction, and quality of care are affected. After reviewing the empirical studies published between 1970 and 1984, Giovannetti (1986) concluded that the findings concerning job satisfaction, patient satisfaction, quality of care, and staffing costs were equivocal.

Whereas some studies noted that primary care was more satisfying to the nurses and led them to perceive more authority, accountability, or autonomy, other studies detected either no difference or an increased frustration with the primary care model. Some evidence exists that nurses on primary care units have increased absenteeism and sick time. Patients were found to experience less anxiety and either no change or an increase in satisfaction. The premise of primary care that nurses would spend more time at the bedside was also challenged. It appears that nurses may spend more time with the patient under the team model, but the daily amount is so small with either method that the difference among modalities may not be that important anyway.

Insofar as cost was concerned, the measures most frequently studied were salaries, number of patient-days, number of beds, extra staff hours, nursing care hours, and turnover. Results from 11 cost-benefit or cost-effectiveness studies conducted since 1975 were analyzed by Fagin and Jacobsen (1985). Again, the results were contradictory and difficult to trust because the research designs were generally weak. Methodological difficulties pertaining to random assignment, case mix adjustment, professional qualifications, organizational support, and salary differences related to tenure are difficult to overcome. However, it seems fair to conclude that staffing costs are highly dependent on unit size, amount of overtime, overall staffing levels, and the relative pay of LPNs and nursing assistants (Hancock et al. 1984). Shukla's studies (1981, 1982, 1983; Shukla and Turner 1984) argue quite persuasively that the competence of the nurses and organizational support are critical variables regardless of the method used.

**Synthesis of Traditional Designs.** In organizations where the functional nursing form predominates, work load concepts are based on tasks, procedures, and routines (Ganong and Ganong 1980). In hospitals where the emphasis is on primary nursing, work load is based on the nursing process of assessing, planning, implementing, and evaluating. Departmental activities and problem resolution are also influenced by prevailing management concepts.

Where an authoritarian management style prevails, managers emphasize classical management functions: plan, organize, staff, direct, and control. At the other end of the continuum, organizations that favor facilitative management value managers who can lead and employees that can plan, implement, and control.

Theory suggests that in circumstances where approaches to problems are well structured, such as in a postsurgical unit for conditions where complications seldom occur, and where the authoritative and medical care styles predominate, there will be a high level of output, rapid processing, and a small number of errors. Yet staff nurses can be expected to report low satisfaction and reject unsolicited innovations. When faced with problems for which no codified answer is applicable, these units will have lower output, slower processing, low-quality solutions, and less creativity. Most experienced managers and organizational change agents can identify a failed change effort that can be explained by the combined effect of trying to solve an ill-structured problem with staff from a unit geared to output and hierarchical structure.

When the organization has poorly structured problems or when patients' needs are diverse and unpredictable, facilitative management and primary nursing should result in high output, rapid processing, high-quality solutions, and a high level of creativity. The process may appear to be disorderly, but it is usually quite functional.

A good example of a poorly structured problem is the recent need to adjust to prospective and limited reimbursement. Executives and managers knew that resources consumed would have to be matched to patient diagnoses, but they did not have a clear enough idea to issue a directive outlining the procedures. Under such circumstances it is not surprising that consultants prescribe facilitative management as the solution of choice.

Just as the authoritarian style will be dysfunctional for complex problems, the approach based on knowledge and problem-solving has its limitations when used with well-structured problems. In such cases, theory predicts lower output, slower processing, and more processing errors, even though the workers will find the work more satisfying and be willing to accept innovative ideas.

Nurses are the largest and most unstable group in the system. Throughout the hospital there is a remarkable division of labor. There exists a high specialization of roles and functions that vary in intensity and extensiveness. Individuals must work together and resolve conflicts through mutual adjustments rather than by relying on formal authority systems and monetary rewards. There is no one best way to plan, organize, staff, direct, and control professional service work, and there are few classification rules that suggest where and under what circumstances one model takes precedence over another.

As a practical matter, an eclectic orientation provides the most flexibility. Most departments are likely to have a mix of systems. Without doubt, the move to primary nursing requires the commitment of the director of nursing to provide leadership with the intersecting problems. However, even if primary nursing were proven to be the most universally desired and cost-effective model, there are not enough RNs for every hospital to adopt the all-RN primary nursing model. For the nursing staff to design a delivery system that is the most amenable to the goals of the organization and the competencies of the staff, management support is critical. Executives and managers are fortunate in that the educational system is sufficiently diverse to allow nurses to adapt to organizational preferences with minimal difficulty.

**Innovative Models.** Some hospitals are experimenting with new designs. At The Johns Hopkins Hospital in Baltimore, three different models have been implemented and evaluated: a contract model, a group practice model, and an operating room practice model (Dear, Weisman, and O'Keefe 1985). Each of the models was based on the primary nursing model. In addition, compensation was by salary rather than hourly wages; two of the models incorporated an incentive plan to stimulate productivity. Decision-making was decentralized, with nurses assuming responsibility for scheduling, standards of practice, and quality assurance. No structural changes were required, but the role of the head nurse was substantially modified away from directing activities to serving as a group facilitator.

The results of each of the models were similar. Job satisfaction increased, turnover decreased, and costs related to recruitment, orientation, and registry use declined. Quality of care, as measured by audits, patient satisfaction surveys, and the number of incident reports, was usually improved. Productivity also dramatically improved. More work was done by the same or fewer nurses without additional incremental labor costs (York and Fecteau 1987).

At St. Mary's Hospital and Health Center in Tucson, Arizona, a program to improve nurses' professional accountability also had impressive results: Job satisfaction increased while job stress and turnover declined; the hospital itself achieved substantial savings. The plan had several elements: a credentialing mechanism for level of practice, extended scope of practice to promote continuity of care, salaried status for the nurses, a spiritual and holistic framework for nursing, an acuity-based billing system using the patient classification system, a decentralized nursing system that extended to the community, and an environment conducive to two levels of nursing practice: case managers and associate RNs (Ethridge 1987).

Barhyte, Counte, and Christman (1987) followed the implementation of a collegial model of practice in a large teaching hospital. At both three and six months, nurses on the experimental units had fewer sick days, and absenteeism was lower.

There is a growing awareness that successful nursing interventions or changes require the support of management and must incorporate practice and reward changes. Neither pay changes nor practice changes alone will improve productivity or retention. Instead, what is needed is better integration of nursing within the hospital, and decentralization combined with better central direction.

## Nursing Units as a Social System

### Experiential Description

Ideally, managers of nurses should experience the world of nursing work by personal observation on different wards throughout several shifts when the work load is light and when it is heavy. Since this is usually not feasible, a brief comment about the "feel" of a medical-surgical unit is indicated. In the usual case, nurses adjust their own schedules and activities around many unscheduled events. Sometimes the nursing unit is hectic; at other times it is quiet. The difference is caused in large part by the changing numbers of nonnursing staff that are on the unit. When patients are sicker and when the therapeutic regime is more complex, there are more interruptions. Technicians from other departments visit to perform procedures or take patients to other departments. Physicians make rounds and leave orders. Both visitors and volunteers circulate freely, although their hours are usually circumscribed. Therapeutic activities are often scheduled for the benefit of individual patients and other departments, with little concern for the overall impact on the nursing unit.

The technical and social aspects of nursing work are affected by requirements that stem from the unscheduled interruptions by professional and laypersons. Although it has not been proved, it is reasonable to assume that the continual readjustments that nurses make to accommodate the flow of strangers lead to inefficiencies and dysfunctional behaviors.

Managers can help minimize such problems by initiating and supporting efforts to minimize distractions, for example by allowing nurses to adjust the schedules and activities of other workers. One hospital reports that nurses can assign housekeeping aides the task of admitting or discharging patients, rather than cleaning rooms, when this would enhance patient flow (Franz 1984). Nursing efficiency has also been increased by giving patients more responsibility for providing care. Patient education can reduce the need for continuing nursing care. Nurses can also shorten hospital stays when they have authority for patient-centered scheduling of diagnostic tests and procedures.

A more radical alternative for decreasing confusion would be to modify physician behavior. Nurses' work load is more predictable when physicians agree on standard protocols and boundaries for autonomous nurse behavior. This may well explain the low nurse-to-patient ratios found in health maintenance organizations (HMOs) and investor-owned hospitals. An appointment system for visiting nonurgent patients, although not a conventional prescription, would also smooth the nursing work load. Alternatives such as this are seldom considered as solutions to problems occurring on nursing units. However, these changes are more likely to occur when a surplus of physicians, a shortage of skilled nurses, and an organizational need to contain costs come together.

The predominant challenge to managers is to understand the tone or culture of the nursing unit, which results from the interaction of patients and their families, staff, and physicians. This milieu affects quality of care, productivity, attitudes, absenteeism, and turnover. Although nurses exert an influence, they do not exclusively determine either the climate on the unit or its potential. Therefore, another major managerial challenge is to identify methods to ameliorate underlying uncertainty and fragmentation resulting from poor interdepartmental coordination.

## Recurring Themes

Three themes appear repeatedly in the nursing management literature: (1) a skilled labor shortage, (2) the need for nurses to have both generalized and specialized competence, and (3) the need to find a balance between strictly defined duties and opportunities for personal initiatives.

**Skilled Labor Shortage.** No organization, hospitals included, can rely exclusively on poorly trained staff or on highly skilled staff. Since it is difficult to predict the degree of skill that will be needed in the future, both categories of workers are important. This suggests that the organization will provide ways for the less skilled to become more skilled and the already qualified to be well utilized.

Upward mobility models exist at all levels in nursing. Nursing aides can receive their education and competency certification in high schools or community colleges, where credit is given toward LPN practical nurse requirements. Likewise, community colleges can link practical nurse education to associate degree (ADN) education. Clear specification of the "second step" (i.e., obtaining the bachelor's degree after either an ADN or diploma in nursing) has been also developed (Lenburg 1979).[3]

However, organizations cite two problems with upward mobility activities. First, there is a fear that the organization will not be able to appropriately employ all the workers as they develop more skills and higher expectations. Second, organizations resist investing in workers who may leave to work in organizations that do not invest in training.

In response to the first objection, the opportunity for advancement often holds more significance than actual participation for many workers (Styskal 1980). It is estimated that only 20% of nurses given the opportunity would advance to the highest step on a professional career ladder (Sovie 1983). A good plan would include a needs assessment enabling management to ascertain potential demand. If anticipated demand is found to exceed the available resources or the ability to place graduates, criteria could be established making the program available only to the individuals most likely to succeed, to work in target programs, or to remain with the organization.

The second objection, that nurses will leave after receiving training, reflects an industry tendency to underinvest in training because of the erroneous assumption that nurses frequently withdraw from the hospital work force. Organizations dependent on skilled and knowledgeable workers must offer education and incentives to remain competitive in the market for talented workers.

The larger question, relative investment among organizations, can be addressed collectively. Through employer associations, areawide programs can be developed to mobilize resources at local colleges, provide industry career mobility opportunities, lobby for career-enhancing reimbursement regulations, and provide visibility for career mobility activities. In this way, employers would benefit from an enriched labor pool without the burden of actively developing programs at all levels—aide to LPN, LPN to RN, RN to BSN, generalist to specialist. These activities offer a bonus advantage of making career lines in hospitals more visible to potential recruits and neophyte workers.

**Staff with General or Specialized Competency.** The growth of specialized nursing staff is encouraged by the proliferation of knowledge and increased skill levels required by advanced technology, medical specialization, increased nursing credentialing, and the increased severity of illness of hospitalized patients. Yet managers cherish the flexibility of a generalized staff that can be assigned patients irrespective of their diagnosis, age, placement, or nursing requirements. Although the specifics of the problem vary across hospitals (teaching hospitals may assimilate a very high proportion of specialists, whereas rural hospitals may require generalists, for example), most hospitals face the dilemma.

Upon graduation, most nurses are generalists. Once they are employed, the institutional and professional incentives, when they exist at all, encourage investing in specialty education. There are few, if any, incentives for maintaining competency in more than one functional specialty, whether it be medical-surgical nursing, obstetrics, pediatrics, or emergency practice. Just as career ladders have been proposed to overcome the shortage of nurses with specialized competencies, so educational programs, pay differentials, and planned unit rotations are prerequisites for developing breadth.

**Strictly Defined Duties Versus Opportunities for Personal Initiative.** Within the constraints of licensing parameters, union contracts, and organization-wide personnel systems, there is much variability and latitude among nurses and between levels of nurses with regard to specific assignments and responsibilities. This is a key issue because managers depend on nurses being flexible in order to adapt to constantly changing physician and patient requirements. Managers cannot afford overly rigid specifications that encourage working "to the rule." Yet hospitals have traditionally needed clear specifications to handle the large numbers of temporary, part-time workers who work all shifts.

There is much potential for managerial intervention in this dilemma. For instance, the design and introduction of bedside terminal systems will automate control of most routine aspects of the nursing plan. Data from management information systems, when configured to present case mix and quality of care feedback at the unit level, will encourage professional controls rather than rules. Any activities that reduce staffing instability on the units lessen the need for rules.

## Technical Mission of the Unit

The technical system of the nursing unit, which consists of tasks and work flows, influences the design of support systems. As general managers are held more accountable for quality of care and costs, they will be under increasing pressure to understand the technical differences among units. Job redesign to improve motivation and job involvement also requires an in-depth understanding of technology and tasks.

### Technology and Structure

Much research has examined the relationship between technology and structure in the belief that the impact of this relationship on organizational functioning is important (Fry 1982). Technology has been defined as the process of transforming inputs into outputs at all organizational levels, but there is little agreement on its theoretical dimensions. Technology involves utilization of knowledge and information transfer as well as machines, tools, computers, procedures, and equipment. Technical knowledge is an important part of technology, one that is different from capital equipment and work flow.

A typology of technologies differentiates them according to the level of interdependence of the task activities or techniques used to achieve an outcome (Thompson 1967). A mass production assembly line, such as those used to process laundry, routine diets, and billing, are hospital examples of a long linked technology, the simplest type. The sequential nature of these tasks allows them to be standardized, repetitive, and predictable. When there is an interdependence between task activities and the object itself, the technology is called an intensive technology. The therapeutic process is an example of an intensive technology. The selection, combination, and sequence of tasks are determined by feedback from the patient. Professionals use a framework of professional expertise to respond to variations in patients' status and the uncertainty of their response to interventions.

Several studies address the technologies of nursing subunits using the usual dimensions of technology: uncertainty, uniformity, and variety. Comstock and Scott (1977) defined technology using a priori dimensions. These dimensions were task predictability (the degree to which raw materials and transformation processes are well understood so that they present few unexpected contingencies to qualified performers) and work flow predictability (the extent to which raw materials and transformation processes associated with the combination of tasks are well understood and nonproblematic for individuals in the unit).

The descending rank order of units according to their work flow predictability was as follows: intensive care, surgical units, medical units, combined medical-surgical units, orthopedic, pediatric, obstetrical, and mental health. The study concluded that it was important to understand both task and work flow, since each had important effects apart from differences attributed to either the size of the organization or the professional attributes of the nurses. Predictable tasks required lesser staff qualifications and greater staff specialization. More predictable work flows increased the bureaucratization and standardization of procedures. Thus, the researchers concluded that technology, rather than tasks, best predicts which type of control system will be successful.

The structure of an organization is defined as the arrangement of people, departments, and other subsystems within the organization. Structure is focused primarily on controlling and coordinating technology both within and between groups of workers. There is growing agreement that complexity (including horizontal and vertical differentiation), formalization, and centralization (including hierarchy of authority and participation) are the major structure dimensions of interest. Specifically, research findings suggest that, as technology moves from routine to nonroutine, subunits adopt less formalized and centralized structures; also, the coordination of interdependencies among organizational levels and other organizations deserves more attention.

Bloom and Alexander (1982) used task conception (number of planned hours of patient care per patient-day) and a task predictability score based on an independent rating of tasks performed in postsurgical units to explore the relationship between technology and structure. They found that the number of planned hours did not match task predictability. On larger units, the nursing team used hierarchical control, but on units where nurses had a high level of professionalism, they used lateral coordination. From these findings the authors concluded that technology does not dictate structure or the measures of coordination.

A study of task interdependence and empirically derived technological factors enabled researchers to describe seven differing nursing units on the basis of these factors (Overton, Schneck, and Hazlett 1977). The technological factors were labeled uncertainty, instability, and variability. Psychiatric units ranked highest in uncertainty and variability, and lowest in instability. Intensive care units also rated high on instability as well as uncertainty, but low on variability. Obstetrical units were low on both uncertainty and variability. Pediatric, rehabilitation, and surgical units were similar in that they were neither high nor low on any of the measures.

This study was replicated with similar results by Leatt and Schneck (1981). Nurse researchers have also explored the relationship between specialization and nursing behaviors. The degree of specialization of units, progressing upward from general medical-surgical, to specialty medical-surgical, to parent/child, to surgical care unit, did not affect role conceptions or role behaviors for new graduate workers. However, the extent of specialization as measured by the quantity and type of procedures and equipment used did make a difference in nursing behavior (Lewandowski and Kramer 1980). There was clear-cut evidence that specialization was positively linked with loyalty to the bureaucratic system as well as to the professional role, self-esteem, and performance ratings. Specialization was negatively related to empathy and change agent activity. A study by Schoonhoven (1981) found that destandardization, decentralization, and professionalization had different influences on effectiveness, as measured by patient deaths and severe morbidity, depending on work flow uncertainty in operating rooms in 17 hospitals. For example, when more than one-third of the operating room work flow was subject to change, the benefits of decentralization were realized, but when uncertainty was low, increasing decentralization was accompanied by decreased effectiveness.

Collectively these studies suggest that, in hospital nursing units as in other organizations, there is little agreement on technology. Without such agreement, it is difficult to argue, as some analysts have, that the technology determines the structure of the unit. It has not been proved that the amount and kind of variability, uncertainty, and instability dictate the extent of decentralization. The relationships between technology and structure are difficult to predict.

The practical inferences that arise from these studies are that:

1.  Since the relationships between technology and organization design are extremely complex and interdependent, a problem-solving approach is appropriate.

2.  Administrators and nurses hold different conceptions of patient care technology; managers emphasize the routine and predictable aspects, whereas nurses emphasize variability and uncertainty.

3.  There is much variability among subunits in the technologies that they employ, the types of coordination they use, and the tasks that are being performed.

4.  Although technology influences design and structure, it does not have an overriding effect.

5.  It is important for hospital managers to become more knowledgeable about the technology of nursing units because they cannot seal off the technical core from client influences as managers in production businesses can.

## Job Design Framework

Task design is an important topic for several reasons. First, job-related concerns have been described as the heart of professional performance (Bechtold, Szilagyi, and Sims 1980). Certainly, from the manager's viewpoint, nothing can be more central than workers performing the task for which they were hired. A second reason is the importance of task redesign in various change interventions to improve productivity and worker morale and to reduce job stress.

Ivancevich and Smith (1982) constructed an index of job difficulty using critical incidents reported by medical-surgical nurses to study the impact of job difficulty. The 29 job difficulty descriptions for nurses clustered into three dimensions: overload, conflict, and supervisory practices. The findings suggest that different aspects of job complexity are related to intrinsic and extrinsic satisfaction, job tension, and performance. The overload factor, which included such items as too many new demands, time pressures, patient demands, too many details, physician demands, and administrative details, was consistently important except for job performance. The implications of the study for job redesign projects were that outcome measures may be affected by one dimension of job difficulty but not another in a particular tenure group.

A study by the Center for the Quality of Working Life (1978) provides valuable insight into the tasks of a nursing unit. Six mutually exclusive but interdependent nursing components were identified in the delivery of patient care on a medical ward in a 250-bed community hospital. These unit operations comprised the technical system of the ward and served as the basis for identifying key problems or variances that the nursing staff either absorb or control. The analysis relied on a systems approach: Patients were seen as raw material that required processing throughout their stay on the unit.

The boundaries were admission to the unit and discharge (i.e., when the patient either was cured, died, or was able to recuperate or died elsewhere). The nursing components, identified by a study team of researchers and nurses, were (1) admission, (2) assessment and initial data collection, (3) diagnosis and development of the nursing care plan, (4) daily care and monitoring, (5) emergency care, and (6) discharge. Within these components, 56 critical disturbances (problems or variances) that occurred in the daily routine of providing care, aside from medical care or ancillary care, were found. Of these 56, the study team identified nine crucial (key) variances, which they linked to one of the 56 critical variances before exploring the interrelationships among them.

The list of problems and components does not apply to every unit and hospital, but it is illustrative:

- Patient acuity (problem on admission)
- Quality and completeness of the care plans (problem during diagnosis)
- Family attitudes (problem at discharge)
- Legal issues (problem during assessment, initial data gathering, and emergencies)
- Staff availability (problem during daily care and at discharge)
- Caliber of staff (problem during daily care and monitoring)
- Census (problem at admission and at discharge)
- Varying amounts of time required by patients (problem during daily care and monitoring)
- Differences in patient morale (problem at discharge)

The dominant job design theory over the past decade has been Hackman and Oldham's (1976, 1980) Job Characteristics Model. This model states that five job characteristics—skill variety, task identity (e.g., entire service rather than just a portion), task significance, autonomy, and feedback—contribute to internal work motivation and positive job attitudes. Nursing has been characterized as an occupation in which the work has low or medium task identity and/or significance, which is similar to the profile of teachers and engineers. However, nurses have less autonomy than the other two groups (Naughton and Outcalt 1988).

Roedel and Nystrom (1988) ascertained that nurses assigned to obstetrics, pediatrics, operating room, emergency room, intensive care, and medical-surgical units perceived differences among skill variety and task identity. They also differed in satisfaction with pay, supervision, and the work itself.

Despite a large body of research, the evidence does not support the hypothesis that changes in objective job characteristics will change job attitudes (motivation and satisfaction) and behavior (performance) (Staw 1984). It seems that the job scope-job performance relationships are modest. They are related to self-rated performance (Stone 1986). The relationship between job characteristics and job satisfaction is moderated by the individual's need for personal growth (Fried and Ferris 1987; Lohrer et al., 1985.)

Attention is now focused on an integrated theory, which incorporates the physical setting, individual attributes, and the social setting to understand the dynamics among the tasks, job, and role of the worker (Campion and Berger 1988; Gardner and Cummings 1988, Quintana, Hernandez, and Haddock 1988; Griffin 1987). In the future, it is likely that there will be a move away from standard measures of task perception, such as the Job Characteristics Inventory, and toward a more systematic consideration of the organizational contexts of jobs and jobholders.

The developmental work system design as outlined by Brousseau (1983) parallels the integrated theory approach. Individuals come to organizations with a career orientation that is influenced by their current needs and abilities, previous job experiences, career stage, and the overall fit between their jobs and preferred developmental sequence. Within the organization, the job-person fit will depend on the organizational context of the job and the worker's longevity in the job. This dynamic model requires a system for placement and movement within organizations based on informed choice. This system in turn depends on data on the characteristics of workers, jobs, alternate job sequences, current and projected job openings, and developmental opportunities, and also a career counseling system.

## Staffing

### Background

It is conservatively estimated that hospitals in the United States spend $19.92 million per year for nursing care (Thompson and Diers 1985). Since labor accounts for almost 54% of total expenses in community hospitals (46% if employee benefits are not included), staffing efficiency is important (American Hospital Association 1987b).

On the other hand, it is also important not to exaggerate the significance of nursing costs. Frequently, nursing costs are not separated from "hotel functions" such as housekeeping and dietary, because hospital accounts treat nursing as a cost center rather than a revenue center. In two medical centers where nursing costs were calculated, direct nursing care accounted for only 11% and 18.5% of the hospital bill (Sandrick 1985). A cost-finding study using four diagnosis-related groups (DRGs) found that direct and indirect nursing costs amounted to between 14% and 20% of hospital charges and between 33% and 40% of room charges (Bargagliotti and Smith 1985). Sovie and Smith (1986) found that variable billing could reduce room rates by 30% (direct nursing costs that were previously included in room costs ranged from 18% to 24%).

Investing in nursing staff may also reduce the number of medical complications among the elderly, shorten length of stay, and prevent revenue loss on Medicare patients. Flood and Diers (1988) estimated that one hospital could have hired an additional 2.68 full-time equivalents (FTEs) with the amount of lost revenue from one understaffed unit.

Nursing departments are now involved with general administrators and physicians in generating DRG-specific allocation statistics and in measuring the intensity of use of nursing resources in routine and special services, to use as a standard for staffing (Thompson 1984). This method may rely too heavily on the medical diagnosis, whereas the previous methods of classifying patients by acuity level relied too heavily on tasks. For example, at Strong Memorial Hospital in Rochester, New York, where there is an identified line item in patient billing for nursing care, individual patients' needs for nursing care are extremely varied; DRGs are not predictive of nursing care needs (Fetter 1988).

The movement toward an increasing proportion of RNs on the nursing staff is more advanced in hospitals that are members of multi-institutional systems (Becker and Foster 1988). RN staffing tends to be low in government hospitals, whereas investor-owned and not-for-profit hospitals are similar in their hiring of RNs. The implications of these findings for quality of care and financial performance are unknown because of the effects of acuity of care, regional wages, and payer mix.

## Policy Initiation and Formulation

Directors of nursing services and human resources management share responsibilities for proposing and drafting new staffing policies for the chief operating officer to consider. Once policies concerning pay levels, skill mix, use of float personnel, number or staff in training, and recruitment have been made, both directors share responsibilities for counseling line managers and monitoring the performance of units in complying with established policies and procedures.

In general, policies for nurses should include retaining valued employees, anticipating nurse requirements, fostering relationships with educational programs, encouraging careers in nursing, and contributing to the attractiveness of the geographic area for nurse employment. These criteria make explicit the dual requirements of organizational survival in the long run and patient care in the short run. To determine success in accomplishing these tasks, managers should ask, "Is the organization relying too heavily on individuals to adjust to uneven work loads?" and "Do the staffing and admitting systems limit nurse adjustments to truly emergency or unpredictable circumstances?"

It should be noted that nurse executives and middle managers have different opinions on what influences nursing hours per patient-day and that managers in teaching hospitals have different opinions than managers in community hospitals (Kirby 1986). For example, middle managers ranked the influence of physician practices low, believing that the availability of nurses was more important. Nurse executives and middle managers in teaching hospitals ranked the impact of support services higher than did their counterparts in community hospitals.

Innovative policy development may be necessary, especially for nurses in high-stress units. For example, nurses on some chronic disease units occasionally attend the funerals of deceased patients as part of their nursing work. More routine measures include a peer support system, a flexible break policy, or a room that can be used for reflection. Staffing is more than a mathematical programming problem to be solved by narrowly focused experts who apply production principles to complex production and service functions. The department of human resources management often has oversight responsibility for position control, initial screening of applicants, and designing job analysis or work load studies. Ideally, the director of nursing services is involved with general administration in overall strategic planning and budgeting. Directors with executive authority manage a staffing budget or exercise position control and coordinate their activities with other departments. The director of nursing services usually delegates shift scheduling, corrective allocations, task assignment, and performance monitoring. In hospitals where the nursing staff is clinically accountable, final hiring decisions are made by the head nurse or a nurse credentialing committee.

Because nursing is a department with many interdependencies, it is unrealistic to expect its effectiveness to be any better than that of the organization itself. In a hospital study in Southern California, for example, the best single predictor of nursing turnover was found to be the separation rate of other employee groups, rather than traditional organizational measures such as staffing mix, costs, work load, or occupancy (Friss 1974). This suggests that there is homogeneity within hospitals, which in turn suggests that departmental success is related to management of the facility as a whole.

An example of these interdependencies is the shortage of critical care nurses in the early 1980s. Patients who could have been cared for in regular units were admitted to critical care units (Myers et al. 1984), because hospitals were reimbursed at higher rates for critical care patients. The apparent shortage of nurses under these circumstances could never be overcome so long as the revenue generated by critical care patients exceeded the costs of staffing the special units. (This is easy to achieve as employers do not pay a significant premium to specialty nurses). Traditional adaptive measures, such as intensive recruiting, more educational offerings, and shift modifications, are palliative investments at best.[4]

Overall, studies support the following imperatives for an effective staffing system:

- Be objective, flexible, and easy to understand.
- Meet the staffing goal.
- Have a built-in justification method when the staffing budget is not met.
- Use personnel effectively.
- Establish a concise audit trail for patterns (Lewis and Carini 1984).

## Staffing Elements

There are four elements to the management of staffing: (1) position control and auditing, (2) selection procedures, (3) presenting problems, and (4) tactical studies.

**Position Control and Auditing.** The number of budgeted positions, including the flexibility to substitute less expensive personnel, is the basic but not the only important, productivity decision made by management. In some organizations this is a responsibility shared with the professional association, as a result of a bargaining agreement.

In community hospitals, 24.3% of all full-time employees (FTEs) are RNs (American Hospital Association 1986). The wide variance in staffing standards among regions (ranging from 2.8 RN hours per patient-day in the South to 4.6 in the Northeast), which cannot be explained on the basis of case mix, leads to the conclusion that the number of FTEs and the staffing mix are a strategic decision rather than a technological imperative (Robinson 1988; Sloan and Elnicki 1980). Staffing decisions are also related to the availability and salaries of nurses at all levels—RNs, LPNs, and nurse aides (Department of Health, Education, and Welfare 1975).

**Selection Procedures.** The more effective selection processes for hospital nurses are, the less need there is for organizational socialization activities. Not only are recruitment costs high—$874 per nurse in 1981—but orientation costs are almost double—$1,563 per nurse (Beyers et al. 1983).

The hospital industry would undoubtedly benefit from more sophisticated recruitment and selection practices. For instance, when hospitals indiscriminately hire young nurses and dismiss mature workers in order to maintain market share, they run the risk that the policy will boomerang when both young nurses and potential nurses become disenchanted with a "use and discard" philosophy. "Flypaper recruiting," catching whoever appears for as long as they stick, is an outdated strategy. In expansionary times, managers argue that they are at the mercy of the supply. During recessionary periods, like the man who failed to fix the roof when it stopped raining, many managers do not take advantage of the opportunity to obtain a desirable proportion of career-committed workers.

**Presenting Problems.** Certain nursing problems wax and wane, thus selectively competing for managers' attention.

*Supplemental Agencies.* Nurses have a long history of using nursing registries as a third party to link nurses to jobs by the day. Originally these were run by professional associations to link individual clients with private-duty nurses and to improve conditions of private-duty work and payment. As more nurses left private-duty nursing during the Great Depression and became hospital employees, these registries almost disappeared.

Today's supplemental agencies, usually provided by commercial companies, are a modification of this original form. They link employers with available nurses and provide employment screening, testing, payroll deductions, and license monitoring. Their mission is to provide employers with a method of meeting variable staffing needs. However, employers are not necessarily relieved of their legal obligations to agency nurses. An Arizona court ruled that an agency nurse injured at a hospital was entitled to workers' compensation because she worked regularly at the hospital, performed ordinary hospital services, and was supervised and controlled like a regular employee (Tammelleo 1985).

The arrangement whereby hospitals use nurses from agencies is referred to as institutionalized individual bargaining. It offers advantages to both hospitals and nurses. Hospitals with unstable occupancy rates can maintain a core staff and hire only as many extra nurses as necessary on a day-to-day basis. Employers can also assess potential employees' skills and personality before hiring them.

Nurses, too, find working through registries advantageous. Agencies are especially attractive to nurses with a spiral or transient career orientation. Steady-state nurses use them to assess the climate of competing hospitals before applying for permanent employment. Nurses using nursing registries gain autonomy over their working hours and are freed from the organizational responsibility of supervising assistants and coordinating hospital activities. Frequently, agency nurses receive a higher per diem rate than the regularly employed nurses with whom they work. As the supplemental agencies have matured, they have begun to offer prorated fringe benefits, training, and career guidance.

One study found that, among nurses, 41% approve of registries, 31% disapprove, and 40% believe nursing will suffer from them (LeRoy 1982). The negative effects for nurses collectively are that fringe benefits are undermined and both upward mobility and full-employment opportunities are lost. Together, the incentives for transitory and spiral careers increase while incentives for steady-state or hierarchical careers decrease.

Organizations also have problems with registries. Managers find it more difficult to control and monitor practice since a portion of the work force is free from both organizational sanctions and rewards. The regularly employed nurses have the extra responsibilities of orienting the supplemental nurses, caring for more complicated patients, and carrying out organizational routines (forms, requisitions, reporting), which lowers their morale when they do not receive extra pay for these added tasks. Although the lack of continuity of care that can result from the use of supplemental nurses could affect the quality of care, there are no studies to prove or disprove this assertion.

The cost to an individual organization of utilizing registry nurses is debatable. The disagreement is over whether saving the costs of longevity (e.g., vacations, pensions, salary increments), fringe benefits (insurance, unemployment compensation), and related administrative costs offset the costs of orientation, low initial productivity, extra coordination, and diminished morale of the regular staff. Many managers choose to use some registry nurses, as they generally believe it is better to hire a few nurses at a higher per diem rate than to raise salaries for all nurses or to have a permanently high number of nurses for the census. Apparently the hospital breaks even as long as the ratio of hospital-based personnel to supplemental service cost per hour is less than the fractional FTE (Thompson 1981). (It takes 1.4 FTEs to fill one position because of vacations, holidays, education time, and fluctuating census levels.)

*Supplemental Nursing Agencies.* Supplemental agencies provide the only wage competition in many areas and were blamed for precipitating and fueling a wage increase spiral in the late 1970s, although the aggregate effect was small (Kehrer, Deiman, and Szapiro 1984). Employers responded by negotiating volume discount rates with the registries and pressuring the agencies to avoid rate competition with one another. Employers also investigated the potential for state regulatory control; this was not productive because states were reluctant to constrain private businesses with a legitimate market niche.

Employers using supplemental agencies (or developing an in-house float pool) need to establish explicit policies addressing orientation, standards of performance, evaluation, assignment criteria, and appropriate use. Appropriate use means not using supplemental agencies to fill regular positions or vacancies caused by poor scheduling decisions and absenteeism.

*Substitutability of Personnel.* State laws, accreditation requirements, federal reimbursement policies, and the supply of personnel set limits on the substitution of one level of personnel for another. Within these limits, hospitals develop policies on downward and upward substitutions based on physician and nurse attitudes, training and experience of personnel, existing staffing, availability of support services, expediency, and patient mix. Since there is usually much variability, especially in case mix, it seems best to allow charge nurses considerable flexibility regarding substitutability (Trivedi 1984).

Performance of medical tasks (as compared with nursing tasks) by nurses should receive more attention than it does. The delegation of medical tasks to nurses was a determinant of nursing turnover in medical centers (Weisman, Alexander, and Chase 1980). In other settings, physicians may attempt to reverse delegation patterns. (The recent change in New York State law concerning nurse practitioners was fueled by an impending legal limit on the number of hours medical residents could work.)

Despite the many staffing studies, universal standards for nursing hours per patient-day and skill mix do not exist. An unofficial formula of 65% licensed nurses and 35% unlicensed personnel has been reported but is now considered obsolete. Although delegating mundane tasks to less-qualified personnel has intuitive appeal, it may not be effective. For example, aides may spend up to 50% of their time receiving instructions and waiting to be told what to do (Franz 1984). In a study of 46 exemplary (magnet) hospitals, the American Academy of Nursing (1983) noted that there was an average of 1.1 RNs per occupied bed. The RN-to-LPN ratio was 10:1, the RN-to-aide ratio was 12:1, and the RN-to-unit clerk ratio was 9:1.[5]

Nationally, substitution is influenced by the availability of educated workers and their wage. The number of FTEs of both RNs and LPNs has been found to be a function of the wage for each category, rather than the pay level of the other occupation (Ehrenberg 1974). That is, if RNs are available and their wage is low, employers will have a richer skill mix. If the LPN wage is low, employers will hire a larger proportion of LPNs. In addition, more RNs are found where there are higher physician-population ratios (Sloan and Elnicki 1980). In markets where there are more neighboring hospitals there are more RNs per bed and more RNs as a percentage of all nurses, and there is a higher use of temporary agency nurses (Robinson 1988).

Experience suggests that prospective reimbursement changes internal management as discussed in Chapter 4. Overall, prospective reimbursement leads to lower payroll expenses and fewer FTEs per patient-day. However, it does not reduce the hospital's payroll expense per FTE. In states where there is prospective reimbursements, the combined impact has been mixed. In New York, where there has been an 11% reduction in payroll, there has been only a 3% reduction in total costs. In Maryland, there has been a 10% decline in both (Kidder and Sullivan 1982). Thus, it appears that even under prospective reimbursement, hospitals contain costs in complex ways; staffing and pay policies are related to other organizational policies in ways we do not understand.

*Staffing Nights and Weekends.* All industries find it more difficult to staff shifts that do not conform to regular life patterns; nursing is no exception. The usual solution is to offer substantial shift pay differentials. Because the premiums offered to nurses who work less desirable shifts (i.e., evenings, nights, weekends, and holidays) do not equal those found in other industries, it seems that hospitals use other techniques to staff difficult shifts. This statement is supported by the finding that among emergency room nurses there were greater differences in perception of work between hospitals than between shifts (Peterson 1985). In another study, extended-shift nurses, who tended to work weekends, were more satisfied with the task requirements, although less satisfied with their professional status, than regular shift nurses (Stanton, Laughlin, and Wheeler 1983).

During recurring shortage episodes there is much publicity over the use of extended shifts and compressed work schedules (such as the three-day, 38-hour week or the four-day, 40-hour week). Managers lobbied and changed state laws eliminating overtime pay for work in excess of eight hours per day and 40 hours per week (Mech, Mills, and Arnold 1984). Thus, in some states nurses lost mandated time-and-a-half or double-time pay for working extended hours.[6]

Data also suggest that, contrary to what is commonly assumed, supplemental nurses are not used more frequently on the difficult shifts. This suggests that staff nurses met the need to staff evenings and nights (Langford and Prescott 1979; Kehrer, Deiman, and Szapiro 1984; Prescott and Langford 1981).

*Management of Turnover.* Turnover among nurses is an important and expensive problem, even though the annual turnover rate has declined to a range of 20% to 30% since 1962 (Institute of Medicine 1983, 192). The wide variance in nursing turnover rates, which is unexplained by the state of the economy, hospital size, location, or ownership within a labor market area, suggests that some hospitals are much more successful than others in managing turnover (Friss 1982a).

It is true that, in some areas, particularly rural areas and inner cities, social forces may be especially compelling in influencing turnover rates. Even here, however, some managers are more successful than others in controlling turnover, probably because they develop professional partnerships even when there are no shortages (Mercer 1987).

Executives and managers control pay and climate policies that determine the internal career structure. A study by Lord (1982) found that nurses with career goals have a greater commitment to nursing. The study further found that those nurses whose supervisors are supportive of career goals also had greater job satisfaction and set more career goals for themselves.

Well-designed nursing studies suggest that marital status, number of children, and family income do not predict nursing turnover (McCloskey 1974; Weisman, Alexander, and Chase 1981; Stuart 1983). As female work force patterns become more like those of males, women can be expected to act more like primary wage earners. That is, they will leave a job for advancement rather than family reasons.

It is particularly important not to confuse age with sex as a predictor of turnover, which is easy to do in hospitals, where the average age of workers is lower than in other industries. Using sexual identification to explain turnover obscures underlying determinants such as career expectations, tenure, and pay. It also leads to less investment in training for women, which in itself can perpetuate turnover among those who want educational opportunities at work.

The turnover rate among females is similar to that among men when similar job levels are compared under similar conditions (Lloyd and Niemi 1979). Young men who enter professional and technical occupations also have high job mobility compared to male workers in general (Pietrofesa and Splete 1975). Thus, it is not surprising that young nurses, who also have had a professional-technical education, have high rates of turnover and mobility. In contrast, mature women have much more predictable career histories than mature men. Generally, the reasons found for turnover depend on how much of the information is consistent with the analyst's personal beliefs and attribution framework (Mowday, Porter, and Steers 1982). An example occurred in Southern California, where separation rates for hospital employees have been obtained by the Hospital Council for two decades. A study suggested that type of ownership rather than the size of the hospital was explanatory of the rate. However, the committee would not change the reporting format because of a firmly held belief that organizational size was a primary determinant.

Effective turnover management rests on the understanding that turnover is a complex phenomenon. Its determinants fall into several categories: the individual, the job, the immediate job situation, the total organization, and off-the-job involvements of workers. Each of these interacts with the others. Therefore, it is highly unlikely that any one determinant will have a completely consistent effect. However, the priorities for policy determination would seem to be (in descending order) the total organization, the job, and the immediate job situation.

Several comprehensive models of turnover have been proposed and have received varying degrees of empirical support (Cotton and Tuttle 1986; Forrest, Cummings, and Johnson 1977; Price 1986; Mobley 1982). The dominant paradigm for explaining the causes and preconditions of turnover has been based on the expectancy theory—what does the worker expect to gain from employment, and how well are these expectations met? Thus, the underlying theme is the fit between the individual and the organization (Caplan 1987a, b). In a nursing study that used the person-environment fit theory, Blau (1987) concluded that the model is useful for predicting job involvement but not organizational commitment, variables that have been found to be precursors of turnover. Organization commitment seemed to be less related to personal factors, such as the Protestant work ethic, than perceived job scope factors. Research also suggests that although women may become committed to their jobs through the same processes as men, their reaction to certain variables differ, specifically sex-role conflict (Chusmir 1982).

Other researchers do not believe that individuals separate their work and professional lives and argue for a model that includes nonwork features (Near, Rice, and Hunt 1980). Again, career concepts can provide executives and managers with a way of thinking about the needs of steady-state workers, the ones most likely to be in short supply.

Nursing turnover studies generally do not present data to evaluate nurse staffing, cost, or client outcomes. In a review of the literature on nursing staff turnover, stress, and satisfaction, Hinshaw and Atwood (1983) concluded that the major weaknesses in the body of research were low explained variances, lack of replication, and the use of different measurements to measure the same constructs. Apparently something is missing from the models; my belief is that the fit between organizational characteristics and career plans needs more attention. Taylor and Covaleski (1985) found that those who changed jobs had career plans inconsistent with the outcomes provided by the employer. Focus on this factor rather than on demographic characteristics of nurses that managers cannot control seems advisable.

Studies also tend to be either hospital- or region-specific, so that generalizing to other hospitals or regions is not warranted. An exception is a study of a sample of hospitals participating in the Commission on Professional and Hospital Activities (Alexander 1988). Alexander found that, when the other factors were controlled for accuracy of evaluation, frequency of patient care conferences, head nurse patient care hours, shift rotation, and the ratio of RNs to patient care total staff were significant determinants; the full-time staff ratio, head nurse decision-making authority, RN influence on unit decisions, explicitness of unit procedures, and staff working contact and communication were not. It seems that a collegial group of professional workers and some degree of organizational stability are necessary to achieve organizational integration and consequently to reduce turnover.

Mobley (1982) suggests that there are four As of turnover management: anticipate, analyze, assess, and actively control.

*Anticipation* includes questioning norms, scanning the environment to detect trends in supply and demand, forecasting, and planning. Anticipation is the activity that managers neglect when supply is adequate. Yet it is during this time that there is the most room for selecting employees carefully, implementing pilot studies, investing in work enhancement projects, and developing departmental capabilities to design and implement a continuing turnover program. This continuing concern can serve management in good stead during the difficult times when some workers must accept shorter hours and layoffs, or longer hours and heavier work loads.

*Assessing* or diagnosing turnover begins by asking the right questions. The question is not, "What is wrong with the nurses?" but, "What is wrong with the organization?" It is not, "What do the nurses want?" but, "What does the organization want and at what cost?" The ideal approach to answering these questions would be to establish a human resource accounting system. Unfortunately, this is probably beyond the capability of most hospitals. When a formal accounting system does not exist to provide a turnover utility analysis, budget policies that facilitate calculation of recruitment, selection, placement, and separation costs are necessary to generate base-line information. Whenever an organization experiences a chronic failure to retain newly trained individuals or mature workers, the recruitment practices, the reward and opportunity structure, and the institution's commitment to the steady-state worker require reexamination.

For proper assessment, both the negative and positive consequences of turnover need to be documented. Negative consequences include decline in morale, disruption of performance and communication, and inability to respond to changed market conditions caused by staff shortages. Positive consequences include the loss of poor performers, a decrease in absenteeism, and reduction of conflicts as well as the immediate dollar savings that come from a low-tenured work force. A central policy for dealing with turnover, rather than ad hoc departmental programs, leads to control strategies that best fit the organization.

The *analyzing* or diagnosing component of turnover management requires policies about measurement of employee attitudes and answering such questions as "What group of workers is affected?" "How does our turnover rate compare to that of other hospitals in the area?" "If it is higher, is it because of special circumstances?" "Is the impact serious enough to warrant investigation?" and "How much of its resources should the organization invest in investigating and remedying the problem?" A comprehensive program would include:

- Comparison of separation rates of similar employee groups with those of comparable employers

- Comparison of both voluntary turnover rates and survival rates internally by career stage, department, Equal Employment Opportunity Commission (EEOC) protected classes, and employee performance and potential

- Assessment of employee perceptions and intentions during employment, upon leaving, and after leaving.

Employers cite many reasons for resisting the installation of a comprehensive turnover reduction program. First, turnover is so high in some hospitals that analysts are overwhelmed by the responses of short-term, usually young employees; trend lines are difficult to establish. Second, exit interviews are believed to be biased. Third, determining who was a valued clinician is difficult. Fourth, the costs of maintaining a system are hard to justify; how does one prove system effectiveness? Fifth, turnover may be lucrative; indeed, managers believe that it may be less expensive to cope with turnover than to prevent it, at least in the short run (Dalton, Todor, and Krackhardt 1982). Sixth, routine assessment of employee attitudes is controversial. Critics argue that it raises unrealistic expectations for change.

There are answers to these objections:

- The very existence of a transient work force demands more investment in turnover management. The military services have pioneered much psychological and personnel research because of similar problems: the need to adjust rapidly to outside events, maintain technological competence, retain highly skilled professionals, and socialize new recruits.

- Attitude surveys can be targeted to those areas where management wants to effect change.

- Exit interviews can be validated by follow-up surveys.

- Supervisors can determine who were valued employees (Lowery and Jacobsen 1984).

- Although justifying a comprehensive system is difficult, other costs are also difficult to justify yet continue to be paid. Management discretion exists in every budget.

- Current estimates are that it costs $20,000 to recruit, orient, and train a new nurse while paying for a temporary substitute (and for advertising, travel, literature, public relations, and a nurse recruiter) (Droste 1987).

- A preference for high turnover may be cost effective in the short run, but it erodes a hospital's competitive position for attracting capable workers in the long run.

*Active control* of turnover aims to encourage turnover when it will have positive organizational and personal consequences, and minimize turnover where the net outcomes are negative. The underlying principle is that there are no panaceas; no single policy will yield a sustained effect. Managers must decide which of the following employment components to emphasize based on the initial analysis and assessment:

Recruitment

Selection

Early socialization

Compensation

Supervision

Working conditions and schedules

Job design.

To expand on these components, a realistic job preview is an essential part of the recruitment and selection process (Popovich and Wanous 1982). Effective selection weeds out individuals unlikely to fit the organization.

A study of organizational socialization among hospital occupations led to three conclusions (Feldman 1976, 1977): First, orientation programs, which were usually short, were found not to be appropriate for the results expected of them. Although socialization affected the general satisfaction of workers and promoted feelings of autonomy and personal influence, job involvement and motivation of employees required redesign of both individual jobs and work groups. Second, hospitals often did not consider all three phases of the socialization process: attraction and recruitment, training and development, and resolution of role conflicts. Finally, organizations relied too heavily on occupational socialization (professional education and norms) rather than on organizational functions—what is expected and how new recruits' professional needs might be met.

Two case studies of nurses are useful in understanding turnover management. The first used the expectancy model of turnover as a basis for measuring the determinants of turnover in university hospitals (Seyboldt 1983). Turnover intentions and work role design were related to employee dissatisfactions and employee tenure. The consistency and equity of organizational policies, role clarity, and feedback from supervisors, co-workers, and clients were identified as key areas for management attention.

The second study based recommendations for turnover management on an areawide study rather than on a sample of hospitals (Price and Mueller 1986). However, some of the recommendations seem to violate affirmative action requirements (e.g., hire more nurses who are married and have children, hire nurses over 30 years old, and recruit more diploma nurses). None of these recommendations are bona fide occupational requirements, but they do reaffirm that older workers, those with family responsibilities, and those without the educational credentials needed to find other employment are less likely to leave. More useful recommendations include the following: (1) Allow voluntary transfers among nursing units, (2) hold regular and brief meetings during working hours, and (3) establish career structures. Managers are also advised to:

- Relate pay to performance and tenure
- Provide new nurses with an adequate orientation
- Hire nurses with a long work history.

*Tactical studies.* Tactical staffing studies cluster around two areas: (1) job satisfaction and turnover and (2) deployment. Rational staffing studies supplement but do not substitute for a career management system.

Job satisfaction is not a good measure of employee attachment and performance. Among hospital employees, satisfaction was found to have no direct effect on turnover (Mobley, Horner, and Hollingsworth 1978). Although satisfaction is most consistently associated with occupational prestige and promotions (Department of Labor 1979), it has been established that satisfaction does not necessarily result in better performance. Satisfaction, however, may well result from good performance (Stone 1978).

Level of job dissatisfaction is a better predictor of turnover during periods of low opportunity (high unemployment rates) than during periods of high opportunity. That is, when opportunity is low and the employee quits, the likely cause is dissatisfaction. When opportunity is high and the employee quits, other reasons in addition to job dissatisfaction are probably the cause (Shikiar and Freudenberg 1982).

Asking individuals whether they intend to leave their jobs is a better way to predict intent to leave than are measures of job satisfaction (Weiland 1969). A measure of organization commitment is also a better predictor than satisfaction. A loyal, dutiful, and self-sacrificing person may or may not be satisfied with certain aspects of work and the organization. Commitment, as contrasted with satisfaction, may be relatively independent of immediate and temporary situational influences (Wiener and Vardi 1980). By the same reasoning, career attachment should also be measured by other, more direct measures, such as job involvement, instead of job satisfaction data.

Although researchers and managers appropriately measure satisfaction during change projects, the emphasis should not be to attempt to create happy workers, as this is a paternalistic approach to labor relations. When used to monitor attitudinal change, the instrument should be well validated and tap multiple facets of satisfaction (Stamps and Piedmonte 1986). Results should be examined carefully to ensure that education, length of service, job level, and reference groups have been adequately considered (Friss 1982b). Since there is a greater likelihood that job dissatisfaction will lead to withdrawal from the labor force among older (30 to 44 years) white women, a high-priority group in hospitals, disaggregation of results by age is especially important (Department of Labor 1979).

Until recently, research on nurse staffing has concentrated on activity analysis and work load prediction at two levels: shift scheduling and corrective allocation (Hershey, Pierskalla, and Wandel 1981). These are key issues to workers, since job assignment is a major determinant of work attitudes and career development (Thompson, Dalton, and Price 1977). Managers must balance efficiency and effectiveness demands with concern for smooth staffing patterns that do not rely on unplanned nurse adjustments to achieve the proper staffing level. Little research has been done on forecasting, monitoring, and coordinating with other hospital activities, although these are also important management staffing functions. Conventional techniques of analyzing nursing activity, such as time study and work sampling, are very expensive and generally have a low level of acceptance among nurses. Further, studies have not established the validity and reliability of time estimates. A recent study based on work sampling in which reliability and validity were addressed suggests that staffing cannot be predicted from the patient care plan (National Center for Health Services Research 1987).

The well-known standards for analyzing hospital efficiency developed by the Commission on Administrative Standards for Hospitals (CASH) are not always trusted. When nurses look at the indices showing the administrative component routinely operating at over 100% efficiency while other departments never achieve 90% efficiency, they suspect that the system is not objective. Nominal group process among RNs and LPNs has been advocated as the best method of reaching agreements on tasks and work load (Trivedi 1982).

Perhaps all hospitals could approach staffing problems more intelligently by heeding the advice of Vaughan and MacLeod (1980), who admonished that there was no need to reinvent the wheel. They were referring to the 20-year history, at an estimated cost of $15 million per year, of patient classification studies that have been the heart of work load measurement. Despite the experience and investment in quantitative nurse scheduling, very few recommendations resulting from these studies have been implemented or accepted (Hershey, Pierskalla, and Wandel 1981). For the foreseeable future, staffing levels and mix apparently will depend on wage rates, the supply of labor, and organizational policy more than on objective work criteria.

## Summary

Nursing departments may be organized by process, by territory, or by product. This chapter identifies various designs of nursing departments—

specifically, unit management by nonnurse personnel (unit managers) and the traditional subunit design are considered. There are five major alternatives for subunit design: case method, functional team nursing (and a variation called modular), primary nursing, and contract nursing. It is suggested that there is no one best way to organize and deliver professional nursing.

The second section of the chapter explores nursing units as social systems. Beginning with a description of a typical medical-surgical unit, three recurring themes are identified: (1) a shortage of skilled labor, (2) the need for a proper mix of generalists and specialists, and (3) the need to balance strictly defined duties and opportunities for personal initiative.

The technical mission of the unit is then explored. Technology is defined to include both nursing and patient care components. The definition includes knowledge utilization and information transfer in addition to machines and tools. As might be expected when dealing with an intensive technology, various studies suggest that there is little agreement about the effects of technology on nursing. The third section concludes with a look at job redesign, which requires managers to assess first their own strengths and weaknesses if a successful result is to be achieved.

The final section addresses staffing, beginning with the social context: prevailing wages and societal attitudes about work and family. Since organizational survival in the long and the short run must be concerned with getting the work done, considerable attention is given to policy formation and procedural initiation.

Four basic staffing elements are presented: (1) position control, (2) selection procedures, (3) presenting problems, and (4) tactical studies. Common presenting problems include the use of supplemental agency personnel, substitution of auxiliary personnel, staffing for night and weekends, and turnover. The four As of turnover—anticipating, assessing, analyzing, and actively controlling turnover—are presented.

The chapter concludes with a review of tactical staffing studies, which cluster around two areas: (1) job satisfaction and turnover and (2) deployment.

## Endnotes

1.  For a concise overview of the nursing service department, refer to the chapter on this subject in Rowland and Rowland (1984).

2.  See Anderson and Choi (1980); Ciske (1977); Durbin (1981); Ellis (1978); Fairbanks (1981); Ferrin (1981); Forster (1978); Ludwig and Waldie (1981); McGreevy and Coates (1980); Nursing Administration Quarterly (1981); Sigmon (1981); and Department of Health and Human Services (1983).

3.  In the New York Regents External Degree Program, a degree is awarded by one institution for learning acquired elsewhere. The program has a nurse faculty committee responsible for developing and monitoring all aspects of the degree. The program is characterized by both standardized written theory tests and performance examinations, which are developed by the Regents College. Outside of New York State, the written test is administered by the American College Testing Program as ACT PEP tests. The objective criterion-referenced performance examinations are offered in testing centers in New York, California, Georgia, and Wisconsin. Students throughout the country can meet graduation requirements through a combination of college courses from accredited institutions, approved military courses, approved non-collegiate-sponsored instruction, or special assessment.

    The program's feature is the requirement of three performance evaluations, which supplement the five written tests. These tests are practice oriented. They even use paid, trained subjects to play the role of clients needing counseling or assistance. Testing centers are available in different regions in the country.

4.  For case examples of improving critical care staffing, see Horsburgh (1988) and Penny (1988).

5.  Detailed studies have been done of subsamples of the magnet hospitals (Kramer 1988; Grimsrud 1987). Although there is wide variance on almost all pertinent elements—number of beds, occupancy, RNs per occupied bed, percentage of nursing staff that were RNs, percentage of RN staff with BSN—very few used supplemental RNs, and the mean years of RN experience in nursing as well as mean years of tenure in the hospital were above average.

6.  Organizations that do not pay overtime rates for all hours worked in excess of 40 hours in each work week are required

by the federal Fair Labor Standards Act, where applicable, to pay overtime rates for 4 hours of every 12-hour shift. However, if overtime is paid for all work hours in excess of 40 each week, no overtime payment is required. State and local laws also apply. Refer to Latack and Foster (1985) for a general review of compressed work schedules.

# References

Alexander, J. 1988. The effects of patient care unit organization on nursing turnover. *Healthcare Management Review* 13(2): 61–72.

American Academy of Nursing. 1983. *Magnet hospitals*. Kansas City, MO: American Academy of Nursing, American Nurses' Association.

American Hospital Association. 1986. *Annual hospital survey*. Chicago: American Hospital Association.

American Hospital Association. 1987a. *Hospital nursing personnel survey*. Chicago: American Hospital Association.

American Hospital Association. 1987b. *National hospital panel survey*. Chicago: American Hospital Association.

Anderson, M., and T. Choi. 1980. Primary nursing in an organizational context. *Journal of Nursing Administration* 10(3): 26–31.

Bargagliotti, L., and H. Smith. 1985. Patterns of nursing costs with capitated reimbursement. *Nursing Economics* 3: 270–275.

Barhyte, D., M. Counte, and L. Christman. 1987. The effects of decentralization on nurses' job attendance behaviors. *Nursing Administration Quarterly* 11(4): 37–46.

Becker, E., and R. Foster. 1988. Organizational determinants of staffing patterns. *Nursing Economics* 6(2): 71–75.

Bechtold, S., A. Szilagyi, and H. Sims. 1980. Antecedents of employee satisfaction in a hospital environment. *Health Care Management Review* 5: 77–88.

Beyers, M., R. Mullner, C. Byre et al. 1983. Results of the Nursing Personnel Survey, Part 1: RN recruitment and orientation. *Journal of Nursing Administration* 13(4): 34–37.

Blau, G. 1987. Using a person-environment fit model to predict job involvement and organizational commitment. *Journal of Vocational Behavior* 30: 240–257.

Bloom, J., and J. Alexander. 1982. Team nursing: professional coordination or bureaucratic control. *Journal of Health and Social Behavior* 23: 84–95.

Brousseau, K. 1983. Toward a dynamic model of job-person relationships: findings, research questions, and implications for work system design. *Academy of Management Review* 8: 33–45.

Burns, L. 1982. The diffusion of unit management among United States hospitals. *Hospitals and Health Services Administration* 27(2): 43–57.

Burns, L. 1985. *Divisionalization and matrix management in hospitals: structure and environment*. Working paper, College of Business and Public Administration, University of Arizona.

Campion, M., and C. Berger. 1988. Conceptual and empirical integration of job design and job evaluation, in *Academy of Management Best Paper Proceedings*, Anaheim, CA: Academy of Management, pp. 268–272.

Caplan, R. 1987a. Person-environment fit theory and organizations: Commensurate dimensions, time perspectives, and mechanisms. *Journal of Vocational Behavior* 31: 248–267.

Caplan, R. 1987b. Person-environment fit in organizations: Theories, facts, and values, in A. Reilly and S. Zaccaro, eds., *Occupational stress and organizational effectiveness*. New York: Praeger, pp. 103–140.

Center for the Quality of Working Life. 1978. *Socio-technical analysis of nursing services*. Los Angeles: UCLA Institute for Industrial Relations.

Christman, L. 1976. The autonomous nursing staff in the hospital. *Nursing Administration Quarterly* 1(1): 37–44.

Christman, L., and M. Counte. 1981. *Hospital organization and health care delivery*. Boulder, CO: Westview.

Chusmir, L. 1982. Job commitment and the organizational woman. *Academy of Management Review* 7: 595–602.

Ciske, K. 1977. Misconceptions about staffing and patient assignment in primary nursing. *Nursing Administration Quarterly* 1(2): 61–68.

Comstock, D., and W. Scott. 1977. Technology and the structure of subunits: distinguishing individual and workgroup effects. *Administrative Science Quarterly* 22: 177–201.

Cotton, J., and J. Tuttle. 1986. Employee turnover: a meta-analysis and review with implications for research. *Academy of Management Review* 11(1): 55–70.

Dalton, D., W. Todor, and D. Krackhardt. 1982. Turnover overstated: a functional taxonomy. *Academy of Management Review* 7: 117–123.

Dear, M., C. Weisman, and S. O'Keefe. 1985. Evaluation of a contract model for professional nursing practice. *Health Care Management Review* 10(2): 65–77.

Department of Health, Education, and Welfare. 1975. *Factors affecting staffing levels and patterns of nursing personnel*. Washington, DC: Government Printing Office.

Department of Health and Human Services. 1983. *The application of primary nursing in a hospital setting*. Washington, DC: Government Printing Office.

Department of Labor. 1979. *Work attitudes and work experience*. Washington, DC: Government Printing Office.

Droste, T. 1987. High price tag on nursing recruitment. *Hospitals* 61(19): 150.

Durbin, E. 1981. Comparison of three methods of delivering nursing care, in T. Kron and E. Durbin, eds., *The management of patient care,* 5th Ed. Philadelphia: W.B. Saunders, pp. 227–232.

Ehrenberg, R. 1974. Organizational control and the economic efficiency of the hospital: the production of nursing services. *Journal of Human Resources* 9: 21–32.

Ellis, B. 1978. The all-RN staff: why not? *Hospitals* 52(20): 107–112.

Ethridge, P. 1987. Nurse accountability program improves satisfaction, turnover. *Health Progress* 68(4): 44–49.

Fagin, C., and B. Jacobsen. 1985. Cost-effectiveness analysis in nursing research. *Annual Review of Nursing Research* 3: 215–238.

Fairbanks, J. 1981. Primary nursing: more data. *Nursing Administration Quarterly* 5: 51–62.

Feldman, C. 1976. A contingency theory of socialization. *Administrative Science Quarterly* 21: 433–452.

Feldman, D. 1977. Organizational socialization of hospital employees. *Medical Care* 15: 799–813.

Ferrin, T. 1981. One hospital's successful implementation of primary nursing. *Nursing Administration Quarterly* 5: 1–12.

Fetter, R. 1988. *Diagnosis related groups (DRGs) and nursing resources.* New Haven, CT: Yale University School of Organization and Management.

Flood, S., and D. Diers. 1988. Nurse staffing, patient outcome and cost. *Nursing Management* 19(5): 34–43.

Forrest, C., L. Cummings, and A. Johnson. 1977. Organization participation: A critique and model. *Academy of Management Review* 2: 586–601.

Forster, J. The dollars and sense of an all-RN staff. *Nursing Administration Quarterly* 3: 41–47.

Franz, J. 1984. Challenge for nursing: hiking productivity without lowering quality of care. *Modern Healthcare* 14(12): 60–68.

Fried, Y., and G. Ferris. 1987. The validity of the job characteristics model: a review and meta-analysis. *Personnel Psychology* 40: 287–316.

Friss, L. 1974. *Labor turnover in hospitals.* Unpublished doctoral dissertation, University of California at Los Angeles.

Friss, L. 1982a. Nursing turnover one more time. *Journal of Health and Human Resources Administration* 5: 209–223.

Friss, L. 1982b. Why RNs quit: the need for management re-appraisal of the "propensity to leave." *Hospital and Health Services Administration* 27(6): 28–44.

Fry, L. 1982. Technology-structure research: three critical issues. *Academy of Management Journal* 25: 532–552.

Ganong, J., and W. Ganong. 1980. Nurse manager's role in cost containment, in E. Turban and J. Tanner, eds., *Cost containment in hospitals.* Germantown, MD: Aspen, pp. 55–59.

Gardner, D. and L. Cummings. 1988. Activation theory and job design. *Resarch in Organizational Behavior.* 10: 81–122.

Giovannetti, P. 1986. Evaluation of primary nursing. *Annual Review of Nursing Research* 4: 127–150.

Griffin, R. 1987. Toward an integrated theory of task design. *Research in Organizational Behavior* 9: 79–120.

Grimsrud, D. 1987. Staffing methods at magnet hospitals. *Hospital Topics* 65(1): 12–14.

Hackman, J., and G. Oldham. 1976. Motivation through the design of work: test of a theory. *Organizational Behavior and Human Performance* 16: 250–279.

Hackman, J., and G. Oldham. 1980. *Work redesign.* Reading, MA: Addison-Wesley.

Hancock, W., P. Flynn, S. DeRosa, et al. 1984. A cost and staffing comparison of an all-RN staff and team nursing. *Nursing Administration Quarterly* 8(2): 45–61.

Hershey, J., W. Pierskalla, and S. Wandel. 1981. Nurse staffing management, in D. Boldy, ed., *Operational research applied to health services.* London, England: Croom-Helm, Ltd., pp. 189–220.

Hinshaw, A., and J. Atwood. 1983. Nursing staff turnover, stress, and satisfaction: models, measures, and management. *Annual Review of Nursing Research* 1: 133–153.

Horsburgh, M. 1988. How we redefined our nursing unit. *Nurse Management* 19(1): 32B–32D.

Institute of Medicine. 1983. *Nursing and nursing education: public policies and private actions.* Washington, DC: National Academy Press.

Ivancevich, J., and S. Smith. 1982. Job difficulty as interpreted by incumbents: a study of nurses and engineers. *Human Relations* 35: 391–412.

Kehrer, B., P. Deiman, and N. Szapiro. 1984. The temporary nursing service R.N. *Nursing Outlook* 32: 212–217.

Kent, R. 1985. *Money talks.* New York: Facts on File, p. 282.

Kidder, D., and D. Sullivan. 1982. Hospital payroll costs, productivity and employment under prospective payment. *Health Care Financing Review* 4: 89–100.

Kimberly, J., P. Leatt, and S. Shortell. 1984. Organization design, in S. Shortell and A. Kaluzny, eds., *Health care management.* New York: Wiley, pp. 291–332.

Kirby, K. 1986. Survey regarding factors influencing nursing hours. *Nursing Economics* 6: 310–313.

Kramer, M. 1988. Magnet hospitals: part I. *Journal of Nursing Administration* 18(1): 13–24.

Kron, T., and E. Durbin. 1981. *The management of patient care,* 5th Ed. Philadelphia: W.B. Saunders, pp. 212–220.

Langford, T., and P. Prescott. 1979. Hospitals and supplemental nursing agencies: an uneasy balance. *Journal of Nursing Administration* 9(11): 16–20.

Latack, J., and L. Foster. 1985. Implementation of compressed work schedules: participation and job redesign as critical factors for employee acceptance. *Personnel Psychology* 38: 75–92.

Leatt, P., and R. Schneck. 1981. Nursing sub-unit technology: a replication. *Administrative Science Quarterly* 26: 225–236.

Lenburg, C. 1979. Emphasis in evaluating outcomes: the New York Regents External Degree Programs. *Peabody Journal of Education* 5: 212–221.

LeRoy, L. 1982. Supplemental nursing agencies. *Health Affairs* 1: 41–54.

Lewandowski, L., and M. Kramer. 1980. Role transformation of special care nurses: a comparative study. *Nursing Research* 29: 170–179.

Lewis, E., and P. Carini. 1984. *Nurse staffing and patient classification.* Rockville, MD: Aspen.

Lloyd, C., and B. Niemi. 1979. *The economics of sex differentials.* New York: Columbia University Press.

Lohrer, B., R. Noe, N. Moeller, et al. 1985. A meta-analysis of the relation of job characteristics to job satisfaction. *Journal of Applied Psychology* 70: 280–289.

Lord, J. 1982. *A study of career goal setting, job satisfaction, career commitment and supervisor support in nursing.* Unpublished doctoral dissertation, University of Texas at Austin.

Lowery, B., and B. Jacobsen. 1984. On the consequences of overturning turnover: a study of performance and turnover. *Nursing Research* 66: 363–367.

Ludwig, C., and D. Waldie. 1981. Primary nursing: a conception that became a reality. *Nursing Administration Quarterly* 5(3): 41–50.

Mauksch, H. 1966. The organizational context of nursing practice, in F. Davis, ed., *The nursing profession: five sociological essays.* New York: Wiley, pp. 109–137.

McCloskey, J. 1974. Influence of rewards and incentives on staff nurse turnover rate. *Nursing Research* 23: 239–247.

McGreevy, M., and M. Coates. 1980. Primary nursing implementation using the project nurse and nursing process framework. *Journal of Nursing Administration* 10(2): 9–15.

Mech, A., M. Mills, and B. Arnold. 1984. Wage and hour laws. *Journal of Nursing Administration* 14(3): 24–25.

Mercer, R. 1987. Solution to nursing shortage involves a change in hospitals' view of nurses. *Modern Healthcare* 17(25): 60.

Mobley, W. 1982. *Employee turnover: causes, consequences and control.* Reading, MA: Addison-Wesley.

Mobley, W., S. Horner, and A. Hollingsworth. 1978. An evaluation of precursors of hospital employee turnover. *Journal of Applied Psychology* 63: 408–414.

Mowday, R., L. Porter, and R. Steers. 1982. *Employee organization linkages: the psychology of commitment, absenteeism and turnover.* New York: Academic Press.

Myers, L., S. Schroeder, S. Chapman, et al. 1984. What's so special about special care? *Inquiry* 21: 103–127.

National Center for Health Services Research. 1987. *Project Nurse (Nurse Utilization Requirements For Staffing Effectiveness): an exploratory study.* Washington, DC: National Center for Health Services Research.

Naughton, T., and D. Outcalt. 1988. Development and test of an occupational taxonomy based on job characteristics theory. *Journal of Vocational Behavior* 32: 16–36.

Near, J., R. Rice, and R. Hunt. 1980. The relationships between work and nonwork domains: a review of empirical research. *Academy of Management Review* 5: 415–429.

Nursing Administration Quarterly. 1981. On the scene: Beth Israel Hospital. *Nursing Administration Quarterly* 5(3): 1–39.

Overton, P., R. Schneck, and C. Hazlett. 1977. An empirical study of the technology of nursing sub-units. *Administrative Science Quarterly* 22: 203–219.

Penny, M. 1988. Recruitment and retention of nurses in critical care. *Nursing Management* 19(2): 72R.

Peterson, M. 1985. Attitudinal differences among work shifts: what do they reflect? *Academy of Management Journal* 28: 723–732.

Pietrofesa, J., and H. Splete. 1975. *Career development: theory and research.* New York: Grune & Stratton.

Popovich, P., and I. Wanous. 1982. The realistic job preview as persuasive communication. *Academy of Management Review* 7: 570–578.

Prescott, P., and T. Langford. 1981. Supplemental agency nurses and hospital staff nurses. What are the differences? *Nursing and Health Care* 2: 200–206.

Price, J., and C. Mueller. 1986. *Absenteeism and turnover of hospital employees.* Greenwich, CT: JAI Press.

Quintana, J., S. Hernandez, and C. Haddock. 1988. Technology and task design: an assessment in hospital nursing units. *Academy of Management Best Paper Proceedings.* Anaheim, CA: Academy of Management, pp. 90–94.

Robinson, J. 1988. Hospital competition and hospital nursing. *Nursing Economics* 6: 116–120.

Roedel, R., and P. Nystrom. 1988. Nursing jobs and satisfaction. *Nursing Management* 19(2): 34–37.

Rowland, H., and B. Rowland, eds. 1984. *Hospital management: a guide to departments.* Rockville, MD: Aspen, pp. 99–194.

Sandrick, K. 1985. Pricing nursing services. *Hospitals.* 59(21): 75–78.

Schoonhoven, C. 1981. Problems with contingency theory: testing assumptions hidden within the language of contingency 'theory.' *Administrative Science Quarterly* 26: 349–377.

Seyboldt, J. 1983. Dealing with premature employee turnover. *California Management Review* 25(3): 107–117.

Shikiar, R., and R. Freudenberg. 1982. Unemployment rates as a moderator of the job dissatisfaction: turnover relation. *Human Relations* 35: 845–856.

Shukla, R. 1981. Structure vs. people in primary nursing: an inquiry. *Nursing Research* 30: 236–241.

Shukla, R. 1982. Nursing care structure and productivity. *Hospital and Health Services Administration* 27(6): 45–58.

Shukla, R. 1983. All-RN model of nursing care delivery: a cost-benefit evaluation. *Inquiry* 20(2): 173–184.

Shukla, R., and W. Turner. 1984. Patient's perception of care under primary and team nursing: revisited. *Research in Nursing Health* 7(2): 83–89.

Sigmon, P. 1981. Clinical ladders and primary nursing: the wedding of the two. *Nursing Administration Quarterly* 5(3): 63–67.

Sloan, F., and R. Elnicki. 1980. Nurse staffing in hospitals. *Industrial Relations* 19: 15–33.

Sovie, M. 1983. Fostering professional nursing career in hospitals: the role of staff development, part 2. *Journal of Nursing Administration* 13: 30–33.

Sovie, M., and T. Smith. 1986. Pricing the nursing product. *Nursing Economics* 4: 216–226.

Spitzer, R. 1981. Alternatives in hospital nursing, in J. McCloskey and G. Helen, eds., *Current issues in nursing*. Boston: Blackwell, pp. 241–250.

Stamps, P., and E. Piedmonte. 1986. Nurses and work satisfaction. Ann Arbor, MI: Health Administration Press.

Stanton, M., J. Laughlin, and C. Wheeler. 1983. Do extended shifts satisfy nurses more? *Nursing Management* 14(10): 49–52.

Staw, B. 1984. Organizational behavior: a review and reformulation of the field's outcome variables. *Annual Review of Psychology* 35: 627–666.

Stone, E. 1978. *Research methods in organizational behavior*. Santa Monica, CA: Goodyear.

Stone, E. 1986. Job scope-job satisfaction and job scope-job performance relationships, in E. Locke, ed., *Generalizing from laboratory to field settings*. Lexington, MA: Lexington Books, pp. 197–206.

Stuart, G. 1983. Nursing role satisfaction: a study of nursing and nursing education. Washington, DC: Institute of Medicine.

Styskal, R. 1980. Power and commitment in organizations: a test of the participation thesis. *Social Forces* 58: 325–343.

Tammelleo, A., ed. 1985. When the "agency's nurse" becomes "hospital employee." *Regan Report on Nursing Law* 26(4): 2.

Taylor, M., and M. Covaleski. 1985. Predicting nurses turnover and internal transfer behavior. *Nursing Research* 34: 237–241.

Thompson, D. 1981. Supplemental staffing: can it be cost effective? *Hospitals* 55(6): 74–77.

Thompson, J. 1967. *Organizations in action*. New York: McGraw-Hill.

Thompson, J. 1984. The measurement of nursing intensity. *Health Care Financing Review* 6(suppl.): 47–55.

Thompson, J., and D. Diers. 1985. DRGs and nursing intensity. *Nursing and Health Care* 6: 435–439.

Thompson, P., G. Dalton, and R. Price. 1977. The four stages of professional careers—a new look at performance by professionals. *Organizational Dynamics* 6(1): 19–42.

Trivedi, V. 1982. Measurement of task delegations among nurses by nominal group process analysis. *Medical Care* 20: 154–164.

Trivedi, V. 1984. Substitution among nurses: its impact on charge nurses' perceptions of quality of care. *Health Care Management Review* 9(3): 59–65.

Vaughan, R., and V. MacLeod. 1980. Nurse staffing studies: no need to reinvent the wheel. *Journal of Nursing Administration* 10(3): 9–15.

Weisman, C., C. Alexander, and G. Chase. 1980. Job satisfaction among hospital nurses: a longitudinal study. *Health Services Research* 15: 341–364.

Weisman, C., C. Alexander, and G. Chase. 1981. Determinants of hospital staff nurse turnover. *Medical Care* 19: 431–443.

Wieland, G. 1969. Studying and measuring nursing turnover. *International Journal of Nursing Studies* 6: 61–70.

Wieland, G., and R. Ullrich. 1981. Changing organizational structures, in G. Wieland, ed., *Improving health care management*. Ann Arbor, MI: Health Administration Press, pp. 209–265.

Wiener, Y., and Y. Vardi. 1980. Relationships betwen job, organization, and career commitments and work outcomes: an integrative approach. *Organizational Behavior and Human Performance* 26: 81–96.

York, C., and D. Fecteau. 1987. Innovative models for professional nursing practice. *Nursing Economics* 5: 162–166.

*Chapter 6*

# Controlling Work

---

> ...controlling the performance of highly skilled technical and professional employees appears contingent on the degree to which organizations can mediate the tensions between the professionals' values, attitudes, and beliefs and the organization's bureaucratic authority and hierarchical control systems.

> (Von Glinow 1983, 73)

The ultimate objective in designing any organization is to increase the fit among tasks, structure, information, decision processes, and reward systems for the purpose of controlling the performance of people (Galbraith 1977). The hospital and its subunits are no exception. On the basis of theory and information presented in the preceding chapters, we can state the following assumptions about hospitals: (1) The operational control system is linked to strategic decision-making, (2) operative value systems influence and are influenced by the staff, (3) client-nursing interaction is a core activity, (4) individual subunits are managed within the existing organization design, and (5) knowledge about career orientation facilitates an understanding of worker motivation. In other words, the organization is both rational and irrational; patient care and service are important; power is dispersed; authority flows up and down; managerial options are present; and an awareness of careers can help leaders achieve organizational goals.

# Trends

Five recent trends in American business are affecting the direction and management of control systems: a convergence of public and professional control, the replacement of rigid reporting systems and narrow productivity projects with sophisticated control systems, the fusion of micro and macro designs, a redefinition of control mechanisms, and an awareness that the personality of executives and managers influences the choice and use of control mechanisms.

## Convergence of Public and Professional Control

In health care the convergence of public and professional control has resulted primarily from increased public financing of medical care. Legislators and bureaucrats cannot simply rely on the word of providers that the public is receiving good value for its health care money when taxes pay for large and increasing expenses. Twenty-five percent of the U.S. population receive Medicare or Medicaid benefits. Outlays of the Health Care Financing Administration, which funds Medicare and Medicaid, are the third highest federal expense after Social Security and defense (Davis 1981). It is therefore understandable that officials require justification that hospitalization was necessary, that the length of stay was appropriate, that the reimbursement did not encourage undertreatment or overtreatment, and that the expenditures were compatible with prevailing views of social justice. External control mechanisms such as utilization review, accreditation standards, and external peer review processes require executives and managers and professionals to take a public perspective and also requires officials to become more knowledgeable about the impact of clinical practices (Scott 1982).

As a rule, governments prefer to control organizations through accounting and statistical systems rather than by interfering with internal arrangements. In a national political climate in which centralized budgeting (per capita reimbursement) is not yet feasible, the continuing need to exert public control over costs is causing governments to overcome this traditional reluctance. The implementing of diagnosis related groups (DRGs), a clinically based measure for prospective payment of Medicare services, is a good example. Prospective payment has altered the traditional managerial role of protecting hospital workers from the outside environment. Managers are experimenting with ways to control practice patterns, and clinicians are involved in designing and implementing better systems for the control of other practitioners' work. This interdependence of managers and professionals will increase as both regulation and competitive pressures increase.

A paradox of the American health care system is that, as a result of trying to preserve fee-for-service medicine for physician and hospital services, providers may now have less autonomy in their treatment of individual patients than before. When outlays are fixed in advance with agreement on the volume of services, governments have less interest in multiple decentralized controls over admissions, discharges, and daily costs. Therefore, controls on the determinants of overall cost (i.e., length of stay, number of admissions, and even cost per case) are less necessary than in a system without fixed outlays.

Present reimbursement systems encourage hospital administrators to increase the patient census to cover fixed costs (or to increase the flow of discretionary revenue once fixed costs have been covered) and hold administrators accountable for many hospital costs over which they cannot exercise effective control. As a result, the three variables that can be managed at the hospital level—resources per case, resource efficiency, and unit prices—are not being adequately controlled, while at the same time the hospital is penalized for adverse changes in its case mix, over which it has far less control (Young and Saltman 1985). This, of course, violates a basic ground rule that individuals should not be held accountable for costs over which they have no control. The danger is that managers under pressure will pass this defect along to the internal control systems.

**Increased Sophistication of Control Systems.** Rigid reporting systems and narrow productivity projects are increasingly being replaced with sophisticated methods of control of the support and core departments, in consultation with them.[1] There is a general acceptance of the principle that an ongoing system will require shared control and acceptance. Productivity is more than the combined skill composition of the workers. "Teaching nurses some management" is a simplistic approach to improving productivity. Since departments are to a large extent interdependent, effectiveness is constrained by the performance of the weakest group. Therefore, control throughout the organization is necessary. Programmed control systems, even for narrowly defined problems, should involve those who will be affected in the design and implementation of the system.

## Fusion of Macro and Micro Designs

A fusion of macro (executive-level) and micro (work unit-level) is more apparent. The tidy separation between the structure at the top of the health care organization and the design of jobs at the bottom of it has diminished (Cummings 1982). Traditional theorists assumed that important information went from the top down and that authority also went down, not up or sideways. The two accepted elements of the control process were a measurable standard and a method for comparing results and changes to correct deviations from standards. These theories were always difficult to apply to hospitals, as hospitals do not have the same kind of line and staff relationships or the task structures that characterized the organizations that inspired the theories. Since professionals are able to exert considerable power to forestall, modify, or subvert industrial engineering or accounting control systems, managers in professional organizations such as hospitals are successful when workers believe that organizational, professional, and personal goals are essentially in harmony.

Changes in both the business and hospital sectors have blurred the distinctions between them. Executives and managers in private industry have learned that production-type controls were ineffective when the number of educated workers with specialized knowledge increased. (Hydebrand foresaw this in 1973 when he called the hospital the prototype of modern work organizations.) In hospitals, the introduction of a measurable standard, the DRGs, enabled executives and managers to measure and compare clinical department performance.

Even so, costs per DRG are not an objective standard like those calculated in industry. Managers must rely on clinicians to make a diagnosis, assign patients an acuity level, and allocate services among patients. This reliance on core staff to provide the input into the control system requires honesty, accuracy, and trust. Disenfranchised, disgruntled, and dissatisfied workers can effectively sabotage control systems. As a result, hospital executives and general managers find themselves less able to distance themselves from the various clinical departments, including nursing.

## Redefinition of Control Mechanisms

Organizational control activities are being given a broader definition than before. Some theorists are using such terms as "feedback" and "information systems" in their definitions of control systems (Dunbar 1981). A major control theory defined control as "any process in which a person or group of persons or organization of persons determines...the behavior of another person, group, organization." (Tannenbaum 1968, 5). Related concepts are power, participation, motivation, leadership, and peer group influence. Much of the management literature in organization behavior acknowledges that encouragement of worker participation is essentially a control mechanism that can substitute for more direct methods, such as negotiation and pay for work performed (Dachler and Wilpert 1978; Kerr and Slocum 1981). This is true in spite of the fact that human relations advocates often avoid explicit reference to social power and its connotations of conflict and authoritarianism.

Organizations depend on training of staff members to facilitate consensus on subjective factors and client complaints. According to Ouchi (1977), a noted expert in the field, real control comes only through changing worker behaviors by selectively rewarding specific outputs. This is most easily accomplished when the training department prepares employees who perform tasks homogeneously and use common scales and language. Ouchi's view of organization behavior as a social control mechanism is not always explicit. Expert practitioners acknowledge that organizational success and survival depend on meeting the organizational needs of employers through worker involvement. Organizational expense on employee development activities is not justified to improve worker satisfaction apart from performance. Appropriate targets for organization development are those areas where individual and organizational goals coincide. Success depends on individualizing rewards to match employer preferences.

Viewing organization development as a control system helps explain why it has had such a difficult time gaining acceptance in hospitals where linkages are weak among governance, tasks, and professional systems (Weisbord 1981). Organization development, as a control system, competes with the accepted professional control system, which has its own tasks, scales and language norms, sanctions, and rewards. In most organization development activities, rewards and the technical and substantive content of the occupation are lost because the emphasis is on managerial or psychosocial concerns. Professionals frequently find training less than credible or irrelevant and manage to subvert organization development activities, even if they do not feel that they are being manipulated by management as the detractors of organization development state.

## Influence of Managers' Personal Attributes

There is an increasing awareness that personal preferences for control mechanisms reflect not only organizational policy and subordinate behavior but also the personal attributes of executives and managers in areas such as leadership (assigning responsibility) and motivation (appealing to self-interest; Kelley and Michela 1980; De Vader, Bateson, and Lord 1986).

The attribution framework for understanding punishment (Podsakoff 1982) suggests that leaders punish workers more for poor performance when they perceive it as resulting from lack of motivation than from lack of ability or task difficulty (Martinko and Gardner 1987). This framework further proposes that supervisors are more likely to punish workers when poor performance is perceived to result from lack of motivation rather than lack of ability or task difficulty. That is, the motivation and perceptions of supervisors may be at least as important for understanding reciprocal expectations and control mechanisms as the motivation of workers.

For example, nursing supervisors disproportionately attribute improperly performed nursing procedures and nonmedical incidents to internal causes, such as a poor work history, rather than external causes, especially when there was a serious outcome. In practice, interventions should focus on the improper behavior, not the seriousness of the outcome in a particular case or past lateness or absenteeism (Mitchell, Green, and Wood 1981).

Sexual biases also play a role in understanding controls. For example, if a task is labeled as feminine, one in which women will excel, it may be perceived as easier to perform (Deaux 1976). Further, if performance is inconsistent with expectations, it may be explained by "ability" if the performer is male, "luck" if female.

Individuals have differing views about the relative importance of individual personalities, the role of the supervisor, and organization policies and procedures. Research suggests that (1) group participation is becoming increasingly important, (2) people with different personalities interpret social influences differently, (3) supervision moderates the effects of technology in relation to the structure, and (4) neither personal factors of workers nor the organizational situation separately explain attitudes or behavior as well as the two together (Blass 1977; Peterson 1983; Hrebiniak 1974).

# Premises

The control system for hospitals is best seen as an integrative device that helps management meet conflicting demands (Khandwalla 1973). This view incorporates two essential premises: (1) a need for management direction and constructive purpose, and (2) a deemphasis of control as manipulation and domination.

There are three basic premises in designing control systems. First, operational control is more effective when desired behavioral sequences are certain to occur and the organization is certain to achieve its desired status (Dunbar 1981). The problem with this proposition is that different constituencies have different goals, the goals may change, and the relative importance of continuing goals may change. A control system tightly tied to identifiable goals may blind executives and managers to changing situations. There is a delicate balance between the need to tie control systems to goals and the need to remain flexible and avoid being overly specific about goals.

A second premise is that control systems do not exist in isolation. Instead, they reflect and perpetuate the prevailing cultural views on worker participation, other values, and strategic plans. Control systems for professionals and highly skilled technicians need to match professional needs, which include attention to maintenance of professional expertise, ethics, collegial maintenance of standards, autonomy, commitment to calling, and peer expectations (Von Glinow 1983).

Third, there is no best control system. Instead, control systems are fragmented, complex, and specialized. They are also constrained by other design choices that have already been made. In hospitals, these include policies concerning nurse-physician relations. Nurses' job satisfaction and productivity cannot be optimized without some control of physician behavior. In a 1987 study, Cox found that 82% of nurses and 77% of directors of nursing service reported verbal abuse by physicians. This abuse accounted for 18% of the turnover among the sample of 1,100 nurses.

Physicians and nurses are fundamentally bonded by their responsibility to address patients' multiple needs. Each of the two professions contributes special knowledge, although in the usual case the physician has greater control over the dissemination and delegation of new knowledge and technology. Nurses have the advantage of a continuing relationship with the patient and the power that comes from being an organizational authority. In spite of this, it is sometimes difficult for nurses to establish a collegial relationship with physicians. Aside from historical female deference to male authority, disparities in income and education separate them. Management has a fundamental obligation to forbid and punish rude and threatening behavior on the part of physicians, just as it forbids and punishes such behavior among its own employees.

If the objective is to reduce the power imbalance between physicians and nurses, then the strategy needs to reduce the social distance between the two in society at large—by promoting more education, use of credentials, and higher income for nurses. This will not guarantee collaboration based on mutual respect, but, given societal values, it is a necessary accompaniment. A less ambitious measure to balance power is the formation of joint committee memberships to deal with shared problems, for example in the areas of quality assurance and continuing education.

## Types

Control systems are based on the monitoring and evaluation of either behavior or output or both. Since performance measures apply only to what can be measured, not the full range of desired outcomes, executives and managers, even in fields where output is easy to measure, design other modes of control. Control systems range from programmed to unprogrammed arrangements to help managers monitor and evaluate performance—to know what is going on. Programmed or impersonal controls include the reporting system (hierarchy), inventory control, auditing, scheduling, task directives, and budgeting. They aim to control uncertainties. The prerequisites for control by formalizing tasks or relying on procedure manuals are that the tasks are predictable and the workers have complete knowledge of the guidelines. Often, tasks and work flow cannot be completely controlled by management; the use of line authority and social (unprogrammed) control then becomes necessary.

Unprogrammed controls include self-control, professional control, and the informal controls that come from task design or group norms. These controls are appropriate when the tasks are too ill-defined or variable to use programmed ones. Organizations need and use both programmed and unprogrammed systems. The former tend to emphasize economics; the latter stem from sociology and psychology. Both arise out of external requirements, organizational values, strategies, and the nature of the work.

A hierarchy of social controls available to managers has been identified by Kerr and Slocum (1981) and Simpson (1985). Role clarification—who does what within the work system—is basic. This explains the universal emphasis on current job descriptions. Beyond role clarification is goal setting, in which supervisors clarify work expectations with employees. The next level involves the leadership structure, feedback, and "stroking" given to individuals. The final and more diffuse options for social control are participative leadership and the administration of punishment and rewards.

Supervisors are advised to choose carefully the approach that best suits their situation. There needs to be consistency between the choice and managerial style; if a manager makes all important decisions without involving subordinates, it would be a mistake to use an internal motivation approach. The control system should also match the culture, structure, and reward system of the organization. The reliability of job performance appraisals determines whether a tight external evaluation and reward system is appropriate. Finally, the supervisor's assessment of employees' career anchors and motivations is important in deciding what incentives employees will respond to.

## Nursing Department

Three primary domains or obligations within the nursing department need control: patient care (quality), system maintenance (productivity), and human resource management (career enhancement). As shown in Table 6-1, each domain is related to core functions. The patient care domain functions are quality assurance for individual patients and accountability to social standards. The system maintenance domain involves adapting to external changes, containing costs, and obtaining resources. The human resource management domain includes the functions of integrating workers into the system and managing the socialization process for all career styles.

### Patient Care Domain—Quality

In addition to meeting organizational goals, patient care preserves social values that ensure ongoing public legitimacy. Nurses are expected to both staff the department and assist in conserving the organization's resources so as to ensure its continuing existence.

**Table 6-1** Control Activities by Function

| Nursing Domain | Domain Function | Programmed | Nonprogrammed |
|---|---|---|---|
| Patient Care | Quality assurance<br>Preserve social<br>  values | Incident reports<br>Client feedback<br>Evaluation studies<br>  (ANA, NLN)<br>Accreditation<br>  (JCAHO)<br>State codes | Peer review<br><br>Laissez-faire<br>Concurrent<br>Retrospective |
| System<br>maintenance | Environmental<br>  adaptation<br>Contain costs<br>Attract resources | Formal structure<br>  and reporting<br>  relationships<br>Utilization review<br>Budget<br>Case-mix<br>  accounting<br>Management by<br>  objectives<br>Management<br>  information systems | Spontaneous<br>  interaction<br>Cooperation<br>Suppression<br>Professional<br>  Self<br><br>Task<br>Peers<br>  Individuals<br>  Group |
| Human resource<br>  management | Integration of<br>  professionals<br>Organizational<br><br>  socialization | Position control<br>Job analyses<br>Job description/<br>  role<br>Performance<br>  evaluation<br>Staffing analysis | Career<br>  management<br>  system<br><br>(Disaggregated) |

**Programmed Systems.** The programmed control systems for patient care include incident reports and routinized patient satisfaction surveys. In addition, each state has continuing education requirements. Evaluation guides for continuing education are provided by the National League of Nursing and the American Nurses' Association (ANA). The ANA standards are generally supported by the Joint Commission on Accreditation of Health Organizations (JCAHO)[2].The JCAHO standards have great influence in equalizing nursing care throughout the United States as they require acuity-based staffing, performance-based job descriptions, and proof of continuing education. In states where the public health codes specify staffing standards, nursing administrators are expected to concurrently evaluate and assess the needs of patients as well as the capabilities of the nursing staff assigned to the unit. This legal responsibility acts to enhance the power, authority, and influence of the nursing service administrator.

Increasingly, as hospitals are held responsible for the quality of care, the nursing department is formalizing the credentialing process to delineate practice privileges and differentiate between levels of practice. (A prime example is St. Mary's Hospital and Health Center in Tucson, Arizona, where there are four defined competency levels with commensurate salaries and a peer review system to oversee the credentialing process. This is combined with a patient acuity billing system based on eight levels of patient classification.) In many hospitals, education, experience, references, license, professional memberships, and practice history are being more rigorously evaluated before a nurse is assigned to specific units and authorized to perform specific procedures than in the past.

**Nonprogrammed Systems.** Peer review is the primary form of nonprogrammed control for nursing. Among the several forms of peer review, the laissez-faire dependence on professionals to provide feedback on quality results is less acceptable today since it is not compatible with professional or accreditation requirements. Four reasons have been given for not depending on audits, feedback, and continuing education to improve quality: (1) Treatment deficiencies stem from inadequate application of knowledge, not inadequate knowledge; (2) feedback is often obtained too late to effect change; (3) participation in continuing education is voluntary, and those who attend sessions may not be the ones with the greatest need; and (4) education may not be relevant to the deficiencies that exist (Scott 1982).

Despite the difficulties with peer review, federally mandated peer review organizations have based their guidelines on the principles of retrospective chart review, comparisons with standards, and feedback. To be effective, the regulatory approach should be limited to situations where outcomes are related to individual actions and where the professionals are subject to control by mutual adjustment (Scott 1982).

Control of quality through concurrent review (review while the patient is still under care) depends on mutual adjustment. The theory of mutual adjustment has been developed for application to professional work where discretion must be preserved to deal with unpredictable events. Nurses advocate the use of concurrent review as part of a quality assurance program.

Since concurrent review provides opportunities for alternative placement and services for the patient, it can be a primary tool to integrate clinical and organizational decision-making; such integration is a desirable goal. Nurses are encouraged to review placement and treatment alternatives that will be appropriate for the health needs of the patient. When this function is supported by the administration and linked with the medical staff, both quality control and cost-effectiveness are enhanced. The opportunity for dialogue among both providers and managers encourages understanding of the difficult cost trade-offs that are necessary. This dialogue, in turn, stimulates clinical workers to propose alternative solutions that can foster both care and cost-effectiveness.

In the new environment, in which hospitals will increasingly be competing on the basis of quality, managers will pay more attention to the quality assurance system to identify where investments are needed. One method is to inventory the various quality measures available in separate departments and post charts comparing clinical units' performance with that of other units and their own past performance. One targeted investment that is needed is in training; another is a differential reward system based on the principle that better performers merit increased pay, promotion, or special commendation. Differential rewards will be accepted more readily by providers when they can see that they are tied to quality enhancement.

## System Maintenance Domain—Productivity

**Programmed Systems.** Programmed control systems for maintaining the organization include formal reporting relationships, utilization review, budgeting based on case-mix accounting, management by objectives (MBO), and management information systems.

Programmed control theory suggests that nursing costs should be measured on the basis of severity of patient illness and that a mechanism should be developed to price nursing services separately from the room charge, so that there can be variable billing among patients. The goal is to provide a picture of the cost of treating patients in comparable disease classes depending on the use of resources (Thompson, Fetter, and Averill 1980). Nursing administration would then be able to use standard financial planning techniques to plan, control, and evaluate nursing as a profit center.

The attractiveness of this method goes beyond increased productivity. According to this approach, "today, nursing would be a cost center; tomorrow, a revenue generating center; next, role clarification and purification as nurses become valued therapeutic commodities; eventually, appreciation of the need for extremely sophisticated nurse clinicians to maximize the progress of select patients; finally, nurses as independently contracted professionals in hospitals" (Joel 1984, 6).

This departure from previous methods of determining nursing costs (i.e., nursing hours per patient-day or FTEs per occupied bed) is controversial and debated among nurses, managers, and policy analysts. The New Jersey Department of Health has conducted studies on allocating nursing costs. From these studies, relative intensity measures (RIMs) have been developed. The use and effects of these have been debated but remain speculative (Grimaldi and Micheletti 1982; Caterinicchio 1983; Ganong and Ganong 1984). Recent data indicating that New Jersey prospective payments to hospitals exceed Medicare reimbursements in other states have already caused concern among Health Care Financing Administration (HCFA) officials.

To accomplish resource-based costing internally, five systems need to be developed: belief, patient classification, staffing, billing, and auditing (Van Slyck 1982). The necessary belief system is one that holds that revenues should be assigned to the department incurring the corresponding costs. That is, there should be no cross subsidy, with one department contributing more to revenues than another. Once this belief system is shared, a patient classification system needs to be developed in order to define and determine the costs of nursing care. Based on the patient classification, the appropriate staffing mix should be developed. Then, patient care costs can be determined based on nursing salaries, fringe benefits, overhead, and contribution to surplus for each activity level. The fifth system is the auditing system, which verifies the accuracy of the documentation, distribution by classification, staffing levels, and quality of care.

Few hospitals are currently able to implement such systems, but some are and more will in the future, according to experts in the field (Lindner and Wagner 1983; American Hospital Association 1985). At Strong Memorial Hospital in Rochester, New York, where nursing became a revenue center instead of a cost center in 1981, the results were improved productivity, more accurate staffing, better budget monitoring and control, and better patient assignment. The study also indicated that DRGs were not predictive of nursing care needs (Sovie et al. 1985; Department of Health and Human Services 1988).[3]

The Division of Nursing at the Department of Health and Human Services is developing a means of identifying nursing costs and revenues (Department of Health and Human Services 1987a, b; 1988b). Participants at a national invitational conference on costing of hospital services convened by the Division of Nursing in 1987 considered several related issues. A consensus exists that patient needs should determine nursing resources, that costing methodologies must be precise, that nursing services must be separated from hospital room and board charges, and that nursing departments should use their patient classification and staffing systems to develop a costing system.

Progress will be hastened if the HCFA incorporates measures of nursing intensity in its prospective payment system. Thompson (1987), who performed the seminal research on DRGs, presented new findings at the conference. He believes that it is possible to encompass variations in nursing intensity in a prospective payment system, with one for routine care and one for special care, and that the measurements made were consistent with clinical judgments. At this time, however, the measurements do not reflect the precision necessary to form the basis for a payment system. Thompson's findings about the relationship between nursing resource utilization (total nursing minutes) and length of stay were generally consistent with the pilot study conducted earlier by the American Nurses' Association (ANA 1985).

The paradigm appropriate for MBO management has shifted from a goal-driven model (management by objectives) to a resource-driven one (Stevens 1985). The contrasting steps are shown in Table 6-2.

Instead of setting goals, the manager must first assess resource availability. The manager then determines the feasible number of goals and the methods to achieve them, rather than deciding how to achieve goals first and then procuring resources. With both methods implementation is followed by evaluation.

The last major programmed method for controlling the system maintenance domain is the health management information system. In Chapter 4, the El Camino medical information system was described. The literature does not give many other examples of using information systems to improve productivity, although an awareness exists that the potential is untapped (Walters and Lincoln 1987).

**Table 6-2**  Operational Steps: MBO and Resource-Driven.

| MBO | Resource-Driven |
|---|---|
| Set the goals. | Assess the resources. |
| Decide how to achieve the goals. | Determine a feasible number of goals. |
| Procure the resources. | Determine the methods. |
| Implement the plan. | Implement the plan. |
| Evaluate success in attainment of goals. | |

Source: Developed from *The nurse as executive*, 3rd ed., by B.J. Stevens, with permission of Aspen Publishers, Inc.© 1985.

**Nonprogrammed Systems.** In a healthy organization, the nonprogrammed control systems that are essential for organizational performance and survival are meshed to a considerable extent with the professional control system. Control of nonclinical activities is characterized by spontaneous interaction among staff members, the relative primacy of cooperation rather than suppression, and professional surveillance. Professional monitoring occurs at several levels: task, individual, and group. Work arrangements, patients, and tasks arising from the patients' problems also exert control over workers. Individual self-control results from the long period of professional education and indoctrination. Peers control one another by one-on-one interaction and through group interaction.

Formal authority systems need to account for the fact that supervisors frequently give advice based on technical knowledge and principles of practice; subordinates take such advice seriously but retain the prerogative to reject it if they cannot justify it on the basis of facts. A superb technique for accomplishing work satisfaction and quality practice is to provide feedback about client outcomes.

To ensure interdepartmental cooperation, managers who have primary responsibility for supplying materials must remain aware of organizational levels. As a simple example, the change from treatment trays set up on the ward to disposable trays created wide-reaching effects. This innovation, which occurred throughout the system 25 years ago, changed how nurses spent their time and also standardized supply use. It is appropriate for managers to identify those areas close to the basic work that could benefit, not necessarily from changed professional control, but from better support systems. Support systems that constrain opportunities for delay, error, or waste may have more impact than the nursing model (Shukla 1981).

## Human Resource Management—Career Enhancement

**Programmed Systems.** Programmed methods for managing careers include position control, job analysis, job description, performance appraisal, and wage and salary administration. If done properly, these combined activities lead to a rational alignment of jobs that workers and managers both perceive as equitable. These activities are usually presented as objective technical systems with codified techniques, although there is a large subjective component in each step of the technique. Tensions between internal equity and external equity are resolved in a manner consistent with the relative power of competing groups. If a shortage of workers exists, or if the workers are unified, managers will make adjustments by upgrading job descriptions or ignoring the market. Affirmative action and the thrust for social equity are making these previously internal activities subject to scrutiny and justification.

The trend toward differentiated practice has focused attention on developing job descriptions for ADN and BSN nurses based on the education competency statements developed by the Western Interstate Commission for Higher Education (1986). Model hospital job descriptions for new ADN and BSN graduates are presented in Appendix 6A. The persistent underlying problem of job descriptions is that they are based on competencies deduced primarily from beliefs and theories about what constitutes effective practice rather than from studies of actual effective practice based on patients' outcome (Gordon 1986). Although this is true of all health occupations, and nursing should not be held to a higher standard than other professions, it remains a problem. Another trend favors performance management rather than performance appraisal. At Presbyterian Intercommunity Hospital in Whittier, California, primary nursing has been combined with departmental decentralization, a performance evaluation system for supervisory personnel, and a method of collecting operations data from each unit (Johnson and Luciano 1983). (Refer to Appendix 6B for a performance summary evaluation form for RN Level I and RN Level II.) Some key elements were that departmental performance indicators were chosen by department heads and supervisors, counseling and coaching of supervisors occurred during the implementation phase, and a merit pay system was established. The performance indicators were attendance, employee turnover, patient-days, salary expense per patient-day, quality assurance compliance, medication error rate, budget variance, and productivity. The appraisal process for supervisors consists of comparing performance against expectations, determining levels of performance reached, and providing performance feedback. Supervisors appraise their own performance monthly; this self-appraisal is followed by formal semiannual and annual reviews.

**Nonprogrammed Systems.** The nonprogrammed method for managing human resources, the career management system, permeates the selection, placement, mentoring, and promotional system. Its purpose is to meet individual career needs for job enhancement or personal enhancement on the job and to relate these needs to the future requirements of the organization. The program should reflect both short- and long-term needs by creating a system that is integrated with existing personnel and supervisory activities. This system is not necessarily a department or even a list of specified activities but a philosophy that pervades the organization. The first step in implementation is an assessment and clarification of managerial attitudes toward career issues (Burack 1983).

Once managers have reached a consensus about career definition and importance, they can develop policies to match career activities with current and future work force needs. This step will stimulate a review of formal personnel activities and job redesign potentials. Several self-assessment tools are available through training departments to assist in determining worker preferences. If the organization is large or can work with other hospitals, formal assessment center programs can be obtained from private consultants. Developing individual career plans not only enlightens managers about the career interests and potentials of workers, but also encourages workers to assess their own potential, limitations, and training needs. The self-selection process prevents many of the problems of unrealistic expectations that managers fear.

As workers develop individual plans, managers have an opportunity to clarify the options and routes available to the workers. Assuming that the hospital is concerned with developing a select core of experienced RNs who will stay in bedside nursing, several activities related to nurses can be highlighted. Among these are:

- Personally tailored reorientation after a leave for personal reasons.

- Rehire at current level upon return from a leave of absence

- Formal system for assignment to other clinical areas

- Extra pay for competence in more than one clinical area

- Opportunity to mentor other nurses

- Participation with physicians in setting and monitoring quality standards

- Guarantee of job security after a specified number of years of above-average performance

- Involvement in administrative activities relating to patient care, training of nursing assistants, and working conditions

- Clinical appointments recognized by the medical staff

- Problem-solving groups to identify, analyze, choose, and implement solutions to problems that influence the quality of care.

Each hospital has unique problems and opportunities that will modify the shape and specifics of the career program. The overriding issue is to develop disaggregated strategies that workers with steady-state, linear, or spiral orientations can perceive and trust. The emphasis on work strategies fostering part-time work and flexible hours needs to be counterbalanced with strategies to attract and retain steady-state and linear nurses.

Career satisfaction for steady-state individuals will be enhanced by a work environment in which professional work is held in high esteem by the employer and is well utilized. Opportunities for personal growth and job challenges that will be valued are those that do not threaten job security. Further, the environment should allow for self-determination of practice issues such as timing, work organization, and staffing. By respecting the individual's professional orientation, using control and authority systems advisedly, and encouraging professional and self-control, executives and managers increase the probability of enhancing both quality of care and productivity. Using professional norms and values will minimize the amount of education and surveillance that the organization has to provide.

# Summary

Controlling the performance of people is the ultimate objective of the organizational design process. Five trends are identified as affecting the direction and management of control systems: (1) a convergence of public and professional control in health care generally, (2) an increase in sophisticated control systems (and a decrease in rigid, narrow ones) in both support and core departments, (3) a fusion of business and medical/ professional theories of management, (4) a broadening of the definition of control activities, and (5) an awareness that the influence of managers is reflected in control mechanisms.

After a discussion of control systems as an integrative device that helps management meet conflicting demands, three basic premises are proposed for the design of control systems:

1. Control is more effective when desired behavioral sequences are certain to occur and the organization is certain to achieve its desired state.

2. Control systems do not exist in isolation.

3. Control systems are complex and situational.

Control systems in hospitals are best understood in relation to the three important domains: patient care, system maintenance, and human resource management. For each domain, programmed (impersonal) and nonprogrammed (individualized and personal) control systems are available. In general, programmed arrangements rely on economics whereas unprogrammed arrangements stem from sociology and psychology. Managers need to monitor and evaluate performance using both impersonal and individualized arrangements.

# Endnotes

1. Nursing productivity has traditionally focused on the work load measurement approach, which was discussed in Chapter 5. Rieder and Lensing (1987) provide a good systems model. The more interesting approach to productivity is to consider it an organization-wide phenomenon based on outcome informa-

tion. Fifield's (1988) study is a good beginning based on financial data. As more good data become available, similar studies should simultaneously consider both revenue and patient results.

2. See Stevens (1980) for a comprehensive discussion of quality assurance and the difference between the JCAHO and ANA approaches to nursing audit.

3. See Stevens (1985) for a discussion of nursing resources, pricing, and productivity, and Department of Health and Human Services (1987a, b) for detailed reports on costing hospital nursing services.

# References

American Hospital Association. 1985. *Medicare payment: per case management.* Chicago: American Hospital Association.

American Nurses' Association, Center for Research. 1985. *DRGs and nursing care.* Kansas City, MO: American Nurses' Association.

Blass, T. 1977. *Personality variables in social behavior.* New York: Wiley.

Burack, E. 1983. *Career planning and management.* Lake Forest, IL: Brace-Park.

Caterinicchio, R. P. 1983. A debate: RIMs and the cost of nursing care. *Nursing Management* 14(5): 36–39.

Cox, H. 1987. Verbal abuse in nursing. *Nursing Management* 18(11): 47–50.

Cummings, L. L. 1982. Organizational behavior. *Annual Review of Psychology* 33: 541–579.

Dachler, H. P., and B. Wilpert. 1978. Conceptual dimensions and boundaries of participation in organizations: a critical evaluation. *Administrative Science Quarterly* 23: 1–39.

Davis, C. 1981. *American Nurse* 13(10): 17.

De Vader, C., A. Bateson, and R. Lord. 1986. Attribution theory: a meta-analysis of attributional hypotheses, in E. Locke, ed., *Generalizing from laboratory field settings.* Lexington, MA: Lexington Books.

Deaux, K. 1976. Special case of judgment. *New Directions in Attribution Research* 1: 335–352.

Department of Health and Human Services. 1987a. *Costing hospital nursing services: a review of the literature.* Washington, DC: Government Printing Office.

Department of Health and Human Services. 1987b. *Costing hospital nursing services: report of the conference.* Washington, DC: Government Printing Office.

Department of Health and Human Services. 1988. Minutes of Secretary's Commission on Nursing, March 4, 1988.

Dunbar, R. 1981. Designs for organizational control, in P. Nystrom and W. Starbuck, eds., *Handbook of organizational design,* Vol. 2. Oxford, England: Oxford University Press, pp. 85–115.

Fifield, F. 1988. What is a productivity-excellent hospital? *Nursing Management* 19(4): 32–40.

Galbraith, J. 1977. *Organization design.* Reading, MA: Addison-Wesley.

Ganong, J., and W. Ganong. 1984. *Performance appraisal in perspective.* Rockville, MD: Aspen, pp. 17–21.

Gordon, D. 1986. Models of clinical expertise in American nursing practice. *Social Science and Medicine* 22: 953–961.

Grimaldi, P., and J. Micheletti. 1982. RIMs and the cost of nursing debate. *Nursing Management* 13(12): 12–22.

Heydebrand, W. 1973. *Hospital bureaucracy.* New York: Dunellen.

Hrebiniak, C. 1974. Job technology, supervision, and work group structure. *Administrative Science Quarterly* 19: 395–410.

Joel, L. 1984. DRGs, RIMs have potential to change nursing. *American Nurse* 16(18): 11.

Johnson, J., and K. Luciano. 1983. Managing by behavior and results—linking supervisory accountability to effective organizational control. *Journal of Nursing Administration* 13(12): 19–28.

Kelley, H., and J. Michela. 1980. Attribution theory and research. *Annual Review of Psychology* 31: 457–501.

Kerr, S., and J. Slocum, Jr. 1981. Controlling the performance of people in organizations, in P. Nystrom and W. Starbuck, eds., *Handbook of organizational design,* Vol 2. New York: Oxford University Press, pp. 116–134.

Khandwalla, P. 1973. Effect of competition on the structure of management control. *Academy of Management Journal* 16: 285–295.

Lindner J., and D. Wagner. 1983. DRGs spur management-related groups. *Modern Healthcare* 13: 160–161.

Martinko, M., and W. Gardner. The leader/member attribution process. *Academy of Management Review* 12: 235–248.

Mitchell, T., S. Green, and R. Wood. 1981. An attributional model of leadership and the poor performing subordinate: development and validation. *Research in Organizational Behavior* 3: 197–234.

Ouchi, W. 1977. Control in organizations. *Administrative Science Quarterly* 22: 95–133.

Peterson, M. 1983. Co-workers and hospital staff's work attitudes: individual difference moderators. *Nursing Research* 32: 115–121.

Podsakoff, P. 1982. Determinants of a supervisor's use of rewards and punishments: a literature review and suggestions for further research. *Organizational Behavior and Human Performance* 29: 58–83.

Rieder, K. and S. Lensing. 1987. Nursing productivity: evolution of a systems model. *Nursing Management* 18(8): 33–38.

Scott, W. 1982. Health care organizations in the 1980s: the convergence of public and professional control systems, in A. Johnson, O. Grunsky, and B. Ravich, eds., *Contemporary health services.* Boston: Auburn House, pp. 177–196.

Shukla, R. 1981. Structure vs. people in primary nursing: an inquiry. *Nursing Research* 30: 236–241.

Simpson, R. 1985. Social control of occupations and work. *Annual Review of Sociology* 11: 415–436.

Sovie, M., M. Tarcinale, A. Van Putte, et al. 1985. Amalgam of nursing acuity, DRGs and costs. *Nursing Management* 16(3): 22–42.

Stevens, B. 1980. *The nurse executive.* Wakefield, MA: Nursing Resources, pp. 360–384.

Stevens, B. 1985. *The nurse as executive*, 3rd ed. Rockville, MD: Aspen, pp. 273–289.

Tannenbaum, A. 1968. *Control in organizations*. New York: McGraw-Hill.

Thompson, J. 1987. Nursing research and practice issues of the Nursing Intensity Project, in Department of Health and Human Services, *Costing hospital services: Report of a conference*. Washington, DC: Government Printing Office, pp. 107–134.

Thompson, J., R. Fetter, and R. Averill. 1980. Case-mix accounting: a new management tool, in S. Levey and T. McCarthy, eds., *Health management for tomorrow*. Philadelphia: J. B. Lippincott, pp. 157–174.

Van Slyck, A. 1982. Models of practice: variable charges for nursing care, in *Professionalism and the empowerment of nursing*. Kansas City, MO: American Nurses' Association, pp. 47–57.

Von Glinow, M. 1983. Incentives for controlling the performance of high technology and professional employees. *IEEE Transactions on Systems, Man, and Cybernetics* 13: 70–74.

Walters, R., and T. Lincoln. 1987. Using information tools to improve hospital productivity. *Healthcare Financial Management* 41(8): 74–78.

Weisbord, M. 1981. Why organization development hasn't worked (so far) in medical centers, in G. Weiland, ed., *Improving health care management*. Ann Arbor, MI: Health Administration Press, pp. 266–284.

Western Interstate Commission for Higher Education. 1986. *Associate and baccalaureate degree nursing graduates: perceptions of and recommendations for their preparation and utilization*. Boulder, CO: Western Interstate Commission for Higher Education.

Young, D., and R. Saltman. 1985. *The hospital power equilibrium*. Baltimore: Johns Hopkins Press.

*Appendix 6A*

# Model Hospital Job Descriptions for New Associate Degree and Baccalaureate Degree Graduates

| Qualifications | | As Provider of Care | |
|---|---|---|---|
| **Associate Degree** | **Baccalaureate Degree** | **Associate Degree** | **Baccalaureate Degree** |
| • Graduate of an approved associate degree nursing program. | • Graduate of an approved baccalaureate degree nursing program. | *Performance Description*<br>Assumes responsibility and accountability for providing nursing care for individual clients and their families. | *Performance Description*<br>Assumes responsibility and accountability for providing nursing care for individuals, families, and groups. |
| • Current state licensure, or in process. | • Current state licensure, or in process. | *Performance Criteria*<br>• Collects data according to established protocols. | *Performance Criteria*<br>• Identifies the need to establish protocols. |
| • Mental and physical health sufficient to meet the demands of the position. | • Mental and physical health sufficient to meet the demands of the position. | • Selects/establishes nursing diagnoses. | • Demonstrates health assessment skills. |
| • Personal and professional qualities commensurate with the position as indicated by credible references and interview. | • Personal and professional qualities commensurate with the position as indicated by credible references and interview. | • Consults with appropriate nurses or members of other health disciplines when client problems are not within scope of own practice. | • Establishes nursing diagnoses and plans of care. |
| | | | • Provides direct client care in accordance with nursing diagnoses. |

**Appendix 6A**, continued.

| Qualifications | | As Provider of Care | |
| Associate Degree | Baccalaureate Degree | Associate Degree | Baccalaureate Degree |
| --- | --- | --- | --- |
| | | • Provides direct client care in accordance with nursing diagnoses. | • Collaborates with other health team disciplines in the care of clients. |
| | | • Participates with other health team members in the care of clients. | • Acts as consultant as appropriate. |
| | | • Participates in evaluation of client's response to care. | • Evaluates client's responses to care. |

*Sources of Evidence/Tools:* nursing or progress notes; assessment or admission forms; discharge planning documents; patient care plans; nurse manager documentation (anecdotal notes; interim evaluations); client feedback (oral and written); nursing audits; and protocol documents (some agencies list names of individuals that were involved in the development of the protocol).

**Appendix 6A**, continued.

| As Client Teacher | | As Planner and Coordinator of Client Care | |
|---|---|---|---|
| Associate Degree | Baccalaureate Degree | Associate Degree | Baccalaureate Degree |
| *Performance Description* Develops/implements short-term teaching plans within the context of established comprehensive teaching plans. | *Performance Description* Formulates and implements comprehensive teaching plans which emphasize health promotion, maintenance, and wellness and are based on long- and short-range goals for individual clients, families, and groups. | *Performance Description* Plans care, with guidance, for assigned clients utilizing resources and other nursing personnel. | *Performance Description* Assumes responsibility for planning and coordinating care for a group of clients. |
| *Performance Criteria* | *Performance Criteria* | *Performance Criteria* | *Performance Criteria* |
| • Identifies client's needs for information. | • Assesses learning needs and readiness. | • Assesses nursing care requirements for assigned clients. | • Analyzes nursing care requirements. |
| • Follows established protocols in collecting data relevant to client need. | • Analyzes support systems, existing and needed. | • Determines priorities for assigned clients. | • Determines priorities. |
| • Implements short-term teaching plans. | • Implements comprehensive teaching plans which emphasize health promotion, maintenance, and wellness. | • Contributes to supportive communication and problem-solving. | • Guides and directs group members in the delivery of client care and discharge planning. |
| • Participates in the evaluation of learning. | • Evaluates learning. | • Participates in cost-effective utilization of available resources. | • Demonstrates supportive communication and problem-solving. |
| • Participates in revision of teaching plans. | | | • Promotes cost-effective utilization of available resources. |

Appendix 6A, continued.

| As Client Teacher | | As Planner and Coordinator of Client Care | |
|---|---|---|---|
| Associate Degree | Baccalaureate Degree | Associate Degree | Baccalaureate Degree |
| | • Revises teaching plans as appropriate. | • Participates in identifying need for changes in delivery of nursing care.<br><br>• Seeks guidance as appropriate. | • Participates in evaluation of group members according to established protocol.<br><br>• Participates in changes within the health care delivery system.<br><br>• Assesses learning needs of health care personnel.<br><br>• Makes provisions to meet learning needs of other health care providers. |

*Source of Evidence/Tools*: nursing or progress notes; assessment or admission forms; discharge planning documents; patient care plans; nurse manager documentation (anecdotal notes, interim evaluations); client feedback (oral and written); protocol documents; teaching documentation forms; and interagency referral forms.

*Sources of Evidence/Tools*: nursing or progress notes; patient care plans; nurse manager documentation (anecdotal notes; interim evaluations); client feedback (oral and written); patient acuity level tools; quality assurance audit sheets which reference patient-care conferences; staff assignment sheets (to document assignments as well as cost-effective use of resources); patient charge documents (to document cost-effectiveness; variable charge for nursing care) performance evaluations of other groups' members; peer review; committee minutes and membership lists (to document participation in change process); self-evaluation and reporting of activities; and division and unit in-service records (to document "makes provisions to meet learning needs").

**Appendix 6A**, continued.

| As Communicator | | As Investigator | |
|---|---|---|---|
| **Associate Degree** | **Baccalaureate Degree** | **Associate Degree** | **Baccalaureate Degree** |
| *Performance Description* Establishes and maintains communication with individual clients and their families and health team members. | *Performance Description* Establishes and maintains communication with individual clients, families, groups, and health team members. | *Performance Description* Demonstrates awareness of the value or relevance of research in nursing. | *Performance Description* Reads, interprets, and evaluates research for applicability to nursing practice. |
| *Performance Criteria* <br>• Uses basic communication skills. | *Performance Criteria* <br>• Uses a variety of communication skills. | *Performance Criteria* <br>• Assists in collection of data. | *Performance Criteria* <br>• Gathers data for refining and extending practice. |
| • Assesses overt verbal and nonverbal communication of individual clients. | • Analyzes overt and covert verbal and nonverbal communication. | • Assists in identifying problem areas in nursing practice. | • Utilizes health-related research as a base for nursing practice. |
| • Reports and records assessments, care plans, and evaluations. | • Establishes/monitors the use of protocols for reporting and recording assessments, care plans, and evaluations. | | • Shares research findings with colleagues. |
| • Modifies personal communication patterns. | • Makes provision for improvement of communication patterns. | | • Identifies nursing problems which need investigation. |
| | | | • Collaborates in designing and completing research relevant to practice. |

*Sources of Evidence/Tools:* nursing or progress notes; assessment forms; patient care plans; nurse manager documentation (anecdotal notes; interim evaluations); client feedback (oral or written); nursing audits. Problem resolution reports (refers to problems related to the institution or interprofessional problems; not client related).

*Sources of Evidence/Tools:* nurse manager documentation (anecdotal notes; interim evaluations); quality assurance documents; nursing audits; peer review; self-evaluation and reporting of activities; patient care conference reports; in-service records (to document sharing of research findings); minutes of research committees and/or staff meetings; and publications and reports.

**Appendix 6A**, continued.

| In the Discipline of Nursing | |
| --- | --- |
| **Associate Degree** | **Baccalaureate Degree** |
| *Performance Description*<br>Demonstrates responsibility and accountability for own scope of nursing practice and as a member of the discipline of nursing. | *Performance Description*<br>Demonstrates responsibility and accountability for own scope of nursing practice and as a member of the discipline of nursing. |
| *Performance Criteria*<br>• Works within established policies and procedures. | *Performance Criteria*<br>• Works within established policies and procedures. |
| • Evaluates own performance against established criteria and with assistance sets goals for improvement. | • Evaluates own performance against established criteria and with assistance sets goals for improvement. |
| • Recognizes and reports policies and procedures which impede client care. | • Functions as a change agent within organizational framework. |
| • Participates in quality assurance programs. | • Participates in quality assurance programs and facilitates needed changes. |
| • Functions as an advocate for clients within the nursing system. | • Functions as an advocate for clients within the health care system. |
| • Serves as a role model. | • Serves as a role model. |
| • Practices within the legal boundaries and ethical framework | • Practices within the legal boundaries and ethical framework. |
| • Participates in maintaining an environment conducive to learning. | • Assumes responsibility for establishing and maintaining an environment conducive to learning. |
| • Assumes responsibility for own continued learning. | • Assumes responsibility for own continued learning. |
| • Volunteers for or accepts assignments for special professional activities. | • Volunteers for or accepts assignments for special professional activities. |

*Sources of Evidence/Tools:* nursing or progress notes; nurse manager documentation (anecdotal notes; interim evaluations); client feedback (oral or written); nursing audit reports; self-evaluation and reporting of activities; feedback from the community; faculty/student feedback; quality assurance and other committee minutes and membership lists; problem resolution reports (refers to problems related to the institution or interprofessional problems; not client related); and continuing education records.

Source: Western Interstate Commission for Higher Education, 1985.

# Appendix 6B

## Performance Summary Evaluation Forms

Presbyterian Intercommunity Hospital, Whittier, California, Performance Summary (Standards for R.N. I)

| | Total |
| --- | --- |
| | Relative Weight |
| | Performance Value |

| Activity | Good (1 Point) | Very Good (2 Points) | Outstanding (3 Points) |
| --- | --- | --- | --- |
| 1. *Nursing Process*<br>a. Assessment | a. Obtains nursing histories from patient and/or others that identify observable variables (e.g., hard of hearing) affecting care and serves as a guide for development of nursing care plans. Reflects this in documentation and charting. | a. Obtains nursing histories from patient and/or others and identifies less common variables (e.g., information not volunteered by patient, "guilt feelings" about illness or trauma) affecting care and serves as a guide for development of nursing care plans. Reflects this in documentation and charting. | a. Obtains nursing histories from patient and/or others and identifies patient problems that include subtle physiological and/or psychosocial needs (e.g., physically or psychologically abused patient). Makes on-going assessment. Relates assessment to clinical diagnosis. Reflects this in documentation and charting. |

**Appendix 6B**, continued.

| Activity | Good (1 Point) | Very Good (2 Points) | Outstanding (3 Points) | Performance Value | Relative Weight | Total |
|---|---|---|---|---|---|---|
| 1. *Nursing Process*, continued. | | | | | | |
| b. Planning | b. Anticipates patient care needs and writes nursing care plan with appropriate, individualized interventions based on assessment data. Utilizes this plan for the daily work schedule. | b. Anticipates patient care needs and writes nursing care plan with appropriate individualized interventions based on assessment data. Anticipates possible outcomes and implements plan of care. | b. Writes individualized nursing care plan based on assessment. Is able to establish priority needs. Anticipates possible outcomes and delivers care based on assessment data. Involves self, patient, family, and other healthcare disciplines in ongoing care and discharge planning. | | | |

**Appendix 6B**, continued.

1. *Nursing Process,* continued.

| Activity | Good (1 Point) | Very Good (2 Points) | Outstanding (3 Points) | Relative Weight | Performance Value | Total |
|---|---|---|---|---|---|---|
| c. Implementation | c. Sets priorities and gives nursing care based on nursing care plan. | c. Sets priorities and gives nursing care based on nursing care plan. Assigns the care given by selected members of the nursing care team. | c. Sets priorities and gives nursing care based on nursing care plan. Supervises the care given by selected members of the nursing team. Coordinates the activities of other disciplines to implement the individual patient care plan. | | | |

**Appendix 6B**, continued.

| Activity | | Good (1 Point) | Very Good (2 Points) | Outstanding (3 Points) | Performance Value | Relative Weight | Total |
|---|---|---|---|---|---|---|---|
| *Nursing Process,* continued. | | | | | | | |
| 1. | | | | | | | |
| d. Evaluation | d. | Evaluates the response of the patient to the nursing intervention. Reflects this in documentation and charting. | d. Evaluates the response of the patient to the nursing intervention and revises goals as they are met. Reflects this in documentation and charting. | d. Evaluates the response of the patient to the nursing intervention. Evaluates and revises goals as they are met or status changes. Reports change to M.D. so as to provide expedient care. Reflects this in documentation and charting. | | | |

**Appendix 6B**, continued.

| Activity | Good (1 Point) | Very Good (2 Points) | Outstanding (3 Points) | Performance Value | Relative Weight | Total |
|---|---|---|---|---|---|---|
| 2. *R.N. Functions List* | Demonstrates knowledge of procedures. May need assistance in assembly and/or use of equipment and/or sequence of events. | Demonstrates knowledge of procedures. Prepares for them by obtaining necessary equipment. (Knows what equipment is needed and where to obtain it.) | Anticipates need for procedures, demonstrates knowledge of procedure, and obtains appropriate equipment and patient consents as necessary. | | | |
| 3. *Intra/interdepartmental Communication Skills* | May ask NUAS/director to help manage inter/intradepartmental interactions. Prefers not to participate in confrontation or negotiation sessions or, if does, plays a passive role in the session. | May ask NUAS/director to help manage inter/intradepartmental interactions but insists on being an active participant in confrontation or negotiation sessions. | Resolves inter/intradepartmental interactions through positive confrontation and negotiation. Does not expect NUAS/director to act as go-between. | | | |

Appendix 6B, continued.

| Activity | Good (1 Point) | Very Good (2 Points) | Outstanding (3 Points) | Performance Value | Relative Weight | Total |
|---|---|---|---|---|---|---|
| 4. *Forecasting and Organization* | Accepts responsibility for additions to or changes in assignment made necessary by sudden increase or decrease in activity or general patient acuity, but wonders why she/he had to do it (i.e., floating, coming in extra prn, and helping others). | Accepts responsibility for additions to or changes in assignment made necessary by sudden increase or decrease in unit activity or general patient acuity. Prepares for sudden increase or decrease in unit or patient acuity by adapting to workload change. Resets priorities while still able to manage previous assignments (i.e., floats, helps others, comes in extra and on other shifts prn when asked). | Accepts responsibility for additions to or changes in assignment made necessary by sudden increase or decrease in unit activity or general patient acuity. Prepares for sudden increase or decrease in unit or patient acuity by adapting to workload change (i.e., floats, helps others, comes in extra and on other shifts prn, sees need and offers.) Sees the "whole picture." | | | |

**Appendix 6B**, continued.

| Activity | Good (1 Point) | Very Good (2 Points) | Outstanding (3 Points) | Performance Value | Relative Weight | Total |
|---|---|---|---|---|---|---|
| 5. *Professional Growth* | | | | | | |
| | a. Attends classes and majority of staff meetings (as verified by attendance record) when assigned. Shares knowledge and information when requested to do so. | a. Attends classes and majority of meetings (as verified by attendance record). Voluntarily shares knowledge and actively participates in discussions. | a. Seeks programs to enhance own professional development and attends majority of staff meetings (as verified by attendance record). Makes opportunity to share knowledge, actively participates in discussions, and offers input to agendas. | | | |

**Appendix 6B**, continued.

| Activity | Good (1 Point) | Very Good (2 Points) | Outstanding (3 Points) | Performance Value | Relative Weight | Total |
|---|---|---|---|---|---|---|
| 5. *Professional Growth*, continued. | | | | | | |
| | b. Is not yet prepared to assume charge position on unit or to do house supervision. | b. Is able to assume charge position on unit. May need assurance or assistance from director. Is not yet prepared to do house supervision. | b. Is able to assume charge position on unit and function effectively. Is prepared to do house supervision. | | | |

Source: Presbyterian Intercommunity Hospital, Whittier, California

**Appendix 6B**, continued.

Presbyterian Intercommunity Hospital, Whittier, California, Performance Summary (Standards for R.N. II)

| Activity | Good (1 Point) | Very Good (2 Points) | Outstanding (3 Points) | Performance Value | Relative Weight | Total |
|---|---|---|---|---|---|---|
| 1. *Nursing Process* <br> a. Assessment | a. Obtains nursing histories from patient and/or others and identifies less common variables (e.g., information volunteered by patient, "guilt feelings" about illness or trauma) affecting care and serves as guide for development of nursing care plans. Reflects this in documentation. | a. Obtains nursing histories from patient and/or others identifying complex patient problems that include subtle physiological and/or psychosocial needs (e.g., physically or psychologically abused patient). Makes ongoing assessment. Relates assessment to clinical diagnosis. Reflects this in documentation and charting. | a. In addition to verbal interview, assembles nursing histories from less obvious resources such as old medical record, physician's office record, etc. Recognizes cultural impact on patient care (e.g., pain tolerance, diet, visitation). Reflects this in documentation and charting. | | | |

**Appendix 6B**, continued.

| Activity | Good (1 Point) | Very Good (2 Points) | Outstanding (3 Points) | Performance Value | Relative Weight | Total |
|---|---|---|---|---|---|---|
| *Nursing Process*, continued. | | | | | | |
| 1. | | | | | | |
| b. Planning | b. Anticipates patient care needs and writes nursing care plan with appropriate, individualized interventions based on assessment data. Anticipates possible out-comes and implements plan of care. | b. Writes individual-ized nursing care plan based on as-sessment. Is able to establish priority needs. Anticipates possible out-comes and deliv-ers care based on assessment data. Involves self, pa-tient, family, and other health care disciplines in ongoing care and discharge plan-ning. | b. Writes individualized nursing care plan based on assess-ment. Able to est-ablish priority needs. Anticipates possible outcomes and delivers care based on assessment data.Involves self, patient, family, and other health care disciplines in on-going care and dis-charge planning. Assures that patient and family recognize and assume ac-countability (e.g., for administration of medicines, crutch-walking). | | | |

**Appendix 6B**, continued.

| Activity | Good (1 Point) | Very Good (2 Points) | Outstanding (3 Points) | Performance Value | Relative Weight | Total |
|---|---|---|---|---|---|---|
| 1. *Nursing Process*, continued. | | | | | | |
| c. Implementation | c. Sets priorities and gives nursing care based on nursing care plan. Assigns the care given by selected members of the nursing care team. | c. Sets priorities and gives nursing care based on nursing care plan. Supervises the care given by selected members of the nursing care team. Coordinates the activities of other disciplines to implement the individual patient care plan. | c. Sets priorities and gives nursing care based on nursing care plan. Supervises the care given by selected members of the nursing care team. Coordinates the activities of other disciplines to implement the individual patient care plan. Ensures that patient and family recognize and assume accountability (e.g., for administration for medications, crutch-walking). | | | |

**Appendix 6B**, continued.

| Activity | Good (1 Point) | Very Good (2 Points) | Outstanding (3 Points) | Performance Value | Relative Weight | Total |
|---|---|---|---|---|---|---|
| 1. *Nursing Process*, continued.<br>d. Evaluations | d. Evaluates the response of the patient to the nursing intervention and revises goals as they are met. Reflects this in documentation and charting. | d. Evaluates the response of the patient to the nursing intervention. Evaluates and revises goals as they are met or status changes. Reports change to M.D. so as to provide expedient care. Reflects this in documentation and charting. | d. Evaluates the response of the patient to the care plan and nursing intervention. Evaluates and revises goals as they are met. Evaluates total interdisciplinary involvement, currently and reflectively, for improvement of this patient's care and records this information for future related cases. | | | |

**Appendix 6B**, continued.

| Activity | Good (1 Point) | Very Good (2 Points) | Outstanding (3 Points) | Performance Value | Relative Weight | Total |
|---|---|---|---|---|---|---|
| 2. *R.N. Functions List* | Demonstrates knowledge of procedures. Prepares for them by obtaining necessary equipment. (Knows what equipment is needed and where to obtain it.) | Anticipates need for procedures. Demonstrates knowledge of procedures and obtains appropriate equipment and patient consents as necessary. | Anticipates need for procedures, and obtains appropriate equipment, making sure it is operable and complete. Knows whom to call and where to obtain equipment and does so independently. Obtains patient consents as necessary to enable assistance with procedure. | | | |

Appendix 6B, continued.

| Activity | Good (1 Point) | Very Good (2 Points) | Outstanding (3 Points) | Performance Value | Relative Weight | Total |
|---|---|---|---|---|---|---|
| 3. *Inter/intradepartmental Communication Skills* | May ask NUAS/director to help manage inter/intradepartmental interactions, but insists upon being an active participant in confrontation or negotiation sessions. | Resolves inter/intradepartmental interactions through positive confrontation and negotiation. Does not expect NUAS/director to act as go-between. | Anticipates potential inter/intradepartmental interactions and resolves them through positive confrontation and negotiations. Does not expect anyone to act as go-between. Is thought of as approachable. This is demonstrated by positive inter/intradepartmental feedback. | | | |

**Appendix 6B**, continued.

| Activity | Good (1 Point) | Very Good (2 Points) | Outstanding (3 Points) | Performance Value | Relative Weight | Total |
|----------|----------------|----------------------|------------------------|-------------------|-----------------|-------|
| 4. *Forecasting & Organization* | Accepts responsibility for additions to or changes in assignment made necessary by sudden increase or decrease in unit activity or general patient acuity. Prepares for sudden increase or decrease in own patient acuity by adapting to workload change. Resets priorities while still able to manage previous assignment (e.g., floats, helps others, comes in extra and on other shifts prn when asked). | Accepts responsibility for additions to or changes in assignment made necessary by sudden increase or decrease in unit and/or patient acuity. Prepares for sudden increase or decrease in unit or patient acuity by adapting to workload change (e.g., floats, help others, comes in extra and on other shifts prn, sees need and offers). Sees the "whole picture." | Accepts responsibility for additions to or changes in assignment made necessary by sudden increase or decrease in unit activity or general patient acuity. Prepares for sudden increase or decrease in unit or patient acuity by adapting to workload change (e.g., floats, helps others, comes in extra and on other shifts prn, sees need and offers). Sees the "whole picture." Demonstrates flexibility to sudden workload or patient acuity change by keeping work and charting current and displaying a positive posture toward assignment change. | | | |

Appendix 6B, continued.

| Activity | Good (1 Point) | Very Good (2 Points) | Outstanding (3 Points) | Performance Value | Relative Weight | Total |
|---|---|---|---|---|---|---|
| 5. *Professional Growth* | a. Attends classes and majority of staff meetings (as verified by attendance record). Voluntarily shares knowledge and actively participates in discussions. | a. Seeks programs to enhance own professional development and attends majority of staff meetings (as verified by attendance record). Makes opportunity to share knowledge, actively participates in discussions, and offers input to agendas. | a. Seeks programs to enhance own professional development and attends majority of staff meetings (as verified by attendance record). Demonstrates knowledge within work area. Is conversant with physicians and peers regarding specialty. | | | |

**Appendix 6B**, continued.

| Activity | Good (1 Point) | Very Good (2 Points) | Outstanding (3 Points) | Performance Value | Relative Weight | Total |
|---|---|---|---|---|---|---|
| 5. *Professional Growth*, continued. | | | | | | |
| | b. Is able to assume charge position on unit. May need assurance or assistance from director. Is not yet prepared to do house supervision. | b. Is able to assume charge position on unit and function effectively. Is prepared to do house supervision. | b. Is able to assume charge position on unit and function effectively. Is a role model. Is prepared to do house supervision. Extends role of competency in work areas other than own unit. | | | |

Source: Presbyterian Intercommunity Hospital, Whittier, California

*Chapter 7*

# Beyond Establishment Views

---

...Policies to raise productivity should proceed on a wide front rather than concentrate on the fad to lead to the promised land.

(Fabricant 1969)

## Interdepartmental Coordination

An integrated human resource system should be part of the strategic and business plan of the hospital. The major goals of any human resource system are to:

- Recognize the importance of human resource assets
- Establish policies for examining the adequacy of systems, proce-dures, and programs
- Help determine the desired and expected return on human assets
- Aid in preparing for change, just as the organization anticipates technology and market demand changes (Boyatzis 1982).

Human resources management is not just the responsibility of a single department, nor is it a technical mastery of personnel functions. Human resources management is the implementation of organizational policies through the coordinated efforts of several departments and individuals. Human resources activities can be improved by being more responsive to

235

merit, more affirmative, more accountable, more capable of supporting long-term careers of excellence, and better informed and guided by a deep and operational expression of values and ethics.

The major components of a hospital's human resource system are the quality assurance and personnel management functions, the core clinical departments, and education. Even though these departments collectively determine quality of care, productivity, and the reward system, their efforts are seldom harnessed to enhance patient service, improve both financial effectiveness and quality of care, and attract and retain competent personnel. The historical legacy of separate domains obscures the vision of the desired future. More broadly, executives should redesign their hospitals to (1) empower workers wherever their efforts can improve either quality of service or financial performance, (2) provide needed training, (3) relate rewards to performance, and (4) measure quality of care, service, and financial outcomes.

No hospital department should be a professional enclave, nor should it be an amalgam of initiatives funded because of vague ideological commitments. Instead, departmental activities should be self-consciously interdependent. Because the education and human resources functions and the clinical departments share responsibility for maintaining the mix of competent workers necessary to provide quality care, departmental performance objectives should enhance patient outcomes. Physician leadership also needs to be mobilized for a synergistic program to work effectively in a hospital. Instead of relying on interpersonal skills or informal relationships, executives and managers need to develop reporting relationships or coordinating mechanisms to handle the continuing professional and administrative dilemmas. The present need to reduce costly inefficiencies between departments to safely shorten length of stay should encourage administrative leadership in creating such relationships and mechanisms.

Hospital managers have primary responsibility for tying the strategic plans of the organization with the activities of several departments so that:

1. Patient care outcomes are the ultimate criteria for spending money

2. Investments in education, pay, and benefits result in the professional career structure needed in the future

3. Valued employees receive the training and rewards that make it worthwhile for them to stay

4. Workers find it worthwhile to make investments in their own education

5. Career structures match the expectations of high school graduates, the primary work force pool

6. Incentives for continued employment match the needs of mature workers.

Interdepartmental committees can coordinate responses to problems that are important to professionals. Time spent in meetings away from the bedside is nonproductive for nurses when the issues are not salient to the members involved or when management support is deficient. However, the past tendency to encourage task performance by nurses at the expense of participation in organizational activities may have contributed to the lack of organizational commitment that has been attributed to many nurses.

There is substantial disagreement among hospital employees about which roles nursing and personnel administration should assume. In an Arizona survey of hospital administrators, personnel directors, and directors of nursing service, the nursing directors wanted personnel directors to place more emphasis on retirements, wage surveys, health insurance, morale opinion surveys, and safety (White and Wolfe 1983). Further, the nursing directors placed less emphasis than administrators did on promotions, wage and salary administration, performance appraisal, and orientation. Of 20 nursing-related activities, the nursing directors ranked performance appraisal 15th in importance and training and development last. Although these findings may not apply to all regions or hospitals, they do suggest that nursing administrators need to rethink their priorities on some of the important components of a career-oriented program, namely, orientation, pay for performance, promotions, and education.

Quality assurance mechanisms are often seen only as an accreditation formality, not as a feedback system that can bring doctors, nurses, and administrators together for the benefit of themselves and their patients. Yet feedback on quality of care along several dimensions has great importance, especially to the steady-state professional workers. External requirements for accreditation can be the stimulus for ongoing interdepartmental arrangements that enhance combined performance. Quality-of-care audits can, for example, provide performance information to clinical departments, target training efforts, and identify individuals or departments deserving a differential reward. External reporting then becomes a spin-off, not an extra burden.

Educational investment choices could be improved if various hospital departments developed joint policies and objectives. Almost all studies indicate that nurses value education. Yet hospitals have been slow to embrace the concept that productivity can be improved by upgrading the competency and education of the work force. Administrators could benefit by capitalizing on the desire of many nurses for education by shaping continuing education to meet organizational needs and promote career attachment for steady-state nurses. Why should administrators focus on paying a competitive entry-level salary and then fail to make the educational investments needed to retain productive career workers? This is not a rhetorical question. Executives who miscalculate by not acting on nurses' desire for education and quality-of-care feedback risk losing their competitive edge in hiring and retaining staff.

A recent study provides a good example of how managers can influence the professional system by increasing clinical feedback and performance visibility while at the same time complying with external requirements (Ravin, Freeman, and Haley 1982). A study of infection control activities, which are mandated by Joint Commission on Accreditation of Health Organizations (JCAHO) guidelines, determined that the infection control nurses evaluated their own efficiency higher when they believed that (1) the infection control committee had authority to act independently and (2) the committee chairperson (a physician) was actively involved. This occurred when the hospital administrator delegated authority to the infection control committee. The nurses in the study were pleased with their position, even though they felt there was limited potential for hospital advancement. The study suggested that a manager committed to enhancing professional practice for nurses could influence the system in several ways:

1. By developing job descriptions (more than half of the nurses did not have them)

2. By increasing instructional opportunities in infection control (even though the nurses already possessed more knowledge than the physician chairperson)

3. By providing education to expand the nurses' options for influencing physicians to conform to standards

4. By developing guidelines with the committee to initiate studies, educational programs, or sanctions related to quality control.

By encouraging these basic measures, administrators would not only increase the attractiveness of the hospital to steady-state nurses but also reinforce the control system, enhance professional practice, and prepare the organization for the accreditation process. Throughout the clinical departments, perceptive managers can uncover situations where a synergistic approach will jointly improve organizational commitment and performance. Examples include enhancing nursing work where it interfaces with physician practice, using external requirements as a stimulus, and formalizing support for nurse autonomy over practice issues.

This is a timely recommendation since JCAHO is granting more frequently than before provisional accreditations based on deficiencies in quality of care. In addition, by 1990 accreditation will emphasize patient outcomes rather than process and documentation alone. The past pattern of leaving quality-of-care issues to the medical staff and nursing departments evaluating quality of care by process criteria is becoming outmoded. To maintain accreditation and public funding, general administrators must extend their reach to clinical areas. Management has not only the legitimate right but also the responsibility to see that performance standards are set and enforced. Increasingly managers will be expected to see that physicians and nurses establish, enforce, and update criteria for quality care. The new leadership will not be impressed by paper compliance. Instead, managers will work with the clinical leadership, which includes physicians and other providers, to meet two bottom lines, the clinical and the financial. Hospital-specific mortality rates may well become the accepted indicator for public accountability—the clinical "bottom line."

## Pay Policy

The process of implementing and maintaining a career management system inevitably involves reconciliation of deeply held beliefs of managers and other employees about the relevant value of pay. People have different attitudes toward pay as a motivator. Some argue that salary attracts workers, but that benefits and working conditions keep them at work. A debate is going on over the impact of financial incentives on quantity and quality of work. A review of laboratory and field studies indicates that financial incentives do not affect performance quality but do have positive effects on performance quantity (Jenkins 1986). In general, relating compensation to goals has been found to be more effective than efforts to increase worker participation or job enrichment.

A national longitudinal study of young women determined that women capable of earning higher salaries were more likely to work throughout their lifetime than those who earned less (Department of Labor 1978). A previous study concluded that, for women in the middle class, the amount of time worked responds to earning capacity more than to the amount of other family income (Department of Labor 1970). Other studies have concluded that the voluntary turnover rate falls when income rises relative to skill level (Mobley 1982). Among employees, pay and benefits has ranked first or second in importance in every job classification for over two decades (Schiemann 1984).

Some hospital employers worry that an emphasis on pay and rewards will reduce intrinsic motivation. Although avoiding an overemphasis on pay is desirable, such a motivational reduction has not been a problem in hospitals, where there is little evidence of enough emphasis. The best theory-in-use suggests that rewards contingent on quality of performance are not injurious and may even enhance intrinsic motivation. The detrimental effects of rewards, according to Ross (1976), are limited to a narrow set of circumstances in which the reward is salient but not related to degree of success. Rewards contingent on quality of performance may enhance intrinsic motivation. This is not to say that people work only for money or that all people respond to money in the same way. Response to money can be modified by different factors. The impact of monetary compensation stems from its being a tangible universal medium of exchange that is also a potent signal from the organization about the worth of employees and their work.

Some economists believe that, when the pay level becomes high enough, workers may also substitute leisure for income, producing a backward-bending supply curve in which further increases in pay actually reduce the number of hours worked. This phenomenon is sometimes used to argue against pay raises for nurses. However, no clear evidence exists that the backward-bending supply curve applies to nurses generally or steady-state nurses in particular (Ezrati 1987).

It is a puzzle why women, even women in lower level jobs, are relatively satisfied with their levels of pay (Varca, Shaffer, and McCauley 1983; Crosby 1982). Several reasons have been offered for this paradox: (1)

Women may be more fatalistic than men over inequitable pay; (2) when external rewards, such as pay and promotion, are extremely low or unrelated to a worker's performance, others may infer the worker's behavior to be intrinsically motivated (Staw 1977) and many women may believe it themselves; (3) the lack of variability in the salary range either within or between community hospitals makes it plausible that nurses cannot detect pay differences; (4) women may expect lower pay than men and thus be more likely to have their expectations fulfilled (Major and Konar 1984); (5) women may self-select themselves into lower paying jobs (i.e., if they were motivated by high salary they would have chosen another career); (6) some women may be trading off higher pay for a job that allows them to meet transient or self-development needs; (7) women in two-income families, where the husband is the chief provider, may see their own salary as supplemental and be less inclined to negotiate forcefully for higher pay, because their livelihood does not depend on it; (8) some nurses (especially steady-state nurses) may accept low pay in the belief that it gives them greater job security.

Pay is important to nurses. Of all hospital employees, nurses indicated the least satisfaction with their level of pay (Hay Associates 1983, 21). One-third of the nurses in another study chose the best-paying job available to them (Munro 1983). However, nurses do not act to get the highest pay and have not been successful in bargaining, either individually or collectively, for pay or benefits. In 1987, after inflation is taken into account, nurses' salaries are lower than in 1977 even though nursing education has increased, technology requires more expert workers, and the case load is heavier (McKibbin 1988).

Comparisons show that nurses are paid less than (1) police officers, who like nurses must provide continuous coverage in their areas and are called on to perform beyond their usual abilities on occasion, although most policemen have less education than nurses; (2) teachers, who work fewer hours per year; (3) engineers, who meld technical skills and knowledge in similar ways; (4) seven careers in the Veterans Administration requiring less than a college education; and (5) hourly workers in an assortment of jobs (including carpenters, printers, and construction laborers) (Friss 1981a,b).

**Table 7-1**  1986 Salary Progression in Various Occupations

| Occupation | Average Starting Salary ($) | Average Maximum Salary ($) | % Salary Progression in Field |
|---|---|---|---|
| Accountants | 21,024 | 61,546 | 192.7 |
| Attorneys | 31,014 | 101,169 | 226.2 |
| Buyers | 21,242 | 41,304 | 94.4 |
| Computer programmers | 20,832 | 42,934 | 106.1 |
| Personnel directors | 39,817 | 75,170 | 88.8 |
| Chemists | 22,539 | 74,607 | 231.0 |
| Engineers | 27,866 | 79,021 | 183.6 |
| Accounting clerks | 12,517 | 21,872 | 74.7 |
| Personnel clerks/assistants | 14,193 | 23,702 | 67.0 |
| Purchasing clerks/assistants | 13,994 | 29,834 | 110.0 |
| Secretaries | 16,326 | 28,051 | 71.8 |
| General clerks | 10,478 | 19,332 | 84.5 |
| Staff registered nurses | 20,340 | 27,744 | 36.4 |

Salary progression figures represent the differences between national average starting and maximum salaries in a given profession or occupation for a certain year, in this case 1986.

Sources: *National survey of professional administrative, technical and clerical pay,* U.S. Department of Labor, Bureau of Labor Statistics, October 1986 (Bulletin 2271), pp. 11-13. Staff nurse salaries from National Survey of Hospital and Medical School Salaries, 1986, University of Texas Medical Branch at Galveston, 29. Reprinted by permission of the American Nurses' Association, 1988.

Table 7-1 provides examples of typical wages for occupations comparable to nursing. It also demonstrates the problem of pay compaction. Even if entry-level salaries were competitive, the overall pay line is short. Nursing has the lowest spread between the average starting salary and average maximum salary of 13 occupations, including clerks, secretaries, and engineers.

Compression of salaries, with a small differential between the top and the bottom, is a hallmark of nursing compensation. The persistence of this compression in nursing contradicts usual market responses, whereby diversity of supply, education, and level of responsibility normally lead to wide pay ranges. Even though nursing is characterized by great diversity in educational preparation, experience, level of responsibility, and place of employment, clinical nurses in 1984 earned only 13.4% more than staff nurses, and administrators earned only 47.3% more than staff nurses—these are considered small differentials (Department of Health and Human Services 1986, 54–55).

One knowledgeable analyst suggests that, if nursing is to remain attractive, salary differentials should allow a nurse with 15 to 20 years' experience and demonstrated competence and motivation to have the opportunity to earn at least twice the salary of a new graduate (Ginzberg et al. 1982). One hospital has outlined a plan that comes close (McDonagh and Sorenson 1988). At this hospital, the ladder provides a potential career gain of 64% for a new nurse, 43% for a 3- to 5-year credentialed nurse, and a 24% increase for a 10- to 15-year credentialed nurse.

The economic return for a baccalaureate degree in nursing is especially modest. In Utah, where three corporations control 26 of the state's 38 nonfederal hospitals, only five hospitals paid a differential for the degree; the differential varied from 19 to 53 cents per hour (Booton and Lane 1985). For the United States as a whole, Link (1987) found that it took the average nurse two years to earn a bachelor of science in nursing (BSN), for a total direct cost of $15,000. For that, the BSN earned $1,400 per year more than an associate degree nurse (ADN). In 1984, all other factors being equal, the diploma nurse earned 3 cents an hour more than the ADN; the baccalaureate earned 78 cents an hour more.

Nurses' generally low salaries are not offset by high benefits. Although data on benefits are not specific to nurses, the U.S. Chamber of Commerce (1988) annual survey indicates that industries spend on average 39.3% of payroll on employee benefits, whereas the health care industry averages 34.2%. In 1985, hospital benefits were 16.1% of total labor expenses and 8.9% of total hospital expenditures (Gardner 1987). In hospitals, the highest percentage of benefits (11.7%) goes for hours not worked (e.g., vacation, sick leave, and holidays), in contrast with the industry average of 10.1%. The percentage devoted to retirement and savings plans in hospitals (4.7%) is below the overall industry average of 6.7%.

Although health care managers are more innovative in developing fringe benefit adaptations, they are a two-edged sword. By attracting young workers with children by means of flexible benefit plans and revised time-off policies, employers encourage the hiring of spiral and transient nurses and overlook strategies, such as retirement programs and tax-shelter plans, that would encourage full-time work by steady-state nurses.

Both economic and noneconomic work incentives are necessary to obtain and retain high-quality nurses. Sometimes, the disagreement over the relative importance of the two types of reward, increased pay and increased noneconomic incentives, is used to resist improving either one. A typical example is when nursing administration minimizes responsibility for changes in the human dimension and argues for salary increases while the human resources staff department resists pay increases, arguing that the nursing department should change worker participation. As the stalemate continues, worker problems get worse as neither pay adjustments nor organization climate problems are addressed.

Citing the changing nature of the work force and the competitive climate, Lawler (1981) identified four major issues for the pay system: First, there needs to be more individualization in the pay system. This is especially true for hospital nurses, as a recent survey indicated that almost half of all community hospitals had only one nursing position level (Beyers et al. 1983); only 3.5% had five or more promotion levels for full-time staff nurses; depending on education, six years of experience in intensive care led to a beginning salary differential of only 11.4% to 12.6%.

Second, executives and managers need to make open and defensible decisions about both pay-setting processes and outcomes. In an industry such as health care, where the norm is to discourage sharing of wage information among employees (but not employers) and where the prerequisite trust usually does not exist, such advice may well sound heretical.

Third, managers need to emphasize performance-based pay. This is difficult to accomplish because the outputs of individual nurses are not easy to measure. A study by Dolan (1983) suggested that, in fact, if performance pay in hospitals means incentive pay, such a policy will benefit those middle managers who have responsibilities for "hotel functions" while other will lag. However, if performance pay were defined more broadly (e.g., to reward nurses with multiple skills, to maximize pay for experience, and to lessen the pay for transitory nurses), steady-state nurses would benefit.

Employee incentive programs should be fair to all workers, fair to the organization, easy to manage and control, based on objective evaluation criteria, and have measurable effects. Since these criteria are difficult for nurses on clinical units to meet, a form of gainsharing may be more appropriate. Under such a system, all workers on clinical units would have a portion of their salary or a bonus tied to improvements in staffing costs adjusted for case mix and monitored for quality changes. (See Kanter [1987] for a full discussion of gainsharing.)

The need for more egalitarian pay systems, the fourth recommendation, focuses attention on the spread between occupations. The trends in nursing are mixed. As mentioned in Chapter 2, the distance between nursing and physician salaries has increased even though nursing practice has become more complex than before. However, the salary distance between practical nurses and nursing aides has decreased (Aiken and Mullinix 1987). Pressures by managers to maintain higher salary differences between themselves and professionals also sets salary limits for advanced nursing practice. Egalitarianism among nurses has been closer to the norm for nurses than for managers. Managers expect and observe large pay differences whereas nurses do not. The nursing profession as a whole is reluctant to encourage pay differentiation because of nurses' dependence on ancillary workers and each other to perform the work and adjust to uneven client demands. However, the current surplus of entry-level managers and management "downsizing," coupled with a growing shortage of nurses willing to work under current conditions, may well conflict with the managers' desires to pay high-performing nurses less than they pay themselves.

In the complex area of pay setting, some employers are surveying nurses' attitudes toward equitable pay (Spitzer and Bolton 1984). At one tertiary hospital, administrators, specialty nurses, and general nurses agreed that nurses should be paid on the basis of education, experience, where that experience was obtained, and public health experience. General nurses wanted pay to be based on tenure. Educators, managers, and administrators, however, wanted nurses' pay to be based on the nature of the nurses' experience, equality of pay for general and intensive care nurses, amount of experience, and good performance. These conflicting views suggest that pay and mobility channels must be jointly considered by nurses and managers using a mix of merit and seniority incentives for the pay base.

## Special Aspects of Motivation

Preconceptions about the various motivational models can influence implementation of the integrated human resources management program in a hospital. When nurses and managers discuss work force problems, there are some common but unspoken themes that can either preclude or facilitate solutions. Although these are seldom addressed explicitly, they are important to consider.

Everyone adheres to one or more models of motivation, depending on the situation. However, the theories a person believes in may not be the ones he or she practices. Practices based on psychological and social motivational theories derive from three models: traditional, human relations, and human resources. The traditional or bureaucratic model suggests close supervision and tight control of subordinates. The human relations model builds on the understanding that limited participation will improve worker morale and enhance cooperation. The human resources model assumes that, given the opportunity, most people will act responsibly to achieve goals when they fully participate in dealing with important problems. Those who advocate the human relations or the human resources model tend to ignore, if not deny, the necessity to administer sanctions on occasion.

In almost all organizations, but especially in governmental or other large organizations, the traditional model with job descriptions, classes, and steps provides the skeleton for human resources management. Although both the human relations model and the human resources model usually "flesh out" a hierarchical system, there is a tendency to ignore the underlying system. Detractors of the traditional model often forget that without the rationality of the bureaucratic system workers would not be as well protected from favoritism, discrimination, or capriciousness.

Motivational research and theory is in a state of disorder (Landy and Becker 1987). Two commonly used models, Herzberg's intrinsic-versus-extrinsic theory (Herzberg, Mousner, and Snyderman 1959) and the Hawthorne's group control of production theory, are appealing because of their simplicity but have serious flaws in that they have not been validated in empirical tests, and reliable scales have been difficult to develop (Acker and Van Houten 1974; Wahba and Bridwell 1976).

The many existing theories of motivation can be grouped in five clusters: need theory, reinforcement theory, balance theory, expectancy theory, and goal-setting theory. Although there is no one "best" theory, each can be used within limits. The two motivational techniques that have produced the most reliable changes in performance are behavior modification and goal setting (Staw 1984). Goal setting has a positive influence on performance when feedback is tied to goals (Latham and Lee 1986). There is agreement that objective feedback has a sizable positive effect (Kopelman 1986).

The following few principles can serve as the cornerstone of work force policies regardless of the underlying theoretical construct (Mitchell 1976):

1. Rewards are more effective than punishment.

2. Both social group processes and the formal reward system can influence behavior.

3. Rewards should be suited to the individual; what is reinforcing, actualizing, or important will be different for different people.

4. Feedback in the form of rewards and punishments should be given frequently and consistently.

An in-depth national study of hospitals with demonstrated success in recruiting and retaining the nurses they need to provide quality patient care demonstrated the following common elements: a participative management style, educated and professionally competent nursing managers, a decentralized structure, competitive salaries, clinical career ladders, responsibility and authority within the scope of practice, and opportunities for professional development (American Academy of Nursing 1983).[1] These hospitals were labeled magnet hospitals.

## Sex Bias

Studies have established that the preponderance of research on management and careers has been examined from the Anglo, middle-class male perspective (Richardson and Kaufman 1983). Three pervasive problems of this biased work have been identified:

- Women are rarely included in the study design even when they are used as subjects for job-related studies.

- Analysis is shaped by sex-biased interpretation. For instance, McClelland (1961, 1975) did not specify that the conclusions of his studies of achievement motivation applied only to men, even though the researchers were aware that sex differences existed and that data from females conformed less reliably to the model (Campbell 1983; Richardson and Kaufman 1983).

- The entire analysis of work is somewhat distorted because certain factors are considered appropriate for either men's or women' work, but not both. The job model, which is used to understand male workers, treats work as a primary independent variable explaining behavior on and off the job. The gender model, which is used to understand female employment, sees employment as deriving from personal characteristics and family relationships (e.g., education, marital status, number and ages of children, husband's income, and husband's attitude toward employment). The end result is "research" that does not present a valid picture of work for either men or women.

There is considerable interest in and speculation about the differences, and resulting dynamics if any, among male and female managers, nurses, and physicians. Differences noted at work between males and females may be real differences, stereotypes, or predictable behaviors of either a token or a powerless person. Token employees are likely to embrace the dominant work culture more vehemently than people already belonging to it (Kanter 1977). Powerless individuals act to enhance their own position by extending whatever authority they have—for example, by enforcing rules and accepting changes slowly. Power is seen as a crucial variable in understanding how women are accepted and move through previously male occupational structures (Hall 1983).[2] Hospital administrators often face special challenges in working with nurse-physician difficulties because of the expert power nurses have over organizational processes and the social status and financial power held by physicians. Managerial actions in such cases are important, since it appears that the attitude and behaviors of women are less important than the behaviors and policies of the organization in explaining differences in authority.

## Leaders, Managers, or Both?

In developing the work force plan and assessing managerial performance, executives need to consider the organizational needs of managers as differentiated from leaders.[3] Executives themselves make a transition from administrative management with its defined operating responsibilities, limited discretion, and set communication channels to being institutional leaders who are primarily expert in the promotion and protection of values. As leaders they are unlikely to confuse survival or personal achievement with success.

Typically, managers emphasize rational assessment and systematic selection of goals, objectives, and processes (Zaleznik 1977). Managers motivate and reward subordinates and avoid solitary activity through transactional power. Their watchwords are "plan, organize, staff, direct, and control." As they marshal resources, they are tough-minded, persistent, and flexible in their use of tactics. For instance, the usual aim of supervisory nurse training programs is to enhance managerial capabilities through exposure to staffing methodologies, budget processes, job description fundamentals, and performance appraisal techniques.

Leaders, according to Zaleznik, are more intuitive and empathetic than managers. They emerge and succeed by using power to profoundly change human, economic, and political relationships. Instead of being systematic and rational, leaders are willing to work from a high-risk position and create disorder. During economically successful times, leaders may be depreciated. There is no known way to train leaders, but some propositions about leaders and followers have emerged.

Heller and Van Til (1982) offered 18 propositions about leaders and followers. The first is that leadership and followership are linked concepts, neither of which can be comprehended without understanding the other. Other propositions suggest that although there are universal management principles, truisms, and activities that apply to managing hospitals and nursing work, continuing performance is linked to leaders understanding workers, who in turn give power to their leaders. This does not mean that leaders are a distinct class of people. In many cases, the follower is a potential leader who chooses not to become active at the time. It is through the dynamics of having followers that good leadership occurs. A common but frequent tragedy is that nurses who prefer to follow are depicted by managers and consultants as being nonassertive or uninterested failures, who need somehow to be either spurred into action or dismissed. Yet if all were to seek to lead (or to follow) there could be no leadership.

## Upward Influence

The literature on individual motivation in organizations has been narrow in both direction and scope because it neglects to take account of the active part workers play in shaping their work by influencing peers, subordinates, and supervisors (Staw 1977; Mechanic 1962). The power of a leader depends upon the willingness of subordinates to accept and support the leader. Management classes seldom address theories of the power of the lower ranking participants in complex organizations. Employees not only desire control, but will often compensate for loss of control (Greenberger and Strasser 1984). Further, these efforts will persist and will follow a hierarchy of responses aimed at restoring the workers' level of control.

Knowledge about methods used by subordinates to influence supervisors is relatively sparse. The following discussion relies primarily on the work of Schilit and Locke (1982). Some methods, such as rational presentations of ideas and appeals to a higher authority, are direct. Rigidly adhering to rules and manipulating the supervisor (e.g., informing and arguing in such a way that the supervisor is not aware of being influenced) are more indirect methods. Another form of indirect influence occurs when a subordinate curries favor, praises the supervisor, or acts humble in an attempt to obtain a favorable exchange. Other methods of upward influence that have been identified are offering a formal (job-related) reward in exchange, forming coalitions, being persistent or assertive, and making threats.

The method of upward influence chosen by the subordinate depends on the desired outcome. For example, an employee whose objective is a better work schedule may combine ingratiation with a formal exchange (e.g., offering to work a difficult shift in order to have a particular day off). When the goal is to initiate change, the common methods are rational argument, persistence, and informal exchange. The methods individuals identified most frequently as successful strategies for initiating change were (1) presenting ideas logically, (2) using organizational rules, (3) being persistent, and (4) trading job-related benefits. Ironically, except for the last one, the same strategies were also identified as unsuccessful strategies for attempting to initiate change.

Although the supervisors and subordinates studied by Schilit and Locke did not agree on the causes of failure of attempts to initiate change, they did agree that logically presenting ideas was the preponderant choice. Using peer group support and threatening to resign or to "go over the supervisor's head" were seldom used and failed about as often as they succeeded. Other emotion-laden tactics were rarely used. This suggests that employees do not resort readily to using embarrassment, asking for favors or pity, applying external pressure, or threatening to take legal action. This study reinforces the commonsense notion that when subordinates want something, they just ask for it. Supervisors are well advised to listen well rather than to attempt to use motivational theories to deal with workers' opposition.

The methods nurses employ to influence their supervisors have not been documented, but the factors that promote physician-administrator cooperation have been explored (Simendinger and Moore 1983) and can be extended logically to nurses. Four factors were found to increase cooperation between physicians and managers when present, or serve as barriers when lacking: (1) honesty and trust; (2) enthusiasm, energy, and hard work; (3) competence; and (4) compatibility. The study demonstrated further that physicians are likely to be "turned off" by supervisors who are incompetent, unfriendly, or lackadaisical; who are habitually opposed to ideas; or who break promises. Competence, enthusiasm, friendly acceptance, and honesty were found to be prerequisites for effective supervision and productivity. Unfortunately, these traits have not received the emphasis they warrant.

# Unions

Union activity has experienced alternating periods of increased and decreased importance in the labor market. This is a timely subject because in September 1988 the National Labor Relations Board identified eight broad categories of employees, including nurses, as appropriate separate bargaining units. This ruling, which was vigorously opposed by the American Hospital Association, effectively eliminates delays caused by fighting over bargaining units. Because management ideology has historically regarded unions negatively, hospital associations exert much influence to prevent union penetration. Yet unions in hospitals can minimize turnover through their emphasis on seniority and grievance handling, which in turn encourages the retention of steady-state nurses—a favorable outcome. Union involvement in job design improvements and in implementing comparable-worth adjustments can be useful.

## The Impacts of Unions

The following impacts of union activity merit study: (1) the economic impact, from the institutional and societal perspective; (2) the impact on administration; (3) work force effects; (4) the effect on quality of patient care; (5) the impact of union activity on the unions themselves.

**Economic Impacts.** Researchers agree that unions raise wages (Miller, Becker, and Kinsky 1979; Becker, Sloan, and Steinwald 1982; Sloan and Steinwald 1980; Feldman and Scheffler 1982; Salkever 1983). The most common estimate is that nurses' wages are raised by 5% per year in a unionized setting (Adamache and Sloan 1982). Unions have had a smaller effect on the wages of RNs than on the wages of nonprofessionals or hospital-specific labor (housekeeping, dietary, etc.). Although unionization of RNs increases the gap between RN wages and nonunionized workers' wages, union contracts for nurses also cause pay compression by lessening the influence of education and experience in determining pay.

Managers believe that the impact of paying union wages on hospital costs is higher than studies suggest. The average increase in patient cost per day and per case is in the range of 3% to 10%. In contrast with many other industries, nurse employers have not increased the productivity of unionized workers to offset the wage gains (Salkever 1983). In states where there is mandatory hospital rate-setting, the pay of nonunion low-wage earners is reduced.

Although economists do not agree on the union effects on wages over time, they do agree that growth of unions has not been an important cause of hospital cost inflation (Sloan and Steinwald 1980; Miller, Becker, and Kinsky 1979; Salkever 1982; Adamache and Sloan 1982).

**Administrative Effects.** As a result of unionization, the hospital personnel function becomes more centralized, formalized, and enhanced. Managers report that physicians and board members are usually not affected. However, relations with other hospitals and third-party payors become more important as managers see an increased need for active cooperation among hospitals, government, and third parties with regard to labor relations and personnel administration (Juris and Maxey 1981). Rarely do hospital managers substitute capital for labor (e.g., by installing automated patient monitoring equipment or bedside terminals) or substitute one level of workers for another. However, these are two responses that could offset the costs of the wage and benefit increases.

**Work Force Effects.** Managers believe that unionized employees are more interested in the hospital than nonunionized ones. They believe, further, that unionization improves employee recruitment and retention. Unionized employees are more interested in transfers, learning more difficult jobs, and obtaining more education (Maxey 1980). Usually in such hospitals, the supervisor receives more training because the job responsibilities are increased, and managers believe that the quality of management and supervision is better. These effects, although noted, are not as pronounced as the administrative changes.

**Quality-of-Care Effects.** There is little agreement and even less documentation on the effect of unions on quality of care. If management perceives that the union limits managerial control, managers are likely to report the impact on performance to be negative. If managers are frustrated at their perceived loss, due to unions, of powers considered essential for the attainment of organizational goals, they may perceive employees as unconcerned, uncooperative, and unproductive. These perceptions will also be associated with beliefs that quality of care has deteriorated (Maxey 1979).

**Anomalies.** The impacts of unions extend to the unions themselves. For instance, when competition for nurses is high, employers may be more willing than union officials to increase nurses' pay. This anomaly occurs when the union also represents other employees, who resent the relatively high pay that they perceive nurses as receiving. For political reasons, then, unions may ask for nursing pay increases that are less than what the market will bear in order to avoid internal dissension. This has the strange result whereby nursing management allies with the staff nurses against the union.

**Extent of Activity.** The U.S. Department of Labor (1980) surveyed 22 major metropolitan areas and found that, in most, hospitals were not heavily organized. Government hospitals were more apt to have unionized employees than private hospitals.

Although one-third of all hospital workers were found to be employed in the 25% of hospitals with bargaining agreements, most of these workers were in large urban hospitals, particularly on the East Coast and in the industrial Midwest (Feldman, Lee, and Hoffbeck 1980; Numerof and Abrams 1984). Most elections to determine union acceptance were held in hospitals with 100 to 200 beds, but proportionately, elections were most common in larger hospitals with 400 or more beds. Service and maintenance units won more elections than professional or service unions, but even they were not successful—the acceptance rate was only 44%. Minorities were found to be overrepresented in union membership; married women and college-educated workers were underrepresented (Feldman, Lee, and Hoffbeck 1980).

In another study (Becker 1983), religious hospitals were found to be less likely to be unionized than voluntary or proprietary hospitals, even though the religious hospitals were no less likely to have an election. The study also showed that union activity is more likely to be successful in large rather than small hospitals, especially if the hospital has a large teaching program. Hospital market share did not predict either the occurrence or the success of an election. Major organizers and blue-collar hospital employees were less likely to win elections than white-collar workers or unions that are not major unionizers in the health care field.

Becker also determined that, among the other fixed components that were positively related to hospital union activity, the important ones were (1) a history and tradition of unionism, (2) the presence of mandatory and regulatory cost-containment agencies, (3) prospective reimbursement, and (4) a high level of Medicaid reimbursement. Cost of living and changes in unemployment levels did not predict success in representation elections (Delaney 1981).

The number of nursing contracts has been slowly increasing. It is estimated that 30.7% of all hospitals had a union in May 1985 (Becker and

Rakich 1988). Three unions—Service Employees International Union (SEIU); the National Union of Hospital and Health Care Employees (District 1199), a division of the Retail Wholesale and Department Store Union (AFL-CIO); and the American Nurses' Association (ANA)—account for 60% of all nursing contracts. (The first two unions belong to the AFL-CIO and have agreed to merge.) Another 20 unions also represent or are soliciting to represent nurses (Numerof and Abrams 1984). Health care unions are 20% more likely to win elections than unions from other industries. Thus, in contrast to the rest of the labor force, where union membership is declining, health care unions have been successful, although unionization of hospital employees and nurses in the 1980s has not continued at the rapid pace of the previous two decades.

Between January 1980 and May 1985 there was a dramatic decrease in the extent of union activity but not in union victory rates (Becker and Rakich 1988). The majority of elections since 1980 have taken place in nonprofit, nonreligious hospitals, which also experienced the highest victory rates, as the for-profit hospitals were very successful in reducing the victory rates of the unions when elections were held. In 1983 and 1984, the number of union elections declined substantially. However, recent trends, if they continue, may encourage more collective bargaining, according to a health care labor-management relations expert (Metzger 1987).

## Contrasts with Other Industries

In spite of many commonalities, hospital worker union agreements were found to differ from contracts in other industries (Juris et al. 1977). In the union security/management rights sections of the agreements, hospital contracts were:

- For a shorter time
- Less likely to include cost-of-living adjustments
- Less likely to include deferred wage increase provisions
- Half as likely to have strong forms of union security
  (e.g., a union shop or a modified union shop)
- One-third as likely to have layoff protection for elected officers
  (although layoffs traditionally have been infrequent in the industry).

Analysis of the contracts' individual and job security provisions, which are the provisions that protect the jobs and earnings of individual members, indicated that management resisted employee demands for security. The contracts were less likely to give seniority the "sole or deciding" weight in allocating scarce job and promotional opportunities. There were relatively few protections against subcontracting work outside the hospital. Comparatively few agreements required severance pay, and supplementary unemployment benefits were nonexistent.

In the due process section of the contracts reviewed, grievance procedures were standard features, as in other industries, but hospital agreements did not specify the offenses against which grievance procedures could be brought and were less likely to provide for final and binding arbitration. This may have resulted from hospital inexperience in contract administration and a low strike rate. In the wage and benefit clauses, pay premiums for less favorable shifts, weekend work, extended schedules, or nonstandard work schedules were not as common as one might expect given the number of workers who work irregular hours. The premium for holiday work tended to be future time off rather than extra pay.

Organizing and strike activity in the 1980s has centered around job security rather than practice issues, reflecting a depressed economy and cost-containment changes. Overall, whatever divergence formerly existed between nurse contracts and those in other industries has probably diminished.

Most analysts conclude that collective bargaining in hospitals is comparable to industrial sector bargaining. This was substantiated in a study of hospitals that experienced collective bargaining—not restricted to unionizing activity—for the first time (Alexander and Bloom 1987). Specifically, collective bargaining occurs with increasing organizational complexity, available community resources, and regulatory intensity. (See Table 7-2 for a comparison of hospital and business union contracts.)

## Professional Practice Issues

The most significant professional practice issue is whether professional associations (e.g., ANA) can continue to represent nurses in the aftermath of a recent circuit court ruling (Lee and Parker 1987). In National Labor Relations Board (NLRB) v. North Shore University Hospital the court found that nursing supervisors' participation in the governance of a professional nurses' association amounted to domination by the supervisors and

**Table 7-2** Comparison of Union Context and Contracts in Hospitals and Businesses.

| Hospitals | Businesses |
|---|---|
| **Industry Characteristics** | |
| Separate unions | Nationwide inclusive unions |
| Craft work, ambiguous product | National product, clearly defined |
| Ideological component | Acceptance of adversary principle |
| High proportion of married females | Male domination |
| **Social Linkages** | |
| History of exclusion from collective bargaining contracts | Bargaining protected by federal law |
| Third-party reimbursement | Disciplined by competition |
| | Wages and benefits connected to productivity |
| **Extent and Scope of Bargaining** | |
| Union security less likely (cost of living, deferred wage increases, and union shop —protection of elective offices) | Union security more likely |
| Job security less likely (security criterion, subcontracting protection, severance pay, supplementary unemployment) | Job security more likely |
| Due process less likely (specification of offenses, binding arbitration) | Due process more likely |
| Shift and holiday pay less likely | Shift and holiday pay more likely |

that the association's attempt to represent a bargaining unit of nonsupervisory nurses involved a conflict of interest and violated the National Labor Relations Act. Since this ruling, however, the NLRB has dismissed more than half a dozen attempts to make an issue of supervisory dominance.

Many professionals in the health care field argue that nurses emphasize professional goals (e.g., quality of care, staffing, and continuing education) over traditional ones (e.g., salary and benefits; Ponak 1981). If this preference does exist, issues such as in-service training, staffing, participation, and performance evaluation require specific attention in union contracts. Management has traditionally viewed such issues and work rule practices as management rights. Although many earlier contracts included language that addressed professional practice issues, management retained advisory authority over such areas as scope and content of education and staffing standards. To allow professional input, committees were formed to guarantee nurse participation in areas such as staffing and scheduling, work assignments, patient care, and nursing practice. (Such jurisdictional overlap among unions and professional associations and the changing ideologies of the work force toward a more calculating involvement are not unique to the United States; the same phenomena have been observed in Canada and England.) Accepting the premise that nurses distinguish between traditional goals and professional goals logically leads to a second premise: The best bargaining agent is the professional association. Conversely, accepting the premise that practice issues are of minor importance to nurses suggests that nurses would not resist other unions. Some individuals believe that the professional association should not be a bargaining agent; this belief is held not only on ideological grounds but also on the practical grounds that the association includes management representatives.

Overall, one study found that contracts negotiated by professional unions, trade unions, and independent unions did not differ substantially on economic issues, but the contracts negotiated by the professional union addressed more professional practice issues (Wakim 1976). Surprisingly, previous bargaining experience was not found to determine the overall inclusiveness of the contract. Other studies have shown that nurses who earned less than professionals in other areas of the hospital had greater salary demands. Yet nurses settled for less than did other hospital employee groups. This suggests that nurses often trade pay for nonpay benefits. However, more militant nurses are less likely to accept such outcomes. These workers frequently do not find their careers satisfying and often are older workers who have shorter tenure.

In spite of the general tendencies discussed above, nurses do not have a monolithic view of collective bargaining. Their behaviors are not consistent with either the collective bargaining model or the professional model to the exclusion of the other. Therefore, for executives to ignore or deny the impact of professional values on nurses joining a union, striking, or alternatively withdrawing from clinical practice in hospitals is a mistake. Interestingly, in a recent study, 68% of a sample of registered nurses felt that nurses needed to be collectively represented, although only 38% actually were. This finding suggests a high level of susceptibility to unionization if employment conditions worsen appreciably (Castiglia, McCausland, and Hunter 1983).

Why do nurses strike? A study of public health nurses is provocative (Bloom, Parlette, and O'Reilly 1980). Even in this educationally homogeneous group of nurses (all had a bachelor's degree), nonstriking nurses had different perceptions than did striking nurses about the reasons for striking; managers' perceptions differed from both. Managers did not seem to understand the needs of either group and could not explain the managerial position to the nurses. To striking nurses, the important issues were (1) solidarity among nurses and other union members, (2) poor communication with management, (3) authoritarian behavior of managers, and (4) a belief in collective bargaining as a way to balance employee and management power. These differ from the concerns, such as economic improvements, pay increases, and job sharing, that managers believed were important to the nurses. The nonstriking nurses believed that strikes were inappropriate for nurses. They were less likely than striking nurses to cite as strike issues such topics as support for other nurses, communication, and the economic costs of lost wages. It seems reasonable to expect that in hospitals where there is more employee diversity and managerial latitude than exists among public health nurses and government managers, differences attributed by different groups would be more, not less, pronounced.

Since hospital management can subcontract for nurses at will, unilaterally determine nurses' job content, use supervisors to perform bargaining unit work, assign the number and type of staff they desire, require long probationary periods, and provide no formal training for promotions, it is only reasonable to ask why nurses have not taken more effective collective action. Several reasons can be given. Nurses are hard to organize, partially because female "balance tippers" (those who would give management a chance) are usually easier to accommodate. In addition, the female labor pool usually has fewer union advocates and fewer malcontents (Foulkes 1980). However, a more fundamental reason for the lack of union impact is that the primary prerequisites do not exist, namely, a homogeneous work force with few alternatives, a common employer, and the perception that concerted effort could result in substantial gains. Nurses are heterogeneous, employed by many employers (who often collaborate to influence the market), have other alternatives, and expect small take-home-pay gains from unionization. As they see little to gain, few sympathizers, no visible adversary, and better jobs and activities available, they simply do not bother to organize. The potential for shaping individual career strategies is much greater.

# Quality-of-Work-Life Interventions

In general hospitals have not embraced quality-of-work-life (QWL) interventions. Yet this integrated technical and social method for improving productivity has potential, especially in critical care units, where job redesign may be essential to avoid employee burnout, high turnover, and shortages. Rice et al. (1985) have developed a conceptual model of organizational work and the perceived quality of life.

The term "quality of work life" encompasses a family of concepts related to work reorganization or restructuring within the organization. These include organization-wide change, behavior modification, incentive plans, flexible hours, autonomous work groups, job restructuring, and participative management. The four common problems that QWL projects have addressed are costs (direct labor costs), productivity (leaner staffing ratios), quality (of patient care), and withdrawal (absenteeism and turnover). Attitudes, such as job satisfaction, may also be defined as a presenting problem.

It is generally agreed that direct attempts to improve worker satisfaction are a mistake. Besides taking a long time, the costs may not be offset by positive changes in the other outcome variables. It is also a mistake to consider QWL projects as a short-term fix for specific attitudinal or behavioral problems of the work force. This does not mean that QWL projects are unconcerned with job satisfaction or the social system as a whole. In fact, just the opposite is so. Social relations at work have more influence than personal psychology (i.e., job satisfaction) and are an integral part of any intervention. Measurement of job satisfaction during a project may be essential for monitoring the progress of an intervention and for modifying plans. However, measuring job satisfaction is not the same as making satisfaction the project goal. Further, it has been well established that job satisfaction and job performance are essentially unrelated (Podsakoff and Williams 1986; Iaffaldano and Muchinsky 1985).

## Principles for Implementing QWL Projects

Three major principles for implementing QWL projects have been suggested. The first is that the activity proposed should address a presenting problem. This discussion assumes that the project's primary purpose is to address an operating problem, not to build social systems in general or to demonstrate the efficacy of a popular solution for problems. Examples of projects that may be solutions in search of a problem (which are advocated by individuals who may have a vested interest, even though they may not be the appropriate intervention) are work standards, courses on team building, management by objectives, and management information systems. The diagnosis should be more than a reflection of management biases, perpetuation of stereotypes, or a premature assumption that a change in nursing (or any other single department) will solve a particular problem. A good diagnosis incorporates both the social and technical components, draws boundaries around it, and provides the information needed to design a solution. Just because a symptom, such as high turnover, poor medical staff relations, or quality deficiencies, occurs on a nursing unit does not invariably mean that the root problem, and hence the solution, will be found on that unit.

The second principle emphasizes that evaluation of design alternatives and of whether the proposed solution is suitable for the problem under discussion should precede the implementation decision. The third principle states that work improvement projects should use data to provide feedback on worker attitudes, behaviors, and work outcomes. Otherwise, managers have no basis for determining the impact of the intervention. That is, the underlying problem may not, for example, be poorly educated or motivated workers but the political or personal orientation of the managers.

Experts have identified other elements that are often present in successful QWL projects (O'Toole 1981). In descending order of agreement, they were:

- Gainsharing (profit sharing)[4]
- Guarantee of job security
- Equal commitment to both economic and human goals
- Workers being given data and training on how to use management data
- Projects structured so that all workers see benefits
- Active participation of a union (when one exists)
- No invidious distinction created between pilot projects and other groups
- Worker participation in all phases of the project
- No time pressures to show early success

- Retraining of managers to act as consultants, negotiators, trainers, and counselors
- Use of an outside consultant
- Beginning with a diagnostic study
- Organizing workers in teams.

These principles are not new or surprising. Therefore, lack of knowledge about them explains either managers' reluctance to initiate QWL projects or the relatively high failure rate of such projects. The barrier to putting knowledge into practice, aside from legitimate risk, has been explained by the unanimous agreement of experts that "many good work-reform projects have been killed by managers who feared they would lose power and control. In many cases control and power are more important to managers than profits or productivity" (O'Toole 1981, 115).

Experts agree that successful programs require that management take the initiative (O'Toole 1981). The irony is that even when projects require a high level of worker participation and promote autonomy over work-related decisions, the use of managerial power and authority is a prerequisite. As a leading nursing educator reminds us, the paradox of modern professional life is that freedom is much greater for professionals who have employers and work in bureaucratic organizations than for those who are in independent practice (Styles 1982, 43).

To be successful, work redesign projects must not be confined to the work itself but also modify opportunity and power structures. Therefore, it is unlikely that managers will be in the vanguard of work reform, since managers tend not to be exposed to worker discontent and are often unclear about how to improve productivity through work changes (Berg, Freedman, and Freeman 1978).[5]

Workers who are interested in new directions lack the authority to affect the top level of management where strategies are initiated. (They do have the power to subvert unacceptable reforms, however.) This need for interest and cooperation by both parties explains why successful projects tend to be found in organizations that already have good relationships and working conditions. Work reform seems to occur where it is needed the least; certainly, QWL projects cannot substitute for a threshold level of working conditions.

Career structures in hospitals can frustrate managerial initiatives in work force reform. Influential nurses with long tenure often control the informal hierarchy. Physician leaders also often have a long association with the hospital and considerable influence over the nursing staff. By contrast, managers' education has frequently not prepared them to be knowledgeable about professional work, or to manage clinicians. When this lack of preparation is coupled with the inexperience of managers often assigned to solve tough clinical problems on nursing units, innovation is unlikely.

Wide-scale testing and adoption of successful QWL projects would be hastened if there were known methods for overcoming managerial resistance to such endeavors. The experience in schools of management does not offer encouragement that this resistance will change. One analysis indicated that, although the expressed values of MBA students were congruent with the QWL paradigm, their actions, based on collective decisions, did not follow therefrom (Jick 1981). This demonstrates that managers are influenced strongly by the prevailing practices of their peers and reaffirms what is known about education: Neophytes can be exposed to comprehensive theories and innovative ideas, but they need reinforcement at work to make changes. Successful change depends on the vision and courage of top managers as well as the enthusiasm of entrants.

Those who want to improve managerial acceptance of the QWL approach will find insights in the literature on decision-making, leadership, and power. It is beyond the scope of this chapter to review this extensive literature, but it comes as no surprise that the nursing literature emphasizes empowerment of nurses. The health care management literature on power, when it concerns clinicians, limits itself to physician rather than employee relationships. Although power relationships may explain the general lack of commitment to human resource development in hospitals, managers also are genuinely reluctant to implement technical changes when the process and the criteria for success are poorly understood. Fortunately, QWL analyses provide a repertoire of solutions and criteria for implementation. Several of these solutions are summarized below.

## Alternatives

Managers wishing to initiate QWL initiatives have a choice of several manipulable variables (Cummings and Molloy 1977). Some of these are organization-wide strategies, which have already been discussed in other contexts. Decentralization, for example, is suited to situations where changes in technology, environment, or hospital policy make existing structures inappropriate. Wage incentive systems are useful when organizations can measure employees' contribution to costs or output (Austin 1973; Groner 1977). The use of flexible working hours is an organization-wide alternative to consider either when tasks do not require continuous staffing by the total work force or when the structure provides the stability required of a continuous operation.

Other initiatives aim to change individual behaviors. Behavior modification programs are relevant when the desired performance is behaviorally determined and measurable. Job-specific training falls in this category, as do new worker orientation, sensitivity training, and career planning. The relevant changes are those at the subunit level rather than organizational or individual interventions. Examples of these work-restructuring projects are job rotation, horizontal job enlargement to increase variety, job extension that increases the number of tasks but not the variety, job enrichment that adds greater scope for achievement and recognition, and semi-autonomous work groups (Wall 1982).

Managers are not limited to one initiative. Indeed, QWL projects frequently make use of several intervention levers. The mix of strategies is usually eclectic, closely related to problem definition as well as hospital-specific constraints. This is true because individuals, units, and organizations are so complex that contingency rules can seldom identify all the potential determinants. Two generalizations can be put forth, however. First, participative management, almost by definition, does accompany autonomous work groups (as well as incentive pay plans and organization-wide changes). Before choosing any one of these strategies, managers can benefit from past experience that suggests that a high level of trust between workers and managers is an essential prerequisite for interventions that require participation.

The second generalization is that aspects of the work itself, especially task variety and supervision, have the strongest statistical relationships with outcome measures (Cummings and Salipante 1976). Task involvement as a motivator is more appropriate for well-defined roles than for cooperation between roles (Galbraith 1977). Task autonomy and challenge are positively related to attitudes and performance and negatively related to withdrawal behavior, such as turnover. Since nurses are task oriented, the assumption is that their job satisfaction stems largely from the job itself. Fortunately, nursing studies that have used technology and task constructs (as discussed in Chapter 5) can help managers clarify subunit design issues in their own hospitals.

The discussion that follows provides an overview of the concepts of technology and job characteristics. Next will be presented the findings of seminal nursing studies, followed by the suggestion of a simple job redesign framework and a few caveats.

The success of employee-management committees depends on good early design. History suggests that a hierarchy of union-management committees can be a powerful vehicle for developing organizational changes (Lawler and Ledford 1981-1982). However, to be successful, such committees must be relatively small, must be placed at the appropriate level in the hierarchy, and must be representative of management as well as other major segments of the work force. Once established, committees should receive the training and consulting assistance necessary to achieve the established goals and objectives. The charge given the committee should be accompanied by clear guidelines about the topics the committee can address as well as realistic expectations. The committee will not increase productivity of itself, but its recommendations for change and support for those changes, once initiated, are the driving force for increased productivity.

Managerial support for QWL projects can be assessed by management responses. Procrastination, forgetting, indecision, discussion with no follow-up, and refusal to alter traditional patterns are signs of management resistance. Positive signs include changed initiatives by managers in key areas of planning, organizing, staffing, directing, and controlling.

Hospitals and nursing departments have not enthusiastically embraced work redesign projects. There are areas, such as critical care units, where work redesign could offer new solutions. Close examination of technical requirements and engineering solutions followed by a social system analysis, including the roles of physicians, would stimulate alternative solutions for pervasive staffing and burnout problems that currently exist. Such projects will be more feasible if nursing salaries increase (and thus make capital substitution justifiable) or if the availability of high-quality workers decreases.

## Summary

Practicing hospital managers are well educated about motivational theories, unionization, and communication. Unfortunately, the concepts they have learned are often outdated or inappropriately applied to the nursing work force, which is diverse, as nurses come from different social classes with different educational experiences and changing expectations about work life.

In this chapter, questions were raised about the applicability of McClelland's hierarchy of needs, Hawthorne's peer control studies, and Herzberg's intrinsic-versus-extrinsic motivation theory. Research on hospital unions was reviewed. We conclude that unions are primarily confined to the public sector, where little growth is anticipated, and their financial impact has not been great. Finally, because of considerable interest in decentralization and participation, the literature on upward influence and quality of working life is discussed. In the current environment managers need to ask new questions, such as, "How do workers influence management?" and "How can management support technical work improvements?"

The single most important responsibility of hospital management is to provide the structural links between departments so that organizational resources can be used to reward quality of care, professional development, and organizational commitment. The challenge is to link quality indicators to nursing units, invest educational money to improve the clinical competence of nurses where needed, reward high-performing nurses with educational opportunities, and provide the executive leadership necessary for redesigning jobs (which will surely be necessary in the future). The most difficult obstacle to overcome will be the resistance of middle managers, whose current value system and managerial methods will likely be ineffective.

## Endnotes

1. *Magnet Hospitals* (American Academy of Nursing 1983) has an extensive list of program material from hospitals in the study. Topics include public relations, professional practice models, collaborative practice, preceptor programs, orientation programs, career ladders, patient care plans, patient education, quality assurance, staff publications, annual reports, governance, survey tools, and benefits.

2. Other good discussions of power include Brief, Aldag, and Russell (1970), House (1988), Mintzberg (1983), McFarland and Shiflett (1979), Stevenson (1982), and Van Wagner and Swanson (1979).

3. For a review of research on leadership in nursing, see McCloskey and Molen (1987) and Van Fleet and Yukl (1986).

4. Neither the productivity literature for hospitals nor nursing management literature discuss this accepted principle of industrial relations.

5. Hospitals have generally not been favorable sites for QWL interventions. A good case study is that by Hanlon, Nadler, and Gladstein (1987).

# References

Acker, J., and D. Van Houten. 1974. Differential recruitment and control: the sex structuring of organizations. *Administrative Science Quarterly* 19: 152–163.

Adamache, K., and F. Sloan. 1982. Unions and hospitals. *Journal of Health Economics* 1: 81–108.

Aiken, L., and C. Mullinix. 1987. The nurse shortage: myth or reality? *New England Journal of Medicine* 317: 641–646.

Alexander, J., and J. Bloom. 1987. Collective bargaining in hospitals: an organizational and environmental analysis. *Journal of Health and Social Behavior* 28: 60–73.

American Academy of Nursing. 1983. *Magnet hospitals*. Kansas City, MO: American Academy of Nursing, American Nurses' Association.

Austin, C. 1973. Wage incentive systems: a review, in W. Cleverly, ed., *Financial management of health care facilities*. Germantown, MD: Aspen, pp. 154–158.

Becker, E. 1983. Structural determinants of union activity in hospitals. *Journal of Health Politics, Policy, and Law* 7: 889–910.

Becker, E., and J. Rakich. 1988. Hospital union election activity. *Health Care Financing Review* 9(3): 59–77.

Becker, E., F. Sloan, and B. Steinwald. 1982. Union activities in hospitals: past, present, and future. *Health Care Financing Review* 3: 1–13.

Berg, I., M. Freedman, and M. Freeman. 1978. *Managers and work reform: a limited engagement*. New York: The Free Press.

Beyers, M., R. Mullner, C. Byre, et al. 1983. Results of the Nursing Personnel Survey, Part I: RN recruitment and orientation. *Journal of Nursing Administration* 13(4): 34–37.

Bloom, J., G. Parlette, and C. O'Reilly. 1980. Collective bargaining by nurses: a comparative analysis of management and employee perceptions. *Health Care Management Review* 5: 25–33.

Booton, L., and J. Lane. 1985. Hospital market structure and the return to nursing education. *Journal of Human Resources* 20: 184–195.

Boyatzis, R. 1982. *Competent manager*. New York: Wiley.

Brief, A., R. Aldag, and C. Russell. 1970. An analysis of power in a work setting. *Journal of Social Psychology* 2: 289–295.

Campbell, P. 1983. Impact of societal biases on research methods, in B. Richardson and J. Wirtenberg, *Sex role research*. New York: Praeger, pp. 197–213.

Castiglia, P., L. McCausland, and J. Hunter. 1983. An alternative conceptual approach to nursing turnover, in B. Bullough, V. Bullough, and M. Soukop, eds., *Nursing issues and strategies for the eighties.* New York: Springer, pp. 55–70.

Chamber of Commerce. 1988. *Employee benefits 1986.* Washington, DC: Economic Policy Division, Chamber of Commerce.

Crosby, F. 1982. *Relative deprivation and working women.* New York: Oxford University Press.

Cummings, T., and E. Molloy. 1977. *Improving productivity and the quality of work life.* New York: Praeger.

Cummings, T., and P. Salipante. 1976. Research-based strategies for improving work life, in P. Warr, ed., *Personal goals and work design.* London: Wiley, pp. 31–41.

Delaney, J. 1981. Union success in hospital representation elections. *Industrial Relations* 20: 149–161.

Department of Health and Human Services. 1986. *National sample survey of registered nurses, 1984: Summary of results.* Washington, DC: Government Printing Office, pp. 54–55.

Department of Labor. 1970. *Dual careers,* Vol. 1 (Manpower Research Monograph No. 21). Washington, DC: Government Printing Office.

Department of Labor. 1978. *Years for decision,* Vol. 4. Washington, DC: Government Printing Office.

Department of Labor. 1980. *Industry wage survey: hospitals and nursing homes, September 1978.* Washington, DC: Government Printing Office.

Dolan, R. 1983. The middle manager's compensation outlook. *Hospital Forum* 26(6): 9–12.

Ezrati, J. 1987. Labor force participation of registered nurses. *Nursing Economics* 5(2): 82–89.

Fabricant, S. 1969. *A primer on productivity.* New York: Random House, p. 191.

Feldman, R., L. Lee, and R. Hoffbeck. 1980. *Hospital employees' wages and labor union organization* (report 03649). Washington, DC: National Center for Health Services Research.

Feldman, R., and R. Scheffler. 1982. The union impact on hospital wages and fringe benefits. *Industrial and Labor Relations Review* 35: 196–206.

Foulkes, F. 1980. *Personnel policies in large non-union companies.* Englewood Cliffs, NJ: Prentice Hall.

Friss, L. 1981a. An expanded conceptualization of job satisfaction and career style. *Nursing Leadership* 4(4): 13–22.

Friss, L. 1981b. Nurse retention recruitment: opposite poles in staffing strategy. *Hospital Progress* 62(8): 54–58.

Galbraith, J. 1977. *Organization design.* Reading, MA: Addison-Wesley.

Gardner, E. 1987. Benefits managers' work to contain costs. *Modern Healthcare* 16(23): 41–51.

Ginzberg, E., J. Patray, M. Ostrow, et al. 1982. Nurse discontent: the search for realistic solutions. *Journal of Nursing Administration* 12(11): 7–11.

Greenberger, D., and S. Strasser. 1984. *Personal control in organizations* (mimeographed). College of Administrative Sciences, Ohio State University, Columbus, OH.

Groner, P. 1977. *Cost containment through employee incentives program.* Germantown, MD: Aspen.

Hall, R. 1983. Theoretical trends in the sociology of occupations. *Sociological Quarterly* 24: 5–24.

Hanlon, M., D. Nadler, and D. Gladstein. 1987. *Attempting work reform.* New York: Wiley.

Hay Associates. 1983. *1982 Hay Health Care Compensation Conference Proceedings.* Philadelphia: Hay Associates.

Heller, T., and J. Van Til. 1982. Leadership and followership. Some summary propositions. *Journal of Applied Behavioral Science* 18: 405–414.

Herzberg, F., B. Mausner, and B. Snyderman. 1959. *The motivation to work.* New York: Wiley.

House, R. 1988. Power and personality in complex organizations. *Research in Organizational Behavior.* 10: 305-357.

Iaffaldano, M., and P. Muchinsky. 1985. Job satisfaction and job performance. *Psychological Bulletin* 97: 251-273.

Jenkins, G. 1986. Financial incentives, in E. Locke, ed., *Generalizing from laboratory to field settings.* Lexington, MA: Lexington Books, pp. 167–180.

Jick, T. 1981. Management and quality of worklife: a clash of values, in G. Dlugos and K. Weiermair, eds., *Management under differing value systems.* New York: Walter de Gruyter, pp. 359–372.

Juris, H., and C. Maxey. 1981. *The impact of hospital unionism.* Washington, DC: National Center for Health Services Research.

Juris, H., J. Rosmann, C. Maxey, et al. 1977. Employee discipline no longer management prerogative only. *Hospitals* 51(9): 67–74.

Kanter, R. 1977. Some effects of proportions on group life: skewed ratios and responses to token women. *American Journal of Sociology* 82: 965–990.

Kanter, R. 1987. From status to contribution: some organizational implications of the changing basis for pay. *Personnel* 64(1): 12–37.

Kopelman, R. 1986. Objective feedback, in E. Locke, ed., *Generalizing from laboratory to field settings.* Lexington, MA: Lexington Books, pp. 138–145.

Landy, F., and W. Becker. 1987. *Motivation theory reconsidered. Research in Organizational Behavior* 9: 1–38.

Latham, G., and T. Lee. 1986. Goal setting, in E. Locke, ed., *Generalizing from laboratory to field settings.* Lexington, MA: Lexington Books, pp. 107–117.

Lawler, E. 1981. *Pay and organization development.* Reading, MA: Addison-Wesley.

Lawler, E., and F. Ledford. 1981–1982. Productivity and the quality of work life. *National Productivity Review* 1: 23–36.

Lee, B., and J. Parker. 1987. Supervisory participation in professional associations: implications of North Shore University Hospital. *Industrial and Labor Relations Review* 40: 364–381.

Link, C. 1987. What does a BS degree buy? *American Journal of Nursing* 87: 1621–1630.

Major, B., and E. Konar. 1984. An investigation of sex differences in pay expectations and their possible causes. *Academy of Management Journal* 27: 777–792.

Maxey, C. 1979. Organizational consequences of collective bargaining: a study of some noneconomic dimensions of union impact. Presented at the 32nd annual meeting of the Industrial Relations Research Association, Atlanta, GA, December 1979.

Maxey, C. 1980. Hospital managers' perception of the impact of unionization. *Monthly Labor Review* 103: 36–38.

McClelland, D. 1961. *The achieving society.* Princeton, NJ: Van Nostrand.

McClelland, D. 1975. *The achievement motive,* 2nd Ed. New York: Halsted.

McCloskey, J., and M. Molen. 1987. Leadership in nursing. *Annual Review of Nursing Research* 5: 177–202.

McDonagh, K., and M. Sorenson. 1988. Restructuring nursing salaries: a mandate for the future. *Nursing Management* 19(2): 39–41.

McFarland, D., and M. Shiflett. 1979. The role of power in the nursing profession, in D. McFarland and N. Shifflett, eds., *Power in nursing*. Wakefield, MA: Nursing Resources, pp. 1–13.

McKibbin, R. 1988. Nurse salaries losing ground. *American Nurse* 20(3): 16.

Mechanic, D. 1962. Sources of power of lower participants in complex organizations. *Administrative Science Quarterly* 7: 349–364.

Metzger, N. 1987. The changing marketplace. *Journal of Health and Human Resources Administration* 10(1): 53–65.

Miller, R., B. Becker, and E. Kinsky. 1979. *The impact of collective bargaining in hospitals*. New York: Praeger.

Mintzberg, H. 1983. *Power in and around organizations*. Englewood Cliffs, NJ: Prentice Hall.

Mitchell, T. 1976. Applied principles in motivation theory, in P. Warr, ed., *Personal goals and work design*. London: Wiley, pp. 163–171.

Mobley, W. 1982. *Employee turnover: causes, consequences and control*. Reading, MA: Addison-Wesley.

Munro, B. 1983. Young graduates: Who are they and what do they want? *Journal of Nursing Administration* 13(6): 21–26.

Numerof, R., and M. Abrams. 1984. Collective bargaining among nurses: current issues and future prospects. *Health Care Management Review* 9: 61–67.

O'Toole, J. 1981. *Making America work: productivity and responsibility*. New York: Continuum.

Podsakoff, P., and L. Williams. 1986. The relationship between job performance and job satisfaction, in E. Locke, ed., *Generalizing from laboratory to field settings*. Lexington, MA: Lexington Books, pp. 241–253.

Ponak, A. 1981. Unionized professionals and the scope of bargaining: a study of nurses. *Industrial and Labor Relations Review* 34: 396–407.

Ravin, B., H. Freeman, and R. Haley. 1982. Social science perspective in hospital infection control, in A. Johnson, O. Grusky, and B. Ravin, eds., *Contemporary health services*. Boston: Auburn House, pp. 139–176.

Rice, R., D. McFarlin, R. Hunt, et al. 1985. Organizational work and the perceived quality of life: toward a conceptual model. *Academy of Management Review* 10: 296–310.

Richardson, B., and D. Kaufman. 1983. Social science inquiries into female achievement: recurrent methodological problems, in B. Richardson and J. Wirtenberg, eds., *Sex role research*. New York: Praeger, pp. 33–48.

Ross, M. 1976. The self-perception of intrinsic motivation. *New Directions in Attribution Research* 1:121–141.

Salkever, D. 1983. Cost implications of hospital unionization. *Advances in Health Economics and Health Services Research* 4: 225–255.

Schiemann, W. 1984. Major trends in employee attitudes toward compensation, in W. Schiemann, ed., *Managing human resources/1983 and beyond*. Princeton, NJ: Opinion Research Survey.

Schilit, W., and E. Locke. 1982. A study of upward influence in organizations. *Administrative Science Quarterly* 27: 304–316.

Scott, W. 1982. Managing professional work: three models of control for health organizations. *Health Services Research* 17(5): 213–240.

Simendinger, E., and T. Moore. 1983. The formation and destruction of physician/administration cooperation. *Hospital Forum* 26: 7–15.

Sloan, F., and B. Steinwald. 1980. *Hospital labor markets: analysis of wages and work force composition*. Lexington, MA: Lexington Books.

Spitzer, R., and L. Bolton, 1984. Attitudes towards equitable pay. *Nursing Management* 15(6): 32–37.

Staw, B. 1977. Motivation in organizations: towards synthesis and redirections, in B. Staw, ed., *New Directions in Organization Behaviour*. Chicago: St. Clair Press, pp. 55–98.

Staw, B. 1984. Organizational behavior: a review and reformulation of the field's outcome variables. *Annual Review of Psychology* 35: 627–666.

Stevenson, J. 1982. Construction of a scale to measure load, power, and margin in life. *Nursing Research* 31: 222–225.

Styles, M. 1982. *On nursing: toward a new endowment*. St. Louis: C.V. Mosby.

Van Fleet, D., and G. Yukl. 1986. A century of leadership research, in D. Wren and J. Pearce, eds., *Papers dedicated to the development of modern management*. Mississippi State, MS: Academy of Management, pp. 12–23.

Van Wagner, K., and C. Swanson. 1979. From Machiavelli to Ms: differences in power styles. *Public Administration Review* 39: 66–72.

Varca, P., G. Shaffer, and C. McCauley, 1983. Sex differences in job satisfaction revisited. *Academy of Management Journal* 26: 353–361.

Wahba, M., and L. Bridwell. 1976. Maslow reconsidered: a review of research on the need hierarchy theory. *Organization Behavior and Human Performance* 15: 212–240.

Wakim, J. 1976. *A comparison of collective bargaining agreements negotiated for registered nurses by different bargaining agents*. Unpublished doctoral dissertation, Indiana University.

Wall, T. 1982. Perspectives on job redesign, in J. E. Kelly and C. W. Clegg, eds., *Autonomy and control at the workplace*. London: Croom Helm, pp. 1–20.

White, H., and M. Wolfe. 1983. Nursing administration and personnel administration. *Journal of Nursing Administration* 13(7/8): 15–19.

Zaleznik, A. 1977. Managers and leaders: Are they different? *Harvard Business Review* 55(3): 69–78.

# Summary of Section II

In Section II, studies relevant to nursing administration conducted by investigators from many disciplines have been organized for discussion into the categories advocated by management theorists. The objective is to encourage executives and managers to articulate a management philosophy appropriate for professional service work while being aware of the contradictions, ambiguities, and limitations of theories and research.

The sequence of topics suggests the order of analysis. First and foremost, nursing is a core hospital department that needs to be integrated into the management structure of the hospital. To manage the three domains— patient care, system maintenance, and career management— hospital and nursing executives need to continually address questions about values and create a compatible culture. The single largest challenge is to coordinate the three systems and balance their competing demands while meeting accountability standards. Research and the characteristics of the magnet hospitals suggest that interdepartmental communication and coordination are essential.

After the decision-making processes and structure have been aligned with the organizational culture, executives need to consider the extent of decentralization that is appropriate for their situation. Although decentralization, participation, and autonomy are often prescribed as a panacea, they may be impossible to implement without a high degree of central direction. Conversely, organizations with the greatest need to decentralize may be least able to achieve decentralization.

Contrary to what the volume of research on nurse staffing would suggest, the direct advantages of one form of departmentation and subunit design over another appear to be modest. Nurses are amazingly adaptable, and there are few data to support the commonsense assumption that nurse staffing levels and differences in subunit design are systematically related to hospital effectiveness. Although more research is needed on the linkage

between nursing and outcome measures, the greatest need is to reconceptu-
alize control processes and link them with organizational and departmental
goals.

Thinking on some issues that affect the workplace has been influenced
more by ideology and tradition than by facts. The role of unions, the nature
of motivation, and the need for hierarchy, as well as the existence and effects
of sex-based discrimination, serve as examples. Available data are presented to encourage managers to clarify their own positions and be alert to
organizational policies and procedures that perpetuate dysfunctional behaviors by managers or workers.

Only when the culture is supportive, the design is appropriate, and
control constraints are understood and accepted should work redesign
projects, which are both more risky and more costly than the previous
actions, be undertaken at the unit level. Successful interventions require
training and reeducation, especially of middle management, whose role will
be changed from one of supervisor to one of coach. Throughout this complex
process, leaders must neither overestimate their own importance nor underestimate the energy and influence of the caregivers, who are aligned with
patients and physicians.

It is traditional to limit management texts to micro issues rather than to
incorporate policy and environmental issues. This emphasis is appropriate
for inexperienced and lower level managers, especially in businesses where
the government does not have a major role in financing education, licensing,
or reimbursing for services. However, hospital executives must deal with
macro issues that influence the operating environment. In the case of
nursing, a dysfunctional system is perpetuated by the interplay of special
interest groups, legislators, and bureaucrats and affects the shaping of
individual hospital careers. This problem, along with some scenarios for the
future, is the subject of Section III.

*Section III*

# Policy Perspectives

---

## Chapter 8

# The Recurrent Hospital Nurse Shortage

---

## Background

One-third of all health workers are nurses. In 1984 there were 984,330 registered nurses (RNs) working full-time in the United States. An additional one-half million nurses were working part-time. Between 1977 and 1984 the number of employed nurses increased by 55% as compared with an 8% growth in the U.S. population. Between 1980 and 1984 there was an increase of 133,351 full-time nurses employed in hospitals (Department of Health and Human Services 1986, 40; Levine and Moses 1982, 487). Hospitals reduced the number of full-time employees (FTEs) between 1983 and 1986 but increased the number of RN FTEs (Aiken and Mullinix 1987). However, the proportion of hospital nurses working full-time was 68.1%, down from 70.6% in 1977 (DHHS 1986, 40; 1982b, 15).

This rapid growth was sustained by an increased number of high school graduates, higher labor force participation by women, higher wages, and educational subsidies. Between 1965 and 1982 the federal government spent $1.6 billion under the Nurse Training Act for institutional and student support (Institute of Medicine 1983, 47). States also invested heavily by establishing RN programs in two- and four-year colleges.

The hospital industry has been described as an oligopolistic industry, one that is dominated by a relatively small number of employers who band together and act as a cartel. Thirty percent of hospitals are in markets comprised of only one or two hospitals. Sixty percent of all hospitals are in markets with fewer than six hospitals (LeRoy 1982). Experts have frequently predicted that 10% of all hospitals will close within the next few years. If this occurs, the concentration of hospitals will increase just as concentration in the airline industry occurred after several years of deregulation.

Hospital labor markets are local, not national. Although there is a highly visible minority of new graduates who move to take advantage of better salaries or career opportunities, mature nurses tend to remain within their own area. Many analysts believe that hospital employers have taken advantage of this immobility to set nurse wages, restrain wage increases, and avoid paying differentials for increased education, experience, or responsibility. The National Academy of Sciences, in a comprehensive study of nursing, found that nurses' wages were not determined by educational degree, years of experience, job position, or age (Institute of Medicine 1983, 295). Yet it is characteristic of white-collar workers to have pronounced variation in earnings within work levels, reflecting size, location, and range of rate plans (Sieling 1982). Even the recent trend toward decentralization, which has encouraged desirable participation in clinical practice issues, has not significantly raised pay for experienced hospital nurses (refer to Chapter 7 for salary data).

The recession of the early 1980s and the adjustment to prospective payment led to a false sense of security about the nursing supply. The current issue is not a shortage of RNs but rather a shortage of full-time working nurses and a decline in nurses enrolling in and graduating from generic baccalaureate degree programs (refer to Chapter 2 for data on graduation trends). Hospitals are experiencing staffing difficulties because the salary structure and working conditions for nurses do not foster either full-time nursing work or college enrollment in nursing programs. The growing dependence on foreign-educated nurses is evidence that the industry is not meeting the threshold requirements of American nurses.

## The Recurrent Cycle of Nurse Shortages

The dynamics of nurse pay and nurse supply are well established (Prescott 1987). Nurses' pay does not respond in a timely fashion to upward market forces. Instead, there is a long period between substantial pay adjustments, with an intervening gradual buildup of pressures for change. The lag is longer and the correction steeper than in other industries, probably because of the employer domination of the local labor markets (Friss 1988). As a result, nurses gradually lose their relative pay position. As after-tax income declines, more nurses work part-time, and the number of new entrants is not enough to meet employers' demands. Since 1960 there has been an inverse relationship between nurses' relative wages and budgeted RN vacancies. Figure 8-1 illustrates the relationship between salaries and reported vacancies.

Belatedly, pay competition returns, and an above-average pay increase occurs to restore the equilibrium (Department of Health and Human Services 1981). Eventually, a 1% increase in the RN wage rate leads to a 1.5% increase in the number of entrants to nursing programs. This cycle of falling behind and catching up in pay, or the "ratchet effect," is the dynamic underlying the recurring shortages of hospital nurses.

During the pressure-building part of the cycle, short-term strategies such as foreign nurse recruitment, use of supplemental agencies, refresher courses, day care centers, and flexible hours are rediscovered. Intense lobbying for increased educational subsidies and relaxed requirements for ancillary workers and foreign-educated nurses occur at all levels of government. New satisfaction and turnover studies rediscover that nurses need more autonomy and participation in decision-making.

Figure 8-2 depicts the relationship among market forces, employer utilization of nurses, and nurse labor force participation. The underpinnings of this cycle have been a limited range of opportunities for career-oriented women, an expanding number of women between the ages of 18 and 25, and government subsidy of entry-level education. Nursing has been exceptional in that it is the only bachelor's degree occupation receiving an educational subsidy greater than that available to all students. This steady "free" supply serves to insulate employers from pressures to increase the efficiency of support systems, tailor reward systems to keep valuable employees, substitute less-skilled workers, develop permanent internship programs, institute real upward mobility ladders, or contribute to the costs of education of vocational workers as do other employers in the community. This strategy is not free to society, however. From 1972 to 1983 it cost the federal government approximately $40,000 to educate each new nurse (Eastaugh 1985). The National Center for Health Services Research concluded that nursing education costs have been even more expensive to society than higher wage costs would have been (Department of Health and Human Services 1982c).

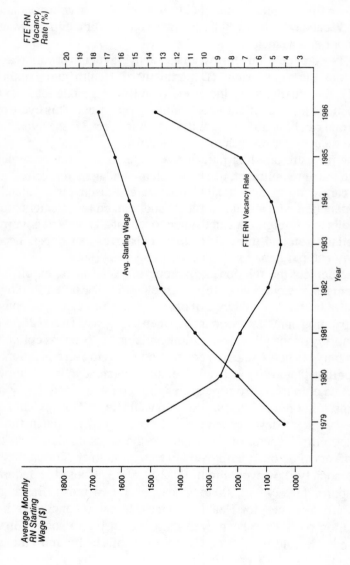

**Figure 8-1.** Registered nurse starting wages and vacancy rates in U.S. hospitals, 1979–1986. Starting wage is the recruiting rate or the going rate normally paid in order to fill vacancies. Data for 1986 are for the week of December 1, 1986. Source: Buerhaus, P. 1987. Not just another nursing shortage. *Nursing Economics* 5: 267–279 (Anthony J. Jannetti, Inc., publisher).

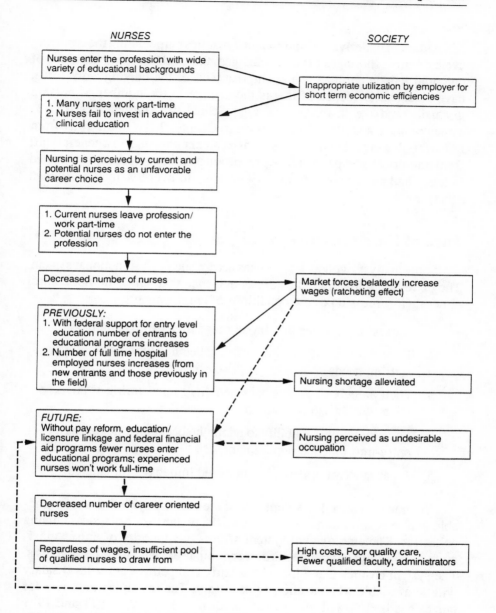

**Figure 8-2.** The self-reinforcing downward cycle of occupational attractiveness. Reprinted with permission from Friss, L. 1988. The nursing shortage revisited. Do we dislike it enough to cure it? *Inquiry* 25: 235.

Although underlying employment dynamics perpetuating the recurring cycle of nurse shortages have not changed, the work force expectations of potential female entrants, who comprise 97% of the nursing work force, have changed. Evidence of this is the decline in the number of nursing graduates and the lower-than-average Scholastic Aptitude Test (SAT) scores of current students as discussed in Chapter 2. The shift away from nursing is due to problems of nursing as a career rather than to a general shift from traditional occupations. The proportion of college freshmen interested in teaching has increased from 4.5% in 1983 to over 7% in 1986 (Green 1987).

## Lack of Nursing Activism

Some analysts wonder why nurses accept such a dysfunctional system. They cite the following indicators as evidence that nurses do not control either their profession or the conditions of employment:

1.  Nurses' acceptance of a broad range of staffing patterns

2.  Their willingness to adjust work schedules to meet employer staffing needs

3.  Their propensity to give back benefits gained during a "crisis" once equilibrium is restored

4.  The profession's inability to adopt the bachelor's degree as an entry-into-practice requirement

5.  An absence of effectively organized initiatives for change.

Yet nurses' collective acceptance of the existing system is understandable. It also enables nurses to perpetuate the pretense of a classless nursing collective. The employment system affords the majority of nurses maximum opportunity to negotiate a career compatible with their life interests. The system ensures that a job with a fairly competitive entry-level salary will be available when desired or necessary. The unemployment rate for nurses has been low–1.9% was the median rate between 1971 and 1981 compared to 6% for all civilian workers (Institute of Medicine 1983, 60).

High educational or certification requirements usually are barriers to employment. Nursing does not have this problem. Because the bachelor's degree is not a prerequisite for licensure, and because certification requirements are rare in hospitals, nurses enjoy flexibility with respect to hours, shifts, and specialties; this flexibility would not exist if the system were changed. For many nurses these trade-offs offset the disadvantages of a compacted salary schedule and limited upward mobility in clinical nursing. This is especially true for those with the least career commitment and for young women, who tend to underestimate their lifetime career attachment.

Other analysts ask why nurses do not unionize to improve their condition. Unionization appeals to some nurses, especially those employed in government hospitals, but for the remainder, the small salary gain unionized nurses get is not worth the required investment of time and energy. Career-oriented nurses with higher aspirations leave hospital nursing for public health, teaching, and management positions.

## Projections

Since 1977 the U.S. Department of Health and Human Services has prepared six reports to the Congress on the supply, distribution, and requirements for nurses, as well as the factors affecting supply and distribution. The department's 1986 *Report on Nursing* concurs with the previous reports and the Institute of Medicine's study of nursing and nursing education (1983) that the aggregate supply of nurses will balance demand for the next decade.

Projections of future requirements are based on two approaches. The historical trend-based model examined requirements for nursing personnel according to the major sectors of the health care system in which RNs and LPNs are employed. The dominant assumption is that historical trends in the health care system will determine future trends. Modifications were made where it appeared that utilization will be affected by cost-containment policies, HMO growth, or the adoption of case management.

The criteria-based model was based on the judgments of a panel of experts from nursing education, employers, and related organizations. They made additional assumptions concerning the mix of aides, LPNs, nurse practitioners, and clinical specialists. They also differentiated among hospitalized patients by severity of illness, a factor that the historical trend model did not specifically include.

In comparing the projections made by both methods, a relative balance of nurses in the year 2000 is forecasted except for the upper-bound estimate of the expert panel. Unless there is wide adoption of case-managed delivery of health care, from about 2006 until 2020 the requirements for FTE RNs will exceed the FTE supply. The shortage of baccalaureate and graduate nurses continues throughout the entire period beginning in the year 2000. Although the two methods used different assumptions concerning LPN utilization, they reached the same conclusions: Requirements will outpace supply, and as time progresses, a wider gap between supply and requirements for licensed personnel will occur.

A business-as-usual approach on the part of the hospital industry, anticipating another passage through the cycle as before, poses significant risk. The underpinnings on which the cycle depends have changed, as evidenced by the following:

- Talented females are choosing male-dominated careers with more opportunities and better working conditions.

- Mature nurses with skills and high career expectations are leaving the hospital setting for other health-related careers, including general management.

- Nurses with expert knowledge and skills, who will be in greatest demand, cannot be produced in as short a time as less-skilled nurses who met previous needs.

- Resistance to immigration by a broad spectrum of Americans militates against the employment of nurses whose first language is not English, even if internal political changes in Thailand, Korea, and the Philippines (the primary international supply sources) do not prevent access to this resource.[1]

- Because of the high cost of nursing education and the lack of student demand, state and local educational funding will be difficult to justify.

In short, nursing is attracting more applicants with less ability who study and work part-time. The pool of nurses who will invest in their own advanced education to become future expert clinicians, teachers, and administrators is in jeopardy. Moreover, the cycle will be more difficult to remedy this time. Not only is there strong resistance to reforming the pay system, but traditional recruitment strategies will be less effective with contemporary women and older workers.

# Needed Changes

A strategy that couples productivity increases with slowed growth in a relatively well-paid work force would be a promising approach to both containing costs and remaining competitive in the occupational choice and career development market. Employers need to focus on reforms that will make hospital nursing attractive, especially to steady-state career nurses, as was discussed in Chapter 1. Individuals who seek a steady-state career are guided by professional norms, they find it worthwhile to invest in their own education, and they seek an environment in which advancement is neither hierarchical, nor self-actualizing in the activist sense, nor entrepreneurial. Although steady-state nurses combine their personal and work lives, their participation is neither erratic nor a springboard for more challenging activities.

A change in management philosophy is required to ensure the career development of a core of clinically oriented nurses. Instead of concentrating on the needs of young women with children, executives and managers will need to concentrate on the career expectations of mature women (Nolan 1985). In the 1990s, the largest number of active nurses will be in their 30s. Their participation, like that of all other workers, will depend on how they are treated in their early career stages. Policies are needed to increase the labor force participation of women aged 25 to 54, the prime working years, to offset the decline in workers aged 18 to 25 years, the primary recruiting pool. This may well be difficult to do for three reasons: (1) The participation rates for older women have changed little over time (Rones 1982); (2) nursing labor force participation rates are already higher at all ages than among the general female population (Buerhaus 1987); and (3) there is a societal trend for older women to work part-time and retire earlier (Personick 1985). It is anticipated that the overall activity rate of nurses will be 72% by the year 2000, compared to a 76.6% rate in 1980 (Department of Health and Human Services 1986, Chapter 10, 55). Later childbearing by career women has the potential for lessening labor force participation even more, but this effect has not been estimated.

Now is the time for assertive innovative management. Several ideas come to mind:

1.  Collectively, employers could lobby for funds or obtain grants for research and demonstration projects that would substitute equipment for labor. Links with architects, biomedical firms,

and systems analysts could revolutionize the design of critical care units, for example.

2. Employers could revamp their technical support systems so that "just-in-time" supplies and equipment would minimize nurse "down-time."

3. Increase pay differentials to encourage the best use of nurses at all levels.

4. Require physicians to develop more standard protocols.

5. Develop extensive internal recruitment and retraining programs.

6. Introduce bedside computerized systems.

The general principle is the one articulated throughout the preceding management chapters. Workers are valuable resources, not disposable ones. The primary function of management is to unleash the potential of workers by reinforcing a professional-service culture, matching organizational design to organizational strategies, staffing appropriately, and fostering a career climate that is supplemented rather than dominated by young, temporary, or part-time workers.

Time is short. The bedside nurse of 1994 has already made a critical career decision—whether to take algebra and chemistry, which are educational prerequisites for a nursing career—in 1989. Neophyte nurses are making career decisions under adverse conditions. Salary increments are lower than before, work loads are heavier, fringe benefits remain below average, givebacks are not uncommon, and the tax outlook is not favorable for two-income families.

Prospective payment resulted in fewer full-time workers and the highest hospital profit margins in history (Reczynski 1986; Guterman and Dobson 1986). Surplus revenues (the difference between income and expenses) more than doubled in 1984. This level of profitability has since been eroded, but the industry lost a window of opportunity when it failed to share gains with productive and career-oriented nurses. Instead, they sowed the seeds for the next cycle of nursing shortage by demonstrating to young nurses that there are no career rewards for long service or performance. Now that profit margins are lower, of course, the problem is more intractable.

## Prerequisites

What is most needed (and most difficult) is to see the employment problems of nurses in organizational and societal terms rather than as a problem of the nursing profession. In the past, many studies concentrated on the characteristics of nurses and never asked why so few nurses over age 35 were working in hospitals. The most common prescriptions exhorted nurses to show their power through either unionization or political action, to put their own house in order (in some unspecified way), to clarify their educational system, to define tasks and scope of responsibility, and to develop a unified position. Although there is an element of reason in each of these prescriptions, they share a propensity to blame the victim and expect nurse initiatives to overcome cultural changes and the lack of organizational incentives. This is unrealistic.

Work satisfaction and participation should not be seen solely as a function of internal events and interactions involving personality and family priorities. Modern occupations are embedded in complex social, political, and economic networks of individuals and groups. Given the reasonable assumption that employment conditions influence the work behaviors of women as well as men, it is time to change the management of women in traditional occupations. Since employers cannot change the number, personality, education, and work expectations of women, executives and managers need to change the employment system, including pay and working conditions.

This assignment is difficult for several reasons:

1.  Current employment practices assume that nursing wages must be kept low enough for all hospitals to survive, regardless of occupancy or clinical outcomes. Incentives are not geared to meet the needs and expectations of mature women. The current system encourages nurses to develop a transient career orientation, working as it fits personal needs or a spiral career, or for self-actualization until a better opportunity arises.

2.  There has been a greater decline in job satisfaction among women in sex-segregated occupations than in mixed-sex ones (Lemkau and Pottick 1984).

3.  Federal policies and schools of nursing are preparing nurses to work in nontraditional modalities, nursing homes, and preventive care.

4.  A countervailing trend of lower labor force participation among mature women already exist.

5.  Competing opportunities attract the most capable potential nurses, leaving a larger residual of nurses who put home and family life ahead of career.

6.  Legislators respond to political pressures by providing nursing scholarships and extending visa requirements, which fuel the cycle.

# Myths

A first step toward changing management philosophy is to reconsider some common assumptions or myths. Myths about turnover, labor force participation, and nursing costs are shared widely and color perceptions of problems and possible solutions (Institute of Medicine 1981). The following observations provide a basis for reexamining assumptions.

**Myth 1:** "I am an expert on what nurses want because I communicate well with one who is a close friend or member of my family."

Individuals often react emotionally to alternative nurse work force policies because almost everyone has some knowledge about nursing education and employment problems based on personal contact with nurses. This tendency to overestimate the value of our own experience occurs whenever we analyze any other group. Because nurses comprise almost 30% of female professional-technical workers, many people have nurse friends and relatives with a strong opinion about what needs to be done. Yet few people understand the multiple facets of nursing work or career options.

Nurses who are career oriented value higher education and tend to aspire to advanced clinical practice. In choosing this objective they must face problems of autonomy, physician dominance, and status. Young nurses frequently depend on the relatively high entry-level salary and the ready availability of nursing jobs as they accommodate their careers to the opportunities available to their mates. Later, easy job accommodation to family life is valued. This group may fear higher education or competency standards, which might restrict their flexibility or job availability. Nurses from traditional working-class families see nursing as a high-status career and treasure stable employment. Many nurses, although eager to learn, are likely to suspect paper credentials such as degrees, which have the potential for pushing them aside.

All of this means that nurses (and their families) come to nursing with divergent expectations and horizons. Employers also need workers with a variety of educational and career backgrounds. In such a complex employment system, it is not realistic to expect simple solutions.

Work force policies for nurses depend on disaggregated solutions rather than single all-encompassing ones to address the career aspirations of nurses from all walks of life.

**Myth 2:** "Nurses have low work force participation."

Nursing labor force participation has been higher than that of women in general and equivalent to that of college-educated women, even though only one-third of nurses have a bachelor's degree (Department of Health and Human Services 1982a; Michelotti 1977). Although 75% of nurses are working, the proportion working part-time is large. Work force analysts conclude that nurses have a high propensity to work, but that wages are not high enough to make a full-time job worthwhile. A concern exists that the participation rate of mature women is less than would be expected on the basis of education and income. This needs closer monitoring.

Among women in the middle or higher income levels, labor force participation decisions respond more to variations in women's own market-earning capacity than to variations in other family income (Department of Labor 1970). To increase the labor force participation of career nurses to the level experienced by professional women in male-dominated fields (lawyers, physicians, business executives), salaries and career structures need to become competitive with those available to other professional women. A managerial challenge for hospitals in the decade ahead is to increase the full-time participation of middle-aged women while keeping the participation edge they already have with young nurses.

**Myth 3:** "Part-time and supplemental agency nurses do not have a commitment to the profession and can only be motivated by salary."

It would be a mistake to impugn the motivation and commitment of individual nurses working part-time. Although earnings potential is one of many determinants of part-time work by married women, this is not the same as saying that part-time workers are less affected by job challenge and complexity than full-time nurses. Part-time workers may simply have a different psychology of work. For example, part-time rehabilitation unit workers have been found to be more satisfied with organization policies, structure, reward systems, level of trust, distribution of power, and the job itself than full-time workers (Eberhardt and Shani 1984). Supplemental agency nurses were found not to differ from staff nurses on measures of job involvement and satisfaction; they were at least as well qualified and experienced (Prescott and Langford 1981; Kehrer, Deiman, and Szapiro 1984).

Enlightened use of part-time workers requires attention to selection, placement, orientation, and reward structure, since these individuals are prone to exit the labor force permanently if their professional needs are neglected. Young part-time workers should be viewed as a pool for future career workers rather than as disposable items to be used to achieve performance targets.

**Myth 4:** "Increases in nurses' salaries cause hospital cost inflation."

Nursing costs comprise about 30% of hospital costs and influence the wages and benefits of other hospital workers (Institute of Medicine 1983, 29). In the aggregate, however, nursing salaries have played a minor role in the hospital cost inflation of the past two decades. Wages have indeed increased; a 10% increase in wages is associated with a 1% increase in hospital expenses. However, "the increase in wages, no matter what the cause, cannot explain the inflation in hospital costs since costs would have increased substantially even if wage rates were held constant" (Abernethy and Pearson 1979).

In community hospitals, inpatient labor expenses increased by 16.4% while payroll increased only by 11.8% from July 1981 to July 1982; overall labor costs increased 39% faster than payroll, suggesting that staffing patterns changed more than pay level (American Hospital Association 1982).

The impact of nurse salaries on costs cannot be ignored. However, the reasonable approach to wage and salary administration and staffing is to differentiate among competency levels, performance, and rewards to obtain the necessary mix of support, technical, and professional personnel.

Moreover, increases in wages paid may be recouped in other ways. A hospital that pay good wages and establishes accountability standards and a responsive control system can attract better-than-average employees, expect more from them, insist on high performance, and refuse to accept anything less than good overall performance. Low wages do not necessarily mean low costs. Nursing productivity does not necessarily improve with task delegation and intensive supervision (i.e., more workers). Nor is it necessary to pay all nurses the same. Productivity depends on administrative systems supporting competent nurses and pay for performance.

**Myth 5:** "Nursing departments are overstaffed."

During the period from 1977 to 1982, the percentage increase in work force hours per patient-day was less for nursing than for all other departments except one—support services (Mistarz 1984). Early staffing data suggest that prospective reimbursement is causing an increase in the proportion of nursing hours per patient-day provided by nurses. However, since hospitals also report an increase in patients' acuity, it is difficult to prove that the increase in nursing days is unjustified (Department of Health and Human Services 1986a, Chapter 10, 28).

**Myth 6:** "Upgrading the educational requirements for professional nurses would lead to a loss of employment opportunities."

Prospective payment and new technologies initially reduced hospital occupancy rates, but the trend is now upward. The segment of the population aged 75 to 85 years will increase to 14 million by the year 2000. The group aged 85 and older will increase even more rapidly. Together, these groups will increase the number of physician visits, nursing home days, and short-stay hospitalizations (Butler 1983; Butz et al. 1982). The U.S. Department of Labor projects that, by 1995, 3.5% of the civilian labor force will be working in hospitals, as contrasted with 2.9% in 1982. This also suggests growth in opportunities rather than decline (Bureau of the Census 1985).

**Myth 7:** "There are not enough nurses. Therefore, we cannot make the bachelor's degree an entry-into-practice requirement."

Linking education to licensure is the only hope for making career lines visible to potential nurses at all levels. Nursing needs to remain competitive for talented high school graduates and have a separate degree and license for nurses (as yet untitled) who want a community college education. It is unreasonable to assume that nursing education and career lines can be isolated from societal expectations for technical-professional education and work. These shared assumptions are that education should relate to the level of responsibility, pay, and opportunities for advancement.

## Summary

The character of new nursing recruits is changing. Future nurses are likely to have lower academic potential on average as bright women choose other careers. The retention of committed, competent nurses will be a problem throughout the next decade, as the nature of the work force is affected by demographic and cultural changes. First, there will be fewer high school graduates, the primary educational pool. Second, women who traditionally chose a career in nursing, especially the most talented, will pursue new, nontraditional career options. (Note that 97% of nurses are women, and the increase of males in the profession is so slow that changes in male career patterns will not have an effect for generations.) Third, currently working nurses are slowly shifting to nonhospital employment. Fourth, employers are not developing initiatives that will keep mature women in the work force. Fifth, nursing is becoming similar to higher status occupations by offering more career options; hospital nursing is likely to become a less attractive alternative. Sixth, federal support for entry-level education is becoming more difficult to obtain, and thus there will be more competition for equally scarce local educational funds. Finally, the demand for hospital nursing will intensify as admitted patients become both older and sicker.

Responsible hospital administrators and associations recognize that long-term survival requires that the industry remain competitive in attracting professional service workers. The days of ready supply of young, technologically expert replacement nurses at low cost (to the hospital) are over. The industry's own long-term best interest is to create career options for mature, talented women. The aggregate supply of day workers with basic skills is not in jeopardy. What is in jeopardy is the core group of steady-state career nurses who provide organizational stability and expert clinical care and serve as the administrators and educators of future steady-state career nurses. Enlightened executives and managers will recognize the futility of waiting for nurses to resolve their problems on their own. They will question the continued reliance on short-run strategies that attract and reward women for part-time, part-life commitment.

## Endnotes

1.  In response to intense lobbying and media efforts, the Immigration and Naturalization Service announced on May 26, 1988, that it would begin granting sixth-year extensions automatically for nurses working on H-1 visas. In addition, regional directors can grant a seventh-year extension on a case-by-case basis in extraordinary cases.

## References

Abernethy, D., and E. Pearson. 1979. *Regulating hospital costs: the development of public policy*. Ann Arbor, MI: Association of University Programs in Health Administration.

Aiken, L., and C. Mullinix. 1987. The nurse shortage: myth or reality? *New England Journal of Medicine* 317: 641–646.

American Hospital Association Office of Public Policy Analysis. 1982. *Trends: community hospital indicators* (mimeographed). Chicago: American Hospital Association.

Buerhaus, P. 1987. Not just another nursing shortage. *Nursing Economics* 5: 267–279.

Bureau of the Census. 1985. *Statistical abstract of the United States: 1986*, 106th ed. Washington, DC: Government Printing Office.

Butler, R. 1983. *A generation at risk*. Austin, TX: University of Texas.

Butz, W., K. McCarthy, P. Morrison, et al. 1982. *Demographic challenges in America's future*. Santa Monica, CA: Rand Corporation.

Department of Health and Human Services. 1981. *The recurrent shortage of registered nurses*. Washington, DC: Bureau of Health Professions.

Department of Health and Human Services. 1982a. *Registered nurse population: an overview*. Washington, DC: Bureau of Health Professions.

Department of Health and Human Services. 1982b. *Statistical profile of registered nurses in the United States 1977–1980*. (DHPA Report No. 82-3). Washington, DC: Government Printing Office.

Department of Health and Human Services. 1982c. *Review and synthesis of research findings on the distribution effectiveness of health professional manpower*. Washington, DC: National Center for Health Services Research.

Department of Health and Human Services. 1986. *National sample survey of registered nurses, 1984: summary of results*. Washington, DC: Bureau of Health Professions.

Department of Health and Human Services. 1988. *Report on nursing: sixth report to the President and Congress on the status of health personnel*. Washington, DC: Public Health Service.

Department of Labor. 1970. *Dual careers, Vol. 1* (Manpower Research Monograph No. 21). Washington, DC: Government Printing Office.

Eastaugh, S. 1985. The impact of the Nurse Training Act on the supply of nurses. *Inquiry* 22: 404–417.

Eberhardt, B., and A. Shani. 1984. The effects of full-time vs. part-time employment status on attitudes toward specific organizational characteristics and overall job satisfaction. *Academy of Management Journal* 27: 893–899.

Friss, L. 1988. Do we care enough to cure the nursing shortage? *Inquiry* 25: 232–242.

Green, K. 1987. What the freshmen tell us. *American Journal of Nursing* 87: 1610–1615.

Guterman, S., and A. Dobson. 1986. Impact of the Medicare prospective payment system for hospitals. *Health Care Financing Review* 7(3): 97–114.

Institute of Medicine. 1981. Myths, realities, and public policy dilemmas in nursing, in *Six month interim report of Committee on Nursing and Nursing Education.* Washington, DC: National Academy of Sciences.

Institute of Medicine. 1983. *Nursing and nursing education: public policies and private actions.* Washington, DC: National Academy Press.

Kehrer, B., P. Deiman, and N. Szapiro. 1984. The temporary nursing service R.N. *Nursing Outlook* 32: 212–217.

Lemkau, J., and K. Pottick. 1984. The declining job satisfaction of white-collar women in sex-segregated and mixed-sex occupations. *Journal of Vocational Behavior* 25: 344–358.

LeRoy, L. 1982. Supplemental nursing agencies. *Health Affairs* 1: 41–54.

Levine, E., and E. Moses. 1982. Registered nurses today: a statistical profile, in L. Aiken, ed., *Nursing in the 1980s.* Philadelphia: J. B. Lippincott.

Michelotti, K. 1977. Educational attainment of workers. *Monthly Labor Review* 100(3): 62–65.

Mistarz, J. 1984. The changing economic profile of United States hospitals. *Hospitals* 58(10): 83–88.

Nolan, J. 1985. Work patterns of midlife nurses. *Nursing Research* 34: 150–154.

Personick, V. 1985. A second look at industry output and employment trends through 1995. *Monthly Labor Review* 108(11): 26–41.

Prescott, P. 1987. Another round of nurse shortage. *Image* 19: 204–209.

Prescott, P., and T. Langford. 1981. Supplemental agency nurses and hospital staff nurses. What are the differences? *Nursing and Health Care* 2: 200–206.

Reczynski, D. 1986. 1985 brings no respite from economic pressures. *Hospitals* 60(9): 166–167.

Rones, P. 1982. The aging of the older population and the effect on its labor force rates. *Monthly Labor Review* 105(9): 27–29.

Sieling, M. 1982. Occupational salary levels for white-collar workers. *Monthly Labor Review* 105: 30–32.

*Chapter 9*

# Future Prospects

---

The business that trusts to luck is bad business.

(Publilius Syrus in Kent 1985, 288)

This chapter begins by discussing three nursing topics likely to be controversial during the next decade. The first is pay pressures, which will be subject to conflicting upward and downward influences. The second topic is differentiated practice and the desire to link nursing education with practice—the "two-tier" movement. In its pure form, this movement would establish the bachelor's degree in nursing as an entry-level requirement for registered nurse (RN) practice. The third topic is the likelihood of union growth among nurses. Increased union power would encourage modest wage increases and reward seniority, but discourage higher pay for merit. This leads to a discussion of the focal role of the director of nursing services to meet these and other challenges previously discussed. After presenting a selection of nationwide data as a base line for analyzing the local nursing employment system, the chapter ends with a discussion of alternative scenarios.

# Pay Pressures

## Downward Pressures

There are many forces exerting downward pressure on nurse wages. The first four are direct whereas the others are indirect.

- The Health Care Financing Administration uses as wage index to calculate routine, special care, and ancillary operating cost reimbursement under Medicare (Federal Register 1988; Prospective Payment Assessment Commission 1985; Fackelman 1985a, b; Greene 1980; Watland et al. 1983). This not only places an upper limit on the amount of money available for hospital operations, but also reinforces relative wage differences from area to area based on 1984 wage data.

- Federal budget pressures make it unlikely that Congress will permit more than marginal increases in diagnosis-related group (DRG) payments for the next few years. The continuing possibility that the rates will be frozen dampens employer willingness to enter into multiyear contracts that include wage increases. Reports that 57% of hospitals received more money than it cost to treat patients during the first year under prospective payment makes it difficult to convince legislators and bureaucrats that hospitals lack funds to increase salaries, even though profit margins are now declining.

- The courts have consistently reaffirmed state laws regulating health care, including costs. When reduced state funding has limited hospitals' abilities to increase wages, the federal courts have ruled that the resulting loss in the employees' bargaining power is not an impermissible attempt to interfere with collective bargaining (Burda 1986).

- State rate commissions interfere with hospital bargaining settlements and limit increases either by use of a formula or by use of a retrospective review of labor settlements (Schramm 1978).

- Internal Revenue Service rulings limit such innovative, individualized approaches as cafeteria benefit and incentive compensation plans (especially in not-for-profit hospitals).

- The tax code penalizes two-family earners (Leuthold 1984). Since the majority of nurses are married, their take-home income is reduced.

- Nursing has been described as a textbook example of a cartelized or monopsonized market (Killingsworth 1986). For instance, in metropolitan areas it is common for hospitals, through their trade association, to share wage information with other hospitals and adopt similar wage practices. This affects community, government, and investor-owned hospitals (Friss 1987). Further, current practices supplant but perpetuate formal wage-setting agreements used until the 1960s. State hospital associations provide similar information for executives. Finally, the American Hospital Association has a history of opposing comparable-worth activity through the activities of a Comparable Worth Task Force formed to counteract such activity.

- Antitrust laws have not been enforced or amended to ensure that employers cannot collude to depress wages. The statute states, "...any combination that tampers with the price structure or pricing mechanism is engaged in an unlawful activity, even absent an agreement on particular prices. The fact that the combination...may have the effect of reducing rather than raising prices will not save the combination or agreement from illegality" (Thompson 1979, 6). Antitrust powers are limited in markets where there is conscious parallel behavior without explicit agreements, as is the usual case in hospital wage-setting.

- Multihospital systems can use profits from one hospital to subsidize hospitals in other areas (General Accounting Office 1983). When this occurs, it is likely that employees in all areas will be led to believe that economic pressures preclude wage increases.

- The federal government is a major employer of RNs in the military services, the Veterans Administration, and the Civil Service. Pay is based, in part, on comparability with the private sector. This is achieved by relating grade level and pay to the private sector. Thus, the federal government adopts and perpetuates the low-pay practices of private employers (Friss 1981).

## Upward Pressures

The many downward pressures on salaries are partially offset by upward pay pressures. The direct pressures are the extension of the Fair Labor Standards Amendments of 1985, unionization, and pay equity, especially comparable-worth activities. An indirect influence is lack of federal funding for basic nursing education.

- The Fair Labor Standards Amendments of 1985 have been extended to government hospitals. As a result, hospitals must pay overtime or compensatory time off for hours worked over 40 per week. The definition of regular work time has been tightened. For example, the time a nurse spends driving to required seminars must be compensated. Because of changes in the Fair Labor Standards Amendments, some salaried positions will need to be changed to hourly positions, with these workers receiving shift differentials and overtime pay. This federal oversight will probably be extended to non-public hospitals (Poulos 1984).

- Union growth among nurses is likely to be gradual rather than explosive (Aronson 1985). Although union activity is unlikely to raise nursing salaries enough to transform nursing into a primary labor market, some pay pressures would be created. The chief advantage of unionization of nurses would be to create the stability that results from rewarding seniority. The chief disadvantage is that pay scales would likely remain compressed because of the difficulty in rewarding individual productivity or merit within collective bargaining units. This prediction, however, could be upset if national bargaining, comparable worth, or pay containment efforts increase.

- Women and men continue to receive unequal treatment with regard to pay. Overall, women earn 60% of male wages. Most studies suggest that no more than half of this difference can be explained by job and individual differences (Treiman and Hartmann 1981). Instead, most of the difference is explained by deeply ingrained social practices and job segregation.

Hospitals also pay men more than women, although education and experience explain much, but not all, of the difference (Muller, Vitali, and

Brannon 1987). It is generally accepted that, although every effort should be made to attract men into nursing, eliminating job segregation is not a realistic solution for today's problems. Activists, who wish to raise the wage rate and overcome the salary compression that has been described as the hallmark of the profession, hope to achieve comparable worth.[1] This means paying workers in female-dominated jobs as much as employers pay workers in male-dominated jobs with equivalent value. Because the job evaluation system in the public sector provides comparative information, most comparable-worth activity has occurred there.

Table 9-1 presents data from a study by the State of Washington documenting that pay was related more closely to the percentage of female incumbents in the class than to the difficulty of the job as it was rated by an employer using traditional job evaluation processes and techniques. This pattern has been found consistently in all studies done by governments.

Nurses in San Jose, California, successfully struck for a substantial pay adjustment based on the comparable-worth argument. In Minnesota the state government initiated a comparable-worth adjustment; the average employee eligible for pay equity will have received $2,200 more in annual salary by the end of the four-year implementation process. Only 12 states (other than the seven with systems already meeting pay equity criteria) have no formal study initiated, ongoing, or completed.

The American Nurses' Association lost a comparable-worth suit in Illinois; lawsuits by nurses generally have not been successful. However, there is no reason to expect that there will be a decline in the number of filings. At the time of this writing, the Service Employees' International Union has a comparable-worth suit pending in Los Angeles.

Four common defenses are used to charges that sex or race was a factor in setting pay: (1) "You can't compare apples and oranges"; (2) the market determines pay; (3) employers cannot afford to correct any inequities that exist; and (4) blame the victim. In the future, such defenses are unlikely to carry much weight.

The apples-and-oranges argument centers around the ability to define job content and evaluate dissimilar jobs. (In truth, apples and oranges *can* be compared on the basis of nutritional content, but not color.) In fact, courts are becoming increasingly knowledgeable about alternative job evaluation and classification plans. They know that responsible employers have for years relied on objective evaluation of the skill, effort, responsibility, and working conditions required by different jobs to determine pay. The trend is to expect and require the employer to defend pay deviations on the basis

**Table 9-1** Comparison of Salaries and Points for Selected Sex-Segregated Positions, State of Washington

| Benchmark Title | Evaluation Points | Monthly Prevailing Rates ($)ᵃ | Prevailing Rate as % of Predictedᵇ | % Female Incumbents |
| --- | --- | --- | --- | --- |
| Automotive mechanic | 175 | 1,646 | 120.4 | 0.0 |
| Civil engineer | 287 | 1,885 | 116.0 | 0.0 |
| Maintenance carpenter | 197 | 1,707 | 118.9 | 2.3 |
| Highway engineer 3 | 345 | 1,980 | 110.4 | 3.0 |
| Correctional officer | 173 | 1,436 | 105.0 | 9.3 |
| Highway engineering technician | 133 | 1,401 | 110.4 | 11.6 |
| Truck driver | 97 | 1,493 | 126.6 | 13.6 |
| Physician | 861 | 3,857 | 128.0 | 13.6 |
| Warehouse worker | 97 | 1,286 | 109.1 | 15.4 |
| Senior architect | 362 | 2,240 | 121.8 | 16.7 |
| Senior computer system analyst | 384 | 2,080 | 113.1 | 17.8 |
| Chemist | 277 | 1,885 | 116.0 | 20.0 |
| Personnel representative | 410 | 1,956 | 101.2 | 45.6 |
| Laundry worker | 105 | 884 | 73.2 | 80.3 |
| Librarian 3 | 353 | 1,625 | 90.6 | 84.6 |
| Licensed practical nurse | 173 | 1,030 | 75.3 | 89.5 |
| Registered nurse | 348 | 1,368 | 76.3 | 92.2 |
| Administrative assistant | 226 | 1,334 | 90.6 | 95.1 |
| Telephone operator | 118 | 887 | 71.6 | 95.7 |
| Data entry operator | 125 | 1,017 | 82.1 | 96.5 |
| Intermediate clerk typist | 129 | 968 | 76.3 | 96.7 |
| Word processing equipment operator | 138 | 1,082 | 83.2 | 98.3 |
| Secretary | 197 | 1,122 | 78.1 | 98.5 |
| Retail sales clerk | 121 | 921 | 74.3 | 100.0 |

ᵃPrevailing rates as of July 1, 1980. Adopted state rates for midpoint of ranges, October 1981.
ᵇPredicted salary from line of best fit = ($2.43) (points) + $936.19; r= 0.8.

Source: Adapted with permission from Remick, H. 1981. The comparable worth controversy. *Public Personnel Management Journal* 10(4): 378.

of a well-managed job evaluation and performance appraisal system. In response to those who argue against installing or updating their job evaluation plan to avoid producing incriminating data, the courts have held that inaction itself is evidence of intent to discriminate.

The market defense is a weak defense, especially for hospitals with a history of wage setting. The U.S. Supreme Court has found that, although an employer may like to take economic advantage of a situation where women would work for less, the labor market cannot serve as a defense of unequal pay for equal work. Extension of this principle to comparable-worth cases is possible (Fogel 1984).

Market wages cannot be ignored, but neither can they be the sole pay determination standard. Although "benchmark pricing" (i.e., pegging salaries to those of key jobs based on surveys) has wide acceptance, it may be a convenient method of perpetuating discrimination rather than providing an objective standard. Employers who use benchmark pricing should include all jobs, including management jobs, and be prepared to prove that discrimination in pay practices does not exist. Arguing that someone else is discriminating is not an acceptable defense (Chi 1984).

Employers need legal advice before they participate in wage-sharing problems, particularly if such programs perpetuate discriminatory pay practices, stem from sex-segregated activities, contain specific pay recommendations, or use biased procedures. Studies conducted by hospital associations are especially suspect.

Many argue that the cost of correcting pay inequities is so high that the economy would be upset if such corrections were imposed. There are difficulties with this argument, however. As one judge noted, the "defendant's preoccupation with its budget pales when compared with the invidiousness of the ongoing discrimination" (AFSCME v. State of Washington 1983). Besides this, cost estimates for implementation may be inflated or inaccurate. In Minnesota, the total cost of achieving pay equity was a 3.7% budget increase. The adjustment affected 8,500 employees in 200 female-dominated classes, including health care workers (Rothchild and Watkins 1987).

The cost of voluntary, phased-in compliance seems to be substantially less than the cost of lawsuits, damages, and low productivity caused by pending suits. One analysis suggests that the cost of achieving comparable worth would be in the 10% to 15% range, far less than advocates anticipate and than employers fear. The correction for nursing is estimated to be 20% (Aldrich and Buchele 1986, 138).

The blame-the-victim argument, which argues that women willingly accept lower wages or should unionize or take other jobs, is also unlikely to impress judges hearing pay discrimination cases. Certainly, it is not a legal defense: "the willingness of women to accept inferior financial reward for equivalent work [is]...precisely the outmoded practice which the Equal Pay Act sought to eradicate" (Loffrey v. Northwest Airlines 1976). Although this reasoning has not been extended to comparable, as opposed to equal, work, it is not an enlightened defense.

Prudent employers must be able to defend pay differences on one of four grounds: (1) a bona fide seniority system, (2) merit, (3) quality or quantity of work produced, or (4) any other factor other than sex (Fulghum 1983). There is no reason to suspect that the trend toward greater pay equity for women will be reversed. Furthermore, employers cannot insulate nurses from broad cultural forces, such as linking education and experience with pay and professional control over work. Only the pace is uncertain. If the health care industry joins with governments to dampen equity pressures artificially, their combined power will reinforce the dysfunctional cycle described in Chapter 8.

An important, but indirect upward influence on pay is the loss of federal funding for entry-level nursing education. In 1980, scholarship support ended after 16 years and $387 million in appropriations. Although federal budget pressures were the precipitating reasons for ending both scholarships and construction grants for schools, there were more fundamental reasons. Several administrations became convinced, after many work force projection studies and the Institute of Medicine study (1983), that no aggregate shortage of nursing existed. The integration of nursing into mainstream higher education had been accomplished, as evidenced by the precipitous decline in diploma schools and the rapid and substantial increase in college nursing programs throughout the United States. Nor was there any compelling justification for extending support to basic nursing education beyond that available to all other students interested in college education.[2] Congress has, however, responded to intense lobbying by the nursing profession and the hospital industry to reinstate nursing scholarships for basic education to address the problem of a high vacancy rate. If these are funded as expected for fiscal year 1989–1990, the monies will fuel the dysfunctional recurrent cycle described in Chapter 8.

## Alternative Pay Possibilities

The following two scenarios offer insight into how the current nursing underpayment problem could unfold in the event that no policy intervention occurs. The first is already beginning to happen; the second is more unfavorable but could happen.

### *Outlook 1*

A precipitous drop in entrants and enrollments in all nursing programs, coupled with social pressures for pay equity, will lead to hospitals being forced to pay all nurses higher wages as the economy expands, the population grows and ages, and nurses have more employment opportunities. Colleges will not expand enrollments for replacement nurses because of a lack of student demand and local and state funding. These trends will lead to a loss of hospital revenues to hospitals without a history of enlightened labor policies.

Many hospitals will find that they are in competition with other employers for local educational monies, entry-level professionals, and experienced clinicians. Rather than invest money in internal career development, hospitals will enrich newspapers via classified advertising. In Los Angeles in 1988, the overall weekly cost of nurse recruitment ads in one major paper was between $400,000 and $450,000. For one special edition, the costs were $900,000 for ads under the nursing heading alone, not including ads listed under medical or hospital sections. Employers will belatedly grant above-average pay increases, which will further undermine their ability to provide career incentives. When it is almost too late, they will develop upward mobility programs for unlicensed nurses, underwrite specialty education for generalist nurses, offer substantial incentives to valued workers, and realign relations between physicians and nurses. In other words, they will either restructure the operating core or become nonviable.

### *Outlook 2*

Prospective prepayment will reinforce and perpetuate the propensity to delay and moderate nursing salary increases. Eventually, state or federal governments will be forced to mandate substantial pay adjustments for nurses to attract enough workers (as has already occurred in New Jersey, where a $9.0 million adjustment was made in September 1987 in response to a 17% RN vacancy rate). These workers will not be among the top quarter of their pool at any level, from aide to Ph.D.

England and Scotland have followed this path. During the first 20 years of the National Health Service, real pay for nurses slumped badly, more than for any other higher occupational group (Smail and Gray 1982a,b). These downward influences in the first 10 years reduced aggregate salaries for health personnel by 12% (Gray and Smail 1982). Concomitantly, the proportion of less-skilled ancillary workers and of part-time nurses increased (Smail and Gray 1982a). To overcome persistent nursing shortages, the government rectified the decline in real pay with special pay awards to nurses. The gains in real wages that occurred were short-lived, however. Although pay for lower nursing grades (e.g., nursing assistants) drew closer to that for licensed nurses, all nurses eventually suffered a substantial fall in income relative to comparable occupational groups (Smail and Gray 1982b).

It is doubtful that such economic solutions to the nursing shortage could be achieved without social unrest in this country, where the majority of nurses do not have the security and pension benefits that accompany civil service employment. Also, the overall decline in talent of the work force would create many more difficulties in the United States, where patients demand more high technology care. More importantly, to effect a similar solution in this country would require a substantial departure from present pay practices in community hospitals.

## Two-Tiered Nursing

Education and licensing will likely be the most critical issues for nurses in the next few years. The American Nurses' Association (ANA) and the National League for Nursing (NLN) endorse a two-level system of nursing practice based on two- and four-year academic programs. Professional nurses with the bachelor's degree in nursing would be the only ones holding the legal title "registered nurse." The American Hospital Association (AHA) and the affiliated Association of Nurse Executives have also endorsed the proposal.

Opponents of restricting the registered nurse title to baccalaureate graduates include the Assembly of Hospital Schools of Nursing, an AHA constituency section, existing diploma programs, and community college faculty. Each of these constituencies are reluctant to give up their identification with professional nursing. The ANA an the NLN may lose members as diploma and community college advocates form new alliances.

The current licensing dilemma is not new to the nursing profession, which has a history of changes in licensing practices. After World War II, the ANA worked to establish examinations and licensing laws for practical nurses (the two-tier nursing solution of that time). If the profession can repeat this success, existing nurses would be "grandfathered in." Generally, nurse duties would be defined by statute or regulation based on models from the pilot projects currently under way.

A task force of the National Council of State Boards of Nursing Examiners is developing testing models. Once a model has been selected, the task force will develop a plan of action, which will result in a decision regarding the need for a new examination and the appropriate job analyses, field tests, test plans, and so forth. Licensed practical nurse (LPN) education and licensure are automatically included in the process, since the board also administers the LPN examinations. In any system, educational linkages to professional nursing could be formalized to prevent the blockage of mobility for many nurses caused by lack of transferable college credits.

Ten major professional associations, including the Health Insurance Association of America, the AHA, and the Business Roundtable, are on the governing board of the National Commission on Nursing Implementation Project. This three-year project, funded by the W. K. Kellogg Foundation, and set up to implement the recommendations of the National Commission on Nursing report, has the responsibility to shape the future of nursing by identifying future trends and taking action (DeBack 1987). The areas for attention are differentiated practice as well as nurse-managed delivery systems, nursing information systems, a process to move nursing education toward preparing two categories of nurse, and public acceptance of nursing research.

Support of such licensing changes by staff nurses is less clear. Individually, many RNs have been enrolling at an impressive rate in second-step and generic programs to obtain their bachelor's degree. Of all students graduating from baccalaureate programs in 1986, 57% were returning RNs (NLN 1988). However, many nurses who have experienced educational barriers remain angry and feel helpless. For example, nearly all nurses educated in diploma schools (the majority of nurses over age 50 as well as many younger ones), did not get the transferable credits necessary for advancement and would have to start at square one to obtain a bachelor's degree.

Employers are also ambivalent about implementation of such standards. Many physicians and administrators prefer nurses who have strong technical skills (such as those taught in diploma schools) rather than analytical skills (such as those emphasized in baccalaureate programs). Employers fear, further, that higher educational requirements will mean higher salaries and a shortage of job opportunities for nurses. However, several studies indicate that when salary differential between BSNs and other RNs is small, employers prefer to hire the baccalaureate nurses. Medical centers already prefer to hire baccalaureate nurses, because educated nurses are apparently able to solve more complex problems and assume more leadership responsibilities than other nurses. A recent survey of hospitals accredited by the Joint Commission on Accreditation of Health Organizations (JCAHO) and home health care agencies in Pennsylvania indicated that the job market for RNs is tightening and that a higher proportion of nursing directors would prefer to hire baccalaureate-prepared nurses rather than diploma or associate graduates (Journal of Nursing Administration 1985).

Clarifying career steps by linking education to licensure and rewarding additional education may be the only ways for the hospital industry to retain its competitive position over nonhospital nurse employers in hiring and retaining nurses at all levels. The challenge is to recruit the best nursing assistants into RN programs, support the best technical nurses in BSN programs, encourage postgraduate education for the academically inclined, and use all levels appropriately.

## Related Social Issues

Two special areas of concern with creating a system with the baccalaureate degree as the cornerstone are (1) providing this level of education to nurses in rural areas and (2) increasing the proportion of minorities in the profession.

### Rural Areas

Rural areas will be especially affected because they may lack easy access to baccalaureate programs. This problem parallels those faced by the field of medicine after the Flexner Report in 1910, when many small medical schools with inadequate resources closed. Nursing's "Flexner Report" (Brown 1948) advocated that nursing be incorporated into the mainstream of college education if it is to keep pace with educational advancements occurring throughout society. The solution to providing rural residents access to professional education rests in adopting the educational innovations rural areas use for all other professions. Nursing is a leader in this area, because a competency-based assessment method of licensure (the New York Regents External Degree Program) allows nurses from around the world to qualify for an upper-division degree, as discussed in Chapter 5.

## Minorities

Minorities are underrepresented in all nursing programs. This is a problem because any profession that provides essential services that are frequently paid for from tax revenues should be broadly representative of the population. Problems of minority education are not unique to nursing, and in fact nursing education's record is better than that of all other health professions except dietitians. During the decade of the 1970s, the minority proportion of RN entrants increased whereas minority enrollment in LPN programs declined (Department of Health and Human Services 1984). Nursing should participate in all targeted initiatives to achieve the goal of minority representation.

Fortunately, nursing does offer a spectrum of careers ranging from nursing aide to positions requiring a Ph.D. Linking education to licensure and differentiating work based on education should not impede minority advancement. What does impede advancement is a system in which educational programs are dead ends and force minorities, who often start at aide and LPN ranks, to start over in order to progress. Nurse educators, in cooperation with local employers, have linked level of practice with education. These levels begin with the nursing aide and include practical, associate, and baccalaureate degree levels. For instance, in Long Beach, California, students can proceed from one level to another without duplicating coursework or having to earn more credits than other students must earn. Students who need to leave school to work can reenter without career progression penalty. Thus, all students, including minorities, progress as their talent and interest dictate. If this model and other similar ones were adapted to local needs, hospitals would become very attractive employers for upwardly mobile workers who have limited resources (Garvey, Castiglia, and Bullough 1983). Indeed, no other major occupation has a model with as much potential for allowing one to combine study and work ranging from one semester in a community college to a doctoral degree.

# Focal Role of Nursing Administrators

## *Responsibilities*

A consensus exists among executives and nurses that the director of nursing services has a central role in the effective management of a hospital and its many related nursing activities (Poulin 1984). A recent study determined that nurse executives have major responsibility for staff development, long-range planning, and collective bargaining (Simms, Price, and Pfoutz 1985). Although nurse executives may be held responsible for financial performance, the researchers found that great variability existed in the development and monitoring of department budgets. Those administrators who participated in overall planning and policy development had more budget authority. Staffing and scheduling were frequently delegated responsibilities.

Clinical practice activities were found to be important functions of the director of nursing services, as were traditional leadership and educational activities. The nurse executives interviewed described major responsibilities in assuring quality, establishing clinical standards, monitoring accidents, handling complaints, and developing policies. These activities involved only limited interaction with physicians, suggesting that nursing has emerged as an autonomous department that uses nursing standards and criteria (as opposed to medical ones).

Further, product line management, which is the management system based on major clinical types, and case-based prospective reimbursement are encouraging organizational restructuring. The director of nursing services is increasingly seen as the executive who can manage and coordinate related departments, such as respiratory therapy, home care, hospice, and skilled nursing care, thus decreasing patient length of stay and increasing hospital operating margins (Watson and Strasen 1987). As a consequence, staff nurses are reabsorbing some of the functions they lost to specialists when such treatments were Medicare- and Medicaid-reimbursable treatments.

## *Tenure*

Directors of nursing services in university-affiliated hospitals were found to have short average tenure and frequent terminations (Freund 1985a). Although some directors stay in their position for 10 years or more,

43% of hospitals surveyed in 1984 had three or more directors within a ten-year period. Whether this is related to the tenure of the chief executive officer or the chief operating officer is not known. In spite of these high rates of mobility, both chief executive officers and directors of nursing report high levels of successful and effective relationships with each other, both past and current. This paradox is not easily explained. The reasons for the combination of high rate of termination and reported job satisfaction need further examination.

## Identified Major Nursing Issues

Nursing service administrators from hospitals (i.e., magnet hospitals) designated as exemplary by the American Academy of Nursing (1983) identified four major nursing issues: (1) nursing practice, (2) payment, (3) education, and (4) colleagueship (Urquhart et al. 1986).[3]

Nursing practice themes included the need to redefine organization-based practice, define quality of nursing while costing out nursing care, and identify the nature of independent and community-based nursing. Problematic reimbursement payment issues included the effects on nurse-patient ratios and skill mix, as well as cost-constraint impacts on nursing education, including continuing education. Major educational issues included concern over reductions in nursing enrollments, the lack of differentiation between formal level of education and practice, and the need for more alternative delivery modes in nursing education programs. Colleagueship issues centered around working with physicians and workers from other disciplines and developing support systems.

Other issues that have been identified include ethical issues and the use of power. A study of all acute care hospitals in one state found that ethical issues in administrative decision-making pose a critical problem for nurse administrators (Sietsma and Spradley 1987). The issues that present the most ethical dilemmas were staffing level and mix decisions, developing and maintaining standards of care, allocation and rationing of scarce resources, and deciding on treatment versus nontreatment for specific patients. In general they relied on administrative colleagues, the CEO and Board of Trustees, nursing colleagues, and the Patient's Bill of Rights in resolving these dilemmas. It is generally recognized that nurse executives, like other executives, must use power effectively and have a keen political sense as well. These issues are covered in detail in del Bueno and Freund (1986).

## Preparation

Within the nursing profession, administration began declining in status during the 1960s, in part because the nursing leadership gave priority to upgrading clinical competence and the practice of nursing over administration. In the 1960s there was a rapid advance in knowledge and an increase in the number of high school graduates going to college. However, there were few nurses with the credentials necessary to teach in accredited colleges. As a matter of necessity, schools of nursing dropped the functional specialties in education and nursing to meet the demands of undergraduate education. Thus, the functional areas lost workers as well as status among nurses.

The result of this shift away from management education was a decline in the percentage of graduations of master's-degree students in nursing administration curricula—from 10.2% of all students graduating in 1967–1968 to 7% in 1978–1979 (Fine 1983). Although many nurse executives are well prepared and competent, in the aggregate, nurse administrators are educationally ill prepared for the diverse and complex responsibilities they are expected to carry (Leininger 1979; Stevens 1978). This decline has been somewhat offset in recent years by the graduation of administrative nurses from nonnursing programs, such as business and public administration schools. Overall, the number of nursing service administrators with master's degrees doubled between 1977 and 1982 (Aydelotte 1984a).

Since then much progress has been made as foundations have sponsored excellent professional development programs, and nursing programs have reinstated the administration/management specialization (Rovin and Ginsberg 1988). In 1976–1977, only 7% of master's program graduates listed administration/management as their area of specialization. In 1985–1986, 16% of graduates majored in administration/management (National League for Nursing 1988, 84).

The integration of the professional component of nursing work and management has been controversial. Many leaders in nursing education argue that advanced professional education for nurses should occur in schools of nursing rather than in schools of management. Many hospital administrators, on the other hand, prefer the reverse. Yet when employers rated the performance of nursing administrators from different programs, educational background was found to be unimportant (Price 1984). Consensus exists among the various factions that general administration, finance, budgeting, computer literacy, and labor relations are valuable components in advanced nursing programs and should be well integrated in such programs, regardless of whether the education occurs in a school of management or a school of nursing (Institute of Medicine 1983, 135; Freund 1985b). Value differences exist between graduate nursing educators and practicing nurse executives. Whether they exist between faculty in management schools and nursing executives is not known (Ulrich 1987).

Recent increases in federal funding for graduate nursing education ensure that an increasing proportion of nurses will have access to management programs in nursing departments. Since there is a shortage of educationally prepared nurse executives, executives can ill afford to denigrate or impede educational efforts by nurses. A more positive approach to ensure a supply of well-educated nurse executives is to encourage management content in nursing programs and to provide internal management development within hospitals. This is a common practice used by many other businesses to meet institutional needs. To ensure high-quality management, employers need also to expect and encourage their directors of nursing services to remain current in such areas as nursing theories, practice, and trends.

## Pay

There is little evidence that the hospital industry is willing to invest in the development of nursing service administrators. Paid internships need to become the norm for nursing administration students, just as they are for generalist administrators. Nursing service administrators' salaries averaged $65,000 in 1987 and varied considerably on the basis of hospital size (Cole and Sizing 1987). Bonuses averaged about 11.3% of base pay for the 10.5% of directors who received incentive compensation. Traditionally, directors have not received pay commensurate with the salaries of administrators in private industry with comparable responsibility (Aydelotte 1984a; American Management Association 1982–1983). In addition, directors work long hours: Only 7% worked 40 hours per week or less and 4% worked over 60 hours per week.

Typically, nursing service administrators supervise the largest single component of both the work force and the budget, and must therefore possess credibility in two professions. Ironically, their average salary ranks below that of nonnurse associate administrators and assistant administrators. Also, the range is more restricted than for other classes. This finding is difficult to explain, as the diversity in education and experience would lead to the expectation of a longer, not a shorter, range (American Management Association 1982–1983). Further, nursing service administrators' salaries do not vary with experience as measured by either age or tenure (Friss 1983). Neither do they correspond to having full responsibility for the nursing budget—an anomalous situation (Aydelotte 1984b).

Oddly enough, nursing administrators may not see themselves as underpaid, since their pay has improved considerably over the past few years. Besides, they not only earn more than staff nurses but also more than their social background had prepared them to expect. Even when they compare themselves to other members of the management team, nursing administrators often accept their salaries as equivalent, although they may have more years of experience or seniority than other members of the team. This perception may prevent them from using the tactic most likely to win a pay increase, namely, to ask for it (Dreher, Dougherty, and Whitely 1988).

Although it is not uncommon to have nursing service administrators whose education, responsibilities, and pay are not aligned with other executives, a trend is developing to treat nurse executives in the same way other senior executives are treated. The legacy stemming from the earlier apprentice education, isolation from decision-making, and stereotypes about the role of females is slowly being eradicated as nurse executives obtain the normal credentials and the same access to management development experiences that other managers have.

## Management Implications

Research has found that competent female managers are not assimilated and given the same rewards as their male colleagues. As a result, they lose friends and access to information, and as a consequence, they often propose extreme solutions to overcoming the disparity (Bartol 1980). This may explain some of the difficulties executives express about working with nursing administrators.

Nursing service administrators probably experience high job stress, even though in at least one study they were in better mental health than normative groups (Cooper, Manning, Poteet, and Hurgley 1988). Scalzi (1988) found, in a sample of nurse executives, that the major causes of role stress were (1) overload, which included conflicting expectations from hospital administration and the nursing departments, too large a span of control, too many expectations for the job, and difficulty in managing personal time; (2) concerns about quality of care; and (3) role conflict—doing things that are accepted by some and not accepted by others.

Hospital executives today are paying the price of their predecessors' neglect in developing depth in nursing management. If circumstances remain unchanged, with a climate of poor financial and career incentives, the pool of qualified executives and managers will shrink, not expand.

To increase the upward mobility of nurses and other female managers in order to upgrade the pool of these workers, executives have been advised to take several actions:

1. Train managers in the use of objective rating scales and specific decision rules.

2. Change the distribution of opportunities and power.

3. Eliminate women's token status.

4. Reduce the salience of gender and associated stereotypes by increasing the amount of information on which decisions are based.

5. Sanction those who block upward mobility of female managers.

6. Give tangible rewards to those who facilitate the advancement of female managers (Riger and Galligan 1980).

Although these activities should help in efforts to attract and retain aspiring managerial nurses, hospitals will have to depend also on the talents and skills of those already in place. Therefore, the challenge to management is to improve the effectiveness of present nursing administrators through management development programs based on the principles that apply to general managers (Forrest 1983; Gleeson, Nestor, and Riddell 1983).

To be most effective, the nursing services director must retain clinical credibility with other professionals. This is a dilemma faced by administrative scientists, engineers, and professors as well. Professional administrators do not need to be expert in every field of clinical practice. Instead, their qualifications and value must be acceptable to their followers.

## Trends

An important trend in the hospital industry is the inclusion of nurses in the corporate structure of multihospital systems. Even though over 30% of all hospital beds are owned, leased, or managed by multihospital systems, there is little literature on the integration of nurses into the corporate structure. Multihospital systems can, however, offer greater mobility and more room for growth for nurses.

There appear to be predictable phases in the development of multihospital systems (Freund and Mitchell 1985). At first, the systems emphasize financing, diversification, and employee benefits (incentives). Later, strategic planning becomes important. The nursing executive can be quite influential at this point. Some of the marketing information and data interpretation activities for which nurses may have responsibility in corporate-level planning are origin of patient population, age groups, sources of current referral services, physician utilization over time and across units, patient volume analysis, and individual nursing unit and program activity (Haddad 1981).

The potential benefits of multihospital systems for nursing include increased financial resources, improved technology, diversification, and increased fringe benefits. Professional benefits could include improved nursing ratios (especially in rural areas), more opportunities for clinical specialists, decentralized organizations, and more upward and geographic mobility. However, concern over constraints is widespread. The potential constraints include:

- Reduced nursing autonomy, especially in governance and diversification

- Reduced quality of care because of reductions in staffing ratios and staff mix

- Decreased morale among staff nurses

- Lack of timely corporate responsiveness to local problems

- Reduction in opportunities for joint ventures, since nursing is not a significant source of capital for multihospital systems.

Another trend is an increase in the social distance between staff nurses and more highly educated administrators and faculty. This phenomenon is not limited to nursing. Instead, it is associated with the complexity of practice, government accountability, and social control of service professions. The distance between the intellectually elite, who establish practice standards (educators and expert practitioners), and administrative clinicians (who enforce standards and allocate resources) and working professionals has been described in detail by Freidson (1984).

When education of staff nurses is linked with licensure and practice expectations, nurse executives will be able to manage more effectively. Professional and managerial leadership is better when workers have a clear understanding of qualifications, tasks, rewards, and opportunities. Formal linkages between practice steps prevent the alienation that arises when mobility is artificially blocked. The existing ambiguity frequently leads workers to attribute supervisors' negative behaviors to prejudice or arbitrary preferences.

## Environmental Assessment of Nursing

Strategic planning for an adequate nursing service begins with an environmental scan. A challenge to executives is to adjust national reimbursement policies and nursing trends to local demographics, educational investments, and wage systems. The generic framework below provides a background for integrating work force planning into the general strategic plan of a hospital. Three major sectors are involved: service, education, and employment.

### Service

To integrate work force planning into their general strategic plan, individual hospitals will need to conform appropriately to national trends. It is generally expected that, in the near future, a larger population, a higher proportion of elderly, and more advanced technology will increase the intensity and possibly the amount of inpatient hospital care.

One prediction is that most hospitals will be converted to critical care units in the 1990s (Flynn 1984). Since more women are working outside the home, there will be fewer women than before to care for the sick and infirm at home or to provide transportation to ambulatory services. In addition, projections by the U.S. Public Health Service indicate that the incidence and prevalence of AIDS are increasing exponentially. The data suggest that this development will impact hospitals in ways that are difficult to foresee. AIDS-related issues include the financial impact on hospitals, involvement in prevention and hospice programs, changed hospital-community interaction, and altered work force training.

The current trend toward restructuring of hospitals into multihospital systems and the increase in prepayment mechanisms will probably lead to consolidation among hospitals; a *Los Angeles Times* (1988) survey suggested that 700 hospitals nationwide may close. In urban areas, personnel and patients will be absorbed by other local hospitals. Certainly, those hospitals expecting to survive and flourish have a vested interest in remaining competitive as employers.

The perceptions held by employees of competing potential employers will determine the number and caliber of workers likely to respond to employment opportunities. This implies that employers need to assess the qualifications, experience, and employment alternatives of current or potential employees in hospitals facing closure or consolidation. Multihospital systems, for example, have some ability to transfer valued employees to other areas. Further, government hospitals, where workers have Civil Service and union protection, many expand in the future and attract additional workers.

Prospective payment should moderate some of the variance in nurse staffing diversity. Still, differences in nurse-to-patient staffing ratios are expected to remain large even for hospitals within a region that are of comparable size and case mix. This is true because nursing is influenced by the same geographic diversity that affects all of medicine, including physician and hospital utilization (Rothberg 1982). Even though prospective payment has been shown to decrease payroll costs and increase productivity (full-time equivalent staff per adjusted patient-day), there are no consistent effects on the skill mix (Kidder and Sullivan 1982). This means that hospitals are more likely to be influenced by local labor market forces, such as the supply of nurses, employer domination, and physician preferences, than by prospective reimbursement. In addition, governments will require more documentation of both appropriateness and quality of care. Therefore, more nurses with higher qualifications will be needed to establish and enforce practice criteria in nursing and medicine.

Experts predict that, in the next several years, direct patient care services will be provided by a proliferation of all types of nursing personnel, from aides to LPNs to RNs with advanced degrees (Ginzberg et al. 1982; Institute of Medicine 1983). They also predict increased support from nursing leaders for raising the required levels of educational preparation to create greater professional independence from physicians. In medical centers, there will likely be a few highly trained, specialized clinical RNs coordinating the care of a defined population of patients. These nurses will be supported by technical nurses and technicians (Institute of Medicine 1983, 32).

## Employment

Since nursing employment is determined primarily by local labor markets, the environmental scan depends on state and local data (which are seldom complete) and on data from local education and business experts. The key criteria center around the supply of applicants, labor force participation by age group, and individual hospital market share of applicants by age pools. Strategic planning should also include a close analysis of local graduation trends from LVN, diploma, ADN, and BSN programs. In states that depend on an influx of graduates from other states, employers should also explore shifts in these "feeder" states. Trend data on Scholastic Aptitude Test (SAT) scores will provide valuable information on the relative attractiveness of nursing to academically superior entrants. National data are reviewed below to provide a comparison for regional findings.

**Supply and Quality of Graduates.** Because nurses come from several educational levels, the resulting ambiguities have generated much debate and raised many questions. Do nurses educated in community colleges, diploma schools, and four-year colleges hold different work-related values? If so, what are the implications for work force management? Some studies indicate the following:

1. More graduates from all three programs work full-time when they are under age 25 and over age 45 than at ages in between.

2. ADN graduates have the highest participation rate among the three for every age group.

3. There is no difference among the three in the amount of time hospital-employed graduates spend in patient care.

4. Bachelor's degree graduates are more mobile and less likely to work in hospitals than are the other two groups (Bauer and Levine 1983).

Together these findings suggest that educational background does not predict which nurses will desire to work part-time in their primary child-bearing years. Neither do they suggest a pattern of nurse utilization within the hospital. However, higher education is associated with expanded career opportunities for nurses.

Compared to other college majors, nursing has a remarkably high retention rate (Rosenfeld 1988). The diploma schools have higher attrition rates than do the BSN and ADN programs. The troublesome fall in admissions is apparently not due to faculty failures.

**Labor Force Participation.** It has been established that nurses follow the labor force participation patterns of other women in professional and technical jobs. Therefore, hospital managers and planners can use U.S. Department of Labor and state statistics to understand general trends and apply them to nurses. National projections for all women workers predict higher participation rates among women 25 to 54 years old, the prime working age group (Department of Labor 1986). Even though nurses have a high rate of labor force participation (at least part-time), many nurses begin dropping their licenses at age 40. Younger workers will be in short supply. The 22- to 44-year-old population will plateau in 1990 for five years and then drop sharply until well after 2004. In 1995 the 15- to 24-year-old cohort will grow sharply until 2007 (Striner 1984).

Hospital employment markets are segmented by type of ownership and control. In 1979, for instance, Catholic hospitals (a large but not all-inclusive segment of religious hospitals) employed 17.39% of full-time equivalent (FTE) nonfederal hospital workers (Fox, Walker, and Unger 1983). State and local government hospitals employed over 20% of nonfederal FTEs. Investor-owned hospitals had 6.29%, leaving non-Catholic community hospitals with only 55%. Religious hospitals have a recruiting and retention advantage for some workers, primarily those with a religious preference and those with a service career anchor, who gravitate toward value-compatible employers.

Government hospitals also have a competitive advantage over other hospitals because they (1) appeal to individuals with technical-functional, security, and identification career anchors, and (2) provide more incentives for a long-term, steady-state career. In communities where there are both religious and government hospitals, community hospitals may be left with a disproportionate share of workers who value variety, creativity, and the autonomous aspects of work, that is, exactly the ones prone to shape spiral careers or participate sporadically in the labor market.

**Salaries.** Executives and managers often base pay scales on entry-level salaries. However, both recruits and incumbents make salary comparisons and base career decisions on their career expectations, long-term earnings potential, and other alternatives. Therefore, executives and managers need to know what salaries and benefits private industry is offering now, and what is the career potential for graduates from each of the primary work force pools: talented high school graduates, college graduates, neophyte employees, and mature women returning to work. Managers would be wise to refine the analysis to include age and educational differences. Otherwise the desired mix of workers may not be available. Such data also are necessary to determine the cost-effectiveness of investments in productivity, such as bedside terminals.

## Education

In most communities the basic supply of new RNs comes from women aged 18 to 25 in the top 25% of the graduating class (Department of Health and Human Services 1981). The largest proportion of these women are high school graduates with college aspirations. A secondary source of new RNs is mature women returning to college prior to establishing a second career. The third source is nursing aides, orderlies, and practical nurses, who are already employed but have upward mobility aspirations. This source has been found to yield the highest proportion of males and ethnic minority employees.

States have the primary responsibility for planning educational investments in nursing to provide the level of nursing services deemed necessary. Unfortunately, few states have ongoing organizational mechanisms for nurse work force planning, but instead rely on special studies (Institute of Medicine 1983, 81). Nursing is not anomalous in this regard. Nationally there is a loose relationship between education and work, with little planning based on need assessment and projections. Indeed, the data available on nursing are relatively ample.

Decisions about the amount of state and local investment in nursing education are influenced by

- The relative cost of providing nursing education programs
- Demands by students for educational opportunities
- The need for specific kinds of workers to meet the competing demands of local employers.

Executives who favor increased educational funding must be aware that nursing programs are expensive to operate. For instance, the low ratio of students to teachers that is required makes nursing students two to three times more expensive to educate than computer specialists or engineers (Holtzclaw 1983). Advocates for expansion of nursing education should anticipate the following questions:

1. Why should the state or locality expand nursing graduations when a high proportion of workers are working part-time, existing nurses are dropping their licenses, a significant proportion of licensed nurses are not working, turnover rates are high, nurses' low salaries and poor working conditions are well publicized, the applicant pool is declining, and graduates often move away for better career opportunities?

2. Do nursing career incentives match those of competing occupations and employers?

3. Will realistic pay differentials by shift, specialty, or day of the week solve the problem?

4. If the shortage is real, why does wage competition not occur?

5. Have enough resources been invested in educational and job upgrading of current employees?

6. What contribution will management make to the cost of education?

Educational planners will generally encourage employers to develop their own upward mobility models and job-related training programs. When this is not possible, planners will urge employers to develop operational definitions of entry-level practice and install an incentive system that will encourage full-time career commitment to nursing. Investment in expensive educational programs is difficult to justify when neither the employers nor already educated employees are willing to commit their own resources.

## Scenarios

Two traditional models used to interpret past events among nurses, physicians, and hospitals are the conflict model and the consensus model. The conflict model emphasizes:

- Physician-nurse disagreements (as evidenced by the AMA's proposal to certify three levels of Registered Care Technologists)
- Oppression of nurses by hospital managers
- Distance between nursing administrators and staff nurses
- A split between nursing theory and practice
- Divided interests on the part of nursing associations
- Home-career conflict on the part of nurses
- Male-female discord in the professions.

If this model is used to understand current problems and design future policies and strategies, there are enough reinforcing currents to produce a self-fulfilling prophecy. Further, there will be an oversupply of physicians to resist upgrading of nurses' status.[4] Administrators will be under more pressures to contain payroll costs and nursing is an easy target for budget cuts. Nurses and nursing associations have conflicting interests because of their diverse constituency. Changes in linking education with practice are virtually impossible without the support of organized medicine, hospitals, and the workers themselves.

The consensus model, however, also explains past events and offers more hope for a health future. Many influential theorists believe that conflict between professionals and bureaucrats has been overstated during the past 20 years. The nursing profession has flourished in hospitals, increasing in size, diversity, and level of responsibility. Individual nurses have negotiated careers so as to combine home and family life in a fashion that many feminists now envy. Hospitals, like other businesses, used the incentives acceptable for the time and in the process were able to provide cost-effective nursing care. Physicians and nurses, despite their difficulties and differences in status, collaborate to provide patient care. No hospital can operate effectively if there is fundamental conflict between physicians and nurses.

Nursing administrators, faculty, and staff nurses do agree on basic nursing program content as evidenced by almost uniform practice entry requirements across the states as well as easy movement of nurses between hospitals. Basic research and models to differentiate levels of practice exist and have been endorsed by national associations of nurses and hospitals.

The crux of current problems surrounding nursing is tied to cultural shifts and new performance demands. Operating efficiently and maximizing the bottom line are not sufficient goals for hospitals. Institutional efficiency that depends on subsidized education, young workers, and transient workers is a suboptimal state of affairs. The real bottom line is that hospitals must operate more responsively as a *system.*

System leaders need to take a long-term career perspective regarding their professional service workers. Since nurses are the largest health care provider group and influence many others, managers can exert the most influence through them.

Specifically, executives and industry leaders need to (1) join with nursing to link education to practice, (2) make the career progression from nursing aide to doctorate, with visible competitive salaries at every level, visible to high school and college students, (3) look for ways to support the slow growth of a relatively well paid work force, (4) restructure nursing services so that assignments and responsibilities are graded to match experience and competence, and (5) foster professional and self-control based on feedback on the quality of care. In short, executives and managers need to treat nurses as a valuable resource rather than as a disposable item.

The heart of obtaining the public support vital to the nursing field as a professional service is the provision of compassionate services. This can be done only if nurses believe that they are being treated fairly. Perceptions of fair treatment depend on community standards and should vary by education and competence rather than age and sex. The compacted nursing career system is a dysfunctional artifact. Nurses are not the only losers. Employers and patients lose as the work force pool becomes unbalanced, with too many using health care organizations and the profession itself to meet personal goals, and too few talented people making career investments in nursing.

At a national policy level:

1. Funds for undergraduate education should be targeted to areas that are underserved and where employers are not collectively dampening free-market forces. Expenses of operating a diploma school of nursing should not be reimbursed by Medicare.

2. Visas should not be automatically extended for foreign-educated nurses. Further, visa eligibility should conform to other professionals, i.e., the foreign national must possess a college degree, or the equivalent of a degree in terms of education and experience, before gaining H-1 status.

3. Reimbursement policies should be developed that encourage differential pay for nurses related to patient acuity.

4. The assumption that wage levels must be kept low enough for every hospital to survive, regardless of occupancy and quality of care, should be abandoned.

5. Any one-time reimbursement awards aimed to increase nursing salaries should be accompanied by reforms that will interrupt the ratchet pay cycle, i.e., minimize emplyer domination of the pay setting process. At the state level, licensure needs to be linked to education with national examinations for both levels.

## Summary

The character of new nursing recruits is changing. In the future, nurses are likely to have lower academic potential on average as bright women choose other careers. The retention of committed, competent nurses will be a problem throughout the 1990s because demographic and cultural changes will affect the nature of the work force. First, there will be fewer high school graduates, the primary educational pool. Second, women who traditionally chose a career in nursing, especially the most talented, will pursue new, nontraditional career options. (The proportion of males is increasing so slowly that their impact will not be felt for generations.) Third, currently working nurses are slowly shifting to nonhospital employment. Fourth, employers are not developing initiatives to keep mature women in the work force. Fifth, nursing is becoming similar to higher status occupations by offering more career options; hospital nursing is likely to become a less attractive alternative. Sixth, federal support for entry-level education is becoming more difficult to obtain, and thus there will be more competition for equally scarce local educational funds. Finally, the demand for hospital nurses will intensify as the patient population becomes both older and sicker.

Responsible hospital administrators and associations recognize that long-term survival requires that the industry remain competitive in attracting professional service workers. The days of a ready supply of young, technologically expert replacement nurses at low cost (to the hospital) are over. It is in the industry's own long-term best interest to create career options for mature, talented women. The problem is not a potential aggregate shortage of nurses. The aggregate supply of day workers with basic skills is not in jeopardy. What is in jeopardy is the core group of steady-state career nurses who provide organizational stability and expert clinical care and can serve as administrators and as educators of future steady-state career nurses. Enlightened executives and managers will recognize the futility of waiting for nurses to "resolve their own problems." They will question continued reliance on short-run strategies that attract and reward women for part-time, part-life commitment.

## Endnotes

1.  For a detailed discussion of comparable worth see Remick (1984), Sape (1985), and Kelly and Bayes (1988).

2.  Funding for nursing clinical research and graduate education has continued because the history of apprentice education has led to administrators and faculty lacking the necessary educational qualifications (master's degrees or doctorates, respectively) of their nonnurse peers. For example, among nursing faculty, only 10% are doctorally prepared, and only 73% have the master's degree as their highest level of preparation. Over 400 positions in baccalaureate and higher degree nursing programs are vacant (National League for Nursing 1985).

3.  See Brown (1981) for a brief but complete overview of the woman manager in the United States.

4.  At this writing, the American Medical Association (AMA) has forwarded a proposal for a new class of health care workers, to be called Registered Care Technologists (RCTs), whose education and credentialing the AMA would control. The proposal is not accompanied by a proposal to pay professionals more for supervising RCTs.

## References

AFSCME v. State of Washington, 33FE cases 808 at 825 n. 22 (W.D. Washington, 1983).

Aldrich, M., and R. Buchele. 1986. *The economics of comparable worth*. Cambridge, MA: Ballinger.

American Academy of Nursing. 1983. *Magnet hospitals.* Kansas City, MO: American Academy of Nursing, American Nurses' Association.

American Management Association. 1982–1983. *Executive compensation service. Hospitals and health care report,* 7th ed. New York: American Management Association.

Aronson, R. 1985. Unionism among professional employees in the private sector. *Industrial and Labor Relations* 38: 352–363.

Aydelotte, M. 1984a. A survey of nursing service administrators—part 1. *Hospitals* 58 (11): 94–100.

Aydelotte, M. 1984b. A survey of nursing service administrators—part 2. *Hospitals* 58: (12) 79–80.

Bartol, K. 1980. Female managers and quality of working life: the impact of sex-role stereotyping. *Journal of Occupational Behavior* 1: 205–221.

Bauer, K., and E. Levine. 1983. *Analysis of career differences among registered nurses with different types of nurse education.* Washington, DC: Institute of Medicine.

Brown, E. 1948. *Nursing for the future.* New York: Russell Sage Foundation.

Brown, L. 1981. *The woman manager in the United States: a research analysis and bibliography.* Washington, DC: Business and Professional Women's Foundation.

Burda, D. 1986. Labor law may create trap for unwary hospitals. *Hospitals* 60(4): 38.

Chi, K. 1984. Comparable worth: implications of the Washington case. *State Government* 57: 34–45.

Cole, B., and M. Sizing. 1987. Nursing managers' salaries vary little. *Modern Healthcare* 17(25): 32–58.

Cooper, C., C. Manning, G. Poteet, and P. Hingley. 1988. Stress, mental health and job satisfaction among nurse managers. *Health Services Management Research* 1(1): 51–58.

DeBack, V. 1987. The National Commission on Nursing Implementation Project. *Journal of Professional Nursing* 3: 226–229.

del Bueno, D., and C. Freund. 1986. *Power and politics in nursing administration.* Owings Mills, MD: Rynd.

Department of Health and Human Services. 1981. *The recurrent shortage of registered nurses.* Washington, DC: Health Resources Administration.

Department of Health and Human Services. 1984. *Minorities and women in the health fields.* Washington, DC: Government Printing Office.

Department of Labor. 1986. *Employment in perspective: women in the labor force* (report 729). Washington, DC: Bureau of Labor Statistics.

Dreher, G., T. Dougherty, and W. Whitely. 1988. Influence, tactics and salary attainment: A study of sex-based salary differentials. *Academy of Management Best Papers Proceedings 1988.* Anaheim, CA: Academy of Management, pp. 346–350.

Fackelman, K. 1985a. Fears about revised wage index draw protests from hospital groups. *Modern Healthcare* 15(8): 60–61.

Fackelman, K. 1985b. Revised wage index won't create expected midwest windfalls—study. *Modern Healthcare* 15(18): 32–34.

Federal Register 53: 190. Sept. 30, 1988. 38493-96, 38540, 38543-75.

Fine, R. 1983. Supply and demand of nursing administrators. *Nursing and Health Care* 4(1): 10–15.

Flynn, K. 1984. Role issues, technology and economics in hospital nursing. *Hospital Topics* 62(3): 27–29.

Fogel, W. 1984. *The Equal Pay Act: implications for comparable worth.* New York: Praeger.

Forrest, I. 1983. Management education and training of nurses: research study. *Journal of Advances in Nursing* 8: 139–145.

Fox, R., W. Walker, and M. Unger. 1983. Changes in full-time equivalent personnel, payroll, and expenses. *Hospital Progress* 64(3): 60–67.

Freidson, E. 1984. The changing nature of professional control. *Annual Review of Sociology* 10: 1–20.

Freund, C. 1985a. The tenure of directors of nursing. *Journal of Nursing Administration* 15(2): 11–15.

Freund, C. 1985b. Director of nursing effectiveness. *Journal of Nursing Administration* 15(6): 25–30.

Freund, C., and J. Mitchell. 1985. Multi-institutional systems: the new arrangement. *Nursing Economics* 3: 24–31.

Friss, L. 1981. Work force policy perspectives: registered nurses. *Journal of Health Politics, Policy and Law* 5: 696–719.

Friss, L. 1983. Organization commitment and job involvement of directors of nursing services. *Nursing Administration Quarterly* 7(2): 1–10.

Friss, L. 1987. External equity and the free market myth. *Review of Public Personnel Administration* 7: 74–90.

Fulghum, J. 1983. The employer's liabilities under comparable worth. *Personnel Journal* 62: 402.

Garvey, J., P. Castiglia, and B. Bullough. 1983. Models for the baccalaureate education of registered nurses, in B. Bullough, V. Bullough, and M. Soukop, eds. *Issues and Strategies for the Eighties*. New York: Springer, pp. 254–265.

General Accounting Office. 1983. *Hospital links with related firms can conceal unreasonable costs and increase administrative burden, thus inflating health program expenditures.* Washington, DC: Government Printing Office.

Ginzberg, E., J. Patray, M. Ostow, et al. 1982. Nurse discontent: the search for realistic solutions. *Journal of Nursing Administration* 9: 7–11.

Gleeson, S., O. Nestor, and A. Riddell. 1983. Helping nurses through the management threshold. *Nursing Administration Quarterly* 7(2): 11–16.

Gray, A., and R. Smail. 1982. *Why has the nursing pay-bill increased?* (paper 01/82). Aberdeen, Scotland: University of Aberdeen Departments of Community Medicine and Political Economy, Health Economics Unit.

Greene, R. 1980. Geographic wage indexing for CETA and Medicare. *Monthly Labor Review* 103(9): 15–19.

Haddad, A. 1981. The nurse's role and responsibility in corporate level planning. *Nursing Administration Quarterly* 5(2): 1–6.

Holtzclaw, B. 1983. Changing student applicant pools. *Nursing and Health Care* 4: 450–454.

Institute of Medicine. 1983. *Nursing and nursing education: public policies and private actions.* Washington, DC: National Academy of Sciences.

Journal of Nursing Administration. 1985. Market demand for diploma, ADN, BSN, and MSN. *Journal of Nursing Administration* 15(6): 5.

Kelly, R., and J. Bayes. 1988. *Comparable worth, pay equity, and public policy.* New York: Greenwood.

Kent, R., ed. 1985. *Money talks.* New York: Facts on File.

Kidder, D., and C. Sullivan. 1982. Hospital payroll costs, productivity, and employment under prospective reimbursement. *Health Care Financing Review* 4: 89–99.

Killingsworth, M. 1986. The economics of comparable worth: analytical, empirical and policy questions, in H. Hartmann, ed., *Comparable worth: new directions for research.* Washington, DC: National Academy Press, pp. 86–115.

Leininger, M. 1979. Territoriality, power, and creative leadership in administrative nursing contexts, in National League for Nursing, *Power: use it or lose it.* New York: National League for Nursing, pp. 6–18.

Leuthold, J. 1984. Income splitting and women's labor-force participation. *Industrial and Labor Relations Review* 38: 98–105.

Loffrey v. Northwest Airlines, In, 5677 2d 429 (DR Con 1976).

*Los Angeles Times.* Up to 700 hospitals may close because of Medicare, study says. June 23, 1988, p. 17.

Muller, A., J. Vitali, and D. Brannon. 1987. Wage differences and the concentration of women in hospital occupations. *Health Care Management Review* 12(1): 61–70

National League for Nursing. 1985. *Legislative challenges for nursing in the '80s.* New York: National League for Nursing.

National League for Nursing. 1988. *Nursing student census with policy implications 1987.* New York: National League for Nursing.

Poulin, M. 1984. Future directions for nursing administration. *Journal of Nursing Administration* 14(3): 37–41.

Poulos, M. 1984. Hospital cutbacks' effects on employee wages. *Health Matrix II* (2): 95–96.

Price, S. 1984. Master's programs preparing nursing administrators. *Journal of Nursing Administration* 14: 11–17.

Prospective Payment Assessment Commission. 1985. *Technical appendixes to the report and recommendations to the secretary, U.S. Department of Health and Human Services, April 1, 1985.* Washington, DC: Government Printing Office.

Remick, H., ed. 1984. *Comparable worth and wage discrimination: technical possibilities and political realities.* Philadelphia: Temple University Press.

Riger, S., and P. Galligan. 1980. Women in management. *American Psychologist* 35: 902–908.

Rosenfeld, P. 1988. Measuring student retention. *Nursing and Health Care* 9: 199–202.

Rothberg, D., ed. 1982. *Regional variations in hospital use.* Lexington, MA: D.C. Heath.

Rothchild, N., and B. Watkins. 1987. Pay equity in Minnesota: the facts are in. *Review of Public Personnel Administration* 7(3): 16–28.

Rovin, S., and L. Ginsberg. 1988. Johnson & Johnson-Wharton Fellows program in management for nurses. *Nursing Economics* 6(2): 78–82.

Sape, G. 1985. Coping with comparable worth. *Harvard Business Review* 85(3): 145–152.

Scalzi, C. 1988. Role stress and coping strategies of nurse executives. *Journal of Nursing Administration* 18(3): 34–38.

Schramm, C. 1978. Regulating hospital labor costs: a case study in the politics of state rate commissions. *Journal of Health Politics, Policy, and Law* 3: 364–374.

Sietsma, M., and B. Spradley. 1987. Ethics and administrative decision making. *Journal of Nursing Administration* 17(4): 28–32.

Simms, L., S. Price, and S. Pfoutz. 1985. Nurse executives: functions and priorities. *Nursing Economics* 3: 338–344.

Smail, R., and A. Gray. 1982a. *The effects of changing hours and holiday entitlements on nursing inputs to Scottish hospitals, 1950–1982* (paper no. 2). Aberdeen, Scotland: University of Aberdeen Departments of Community Medicine and Political Economy, Health Economics Unit.

Smail, R., and A. Gray. 1982b. *Nurses' pay in the NHS* (paper no. 3). Aberdeen, Scotland: University of Aberdeen Departments of Community Medicine and Political Economy, Health Economics Unit.

Stevens, B. 1978. Education in nursing administration: where are we and where should we be? in *The education and roles of nursing service administrators.* Battle Creek, MI: W. K. Kellogg, pp. 21–38.

Striner, H. 1984. Changes in work and society 1981–2004: impact on education, training, and career counseling, in N. Gysbers, ed., *Designing careers.* San Francisco: National Vocational Guidance Association.

Thompson, M. 1979. *Antitrust and the health care provider.* Germantown, MD: Aspen.

Treiman, D., and H. Hartmann, eds. 1981. *Women, work, and wages.* Washington, DC: National Academy Press.

Ulrich, B. 1987. Value differences between practicing nurse executives and graduate educators. *Nursing Economics* 5: 287–291.

Urquhart, A., G. Wooding, K. Budinger, et al. 1986. Perspectives on nursing issues and health care trends. *Journal of Nursing Administration* 16: 17–23.

Watland, A., B. Morgan, J. Diviney, et al. 1983. Study shows adverse effect on hospital reimbursement. *Hospital Financial Management* 13(8): 32–35.

Watson, D., and L. Strasen. 1987. The integration of respiratory therapy in nursing: reorganization for improved productivity. *Hospitals and Health Services Administration* 32: 369–379.

# Summary of Section III

Section III has identified the dynamics that produce the recurring cycle of nursing shortages. In career terms, the employment system in which nurses participate, which is organized to ensure survival of all hospitals regardless of occupancy, has created a surplus of nurses oriented to transitory and spiral careers and a dearth of nurses pursuing steady-state careers. As a result, the quality of applicants is declining. If the cycle is not interrupted, the public will be paying more for less able nurses, and health care organizations will still be subject to persistent shortages that require above-average wage adjustments for all nurses regardless of education, competence, or responsibility.

The new paradigm treats all hospital workers with dignity, if for no other reason than that patients cannot be cared for with dignity by workers who do not experience it themselves at work. Next, the paradigm recruits workers and assigns them to tasks based on organizational needs and worker education and performance. These differential assignments are linked with both salary differences and increased participation in the control process. This differentiation at work needs to be formalized by linking education with licensure. Together these actions provide a career structure that is compatible with cultural norms, understandable to many upwardly mobile workers from all social backgrounds, and sustainable.

It is not too late to avoid the fate of government pay adjustments and gradual erosion of the caliber of the work force. However, the obstacles are many. The first step, accepting the roots of the problem—education not linked to licensure and pay not linked to education, experience, and performance—is almost impossible for some to take. They insist that either nursing education or the employment system can be reformed apart from the other. Once the synergism of education and employment is accepted, leaders will find that political constituencies within and without nursing resist changes that threaten the viability of either their local nursing schools or their hospitals. Politicians, under pressure from well-funded lobbying groups, find it easier to fund entry-level education and encourage foreign immigration; these responses merely fuel the cycle and fail to encourage competition in an industry that prefers regulation and a managed pay system.

Fortunately, there are an abundance of strong leaders in nursing, hospital management, and medicine. We can only hope that they will channel their energies to make hospital nursing as attractive a career for steady-state nurses as it is for nurses with transient and spiral career orientations.

# *Index*